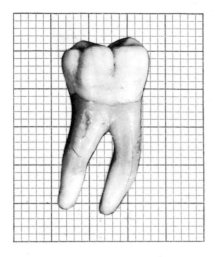 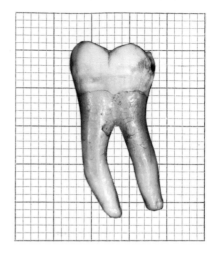

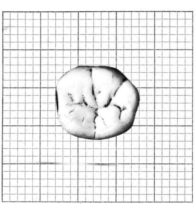

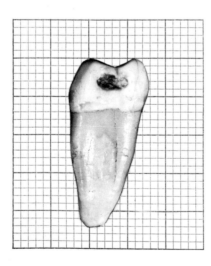 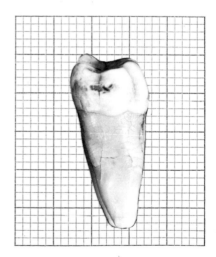

"ART AND SCIENCE HAVE THEIR MEETING POINT IN METHOD" — BULWER

Photographs of a natural specimen of a mandibular first molar, taken with a lens capable of two diameter registrations. Cut-outs of these photos were placed on graphs depicting squared millimeters. The result is an accurate graph in millimeters of tooth outlines from five aspects. See Chapter I, page 16.

4th EDITION

A TEXTBOOK OF
Dental Anatomy and Physiology

RUSSELL C. WHEELER, D.D.S., F.A.C.D.

WASHINGTON UNIVERSITY SCHOOL OF DENTISTRY
Instructor, Crown and Bridge Prosthesis, 1924–1927
Instructor, Dental Anatomy and Prosthetic Art, 1927–1935
Assistant Professor, Oral Anatomy, 1936
ST. LOUIS UNIVERSITY SCHOOL OF DENTISTRY
Associate Professor of Dental Anatomy, Human and Comparative,
Chairman of Department, 1937–1944
WASHINGTON UNIVERSITY SCHOOL OF DENTISTRY
Associate Professor of Anatomy, 1945–1951

ILLUSTRATED

W. B. SAUNDERS COMPANY,
Philadelphia and London

W. B. Saunders Company: West Washington Square
Philadelphia, Pa.   19105

12 Dyott Street
London, WC1A   1DB

1835 Yonge Street
Toronto 7, Ontario

A Textbook of Dental Anatomy and Physiology   SBN 0-7216-9261-3

Print No.:   10   9   8   7

DEDICATED TO

Those interested in establishing the
highest standards
for Operative and Restorative Dentistry,
keeping it abreast of other branches of Dental Science
through practice and research.

PREFACE TO THE
FOURTH EDITION

Twenty-five years have elapsed since this book went to press for the first time. Increased public interest in dentistry has stimulated new developments in dental education since then. Dentistry is recognized as a major division of the complete health service, and dental schools and complete dental clinics are being included as functioning departments of medical centers.

It is the author's opinion, however, that although this situation is satisfying, there is some danger that students of dentistry may forget their primary duties and the way in which they will become most valuable to the public in their future life in dentistry. With the present emphasis on research in teaching, students tend to pursue attractive "mirages" of subjects usually associated with the practice of various fields of medicine.

Actually, in recent years the dental profession has come to realize that no other group enjoys a more advantageous position in scientific pursuit, now or in the future. Graduate students and undergraduate students should accept this truth also: there is no other profession capable of assuming the duties involved in the diagnosis and treatment of dental problems. Basically, these duties involve care during development as well as the maintenance of the normal function of the teeth and jaws after maturity. The teeth and jaws are the foundation tissues of the oral cavity.

It is now common knowledge that the health and welfare of the human being must wait upon the health and welfare of the "portal" of his body, his mouth. This fact promotes emphasis on the most important single subject in the dental curriculum: Dental Anatomy and Physiology.

Teeth are unique in that their static outside form is functional. They are incapable of readaptation in case of wear or accident; neither are they capable of recovery when they are partially destroyed by disease. Any dental treatment, general or specialized, requires an intimate and detailed knowledge of dental anatomy and physiology. Only dentists, among those in the health sciences, have the knowledge or the skills needed to care for the mouth; they must therefore apply themselves dutifully to this basic need.

Each new edition of this book was revised to keep up with the times and to cooperate with those who were interested enough to contribute constructive criticism. In this fourth edition, more changes in text and illustration have been made than in any previous revision.

The overall teaching plan has not been changed except to include the chapter on deciduous teeth within the first three chapters; these chapters are considered elementary instruction. It was thought that instruction in development, calcification and eruption should be closely followed by information concerning the deciduous dentition; that all of this information was really one phase of instruction.

The first twelve chapters are intended for first year work in dental school, with portions of Chapter XVI (the last chapter) on occlusion to be assigned at the instructor's discretion. The major portion of the material in the last four chapters, XIII to XVI, is intended for more advanced students and for postgraduate instruction.

If separate instruction in drawing and carving of teeth is required for laboratory reference, it is recommended that the student obtain "An Atlas of Tooth Form" (W. B. Saunders Co.), a book designed for that purpose. It is a useful companion to this text.

The new frontispiece of the textbook illustrates graphically the principles followed in making new half page figures for chapters VI through XII. These figures are enlargements of photographs of specimens of the permanent dentition, illustrating true anatomy from five aspects, obviating misrepresentation or errors in observation which might be registered in artist's drawings. Most of the illustrations in the seven chapters are new reproductions from new prints and photographs. An additional feature is the inclusion of full page figures of graph drawings facing full page figures of shaded drawings with three dimensional quality. These illustrations represent the eight typical tooth forms.

There has been some criticism from instructors that there was too much descriptive detail in the text. The author understands such criticism, but insists that there will always be a need for reference works in dental anatomy and physiology. Elaborate detail is necessary in a subject of this sort; this is true of most scientific disciplines! Let the student absorb as much as he can, for what he does retain may be the foundation for his success in practice.

Chapter XIII on pulp cavities in permanent teeth is probably more complete in anatomical description and illustration than material found in any other textbook at present writing. All illustrations are actual photographs of sectioned teeth or illustrations copied from photographs. Illustrations of cross sections which portray angles which cannot be obtained in radiographic examination are so labeled. This chapter should be of interest to endodontists in practice as well as upper classmen in dental school.

Particular attention should be paid to Chapter XIV on dento-osseous structures. Description of the maxilla and mandible must include the normally developed framework encompassing the teeth in complete dental arches. *This establishes the teeth as foundation tissues to be included with the bones for proper jaw relations and as integral parts of the important framework which supports the mobile portion of the face.* The size and angulation of the root forms of the teeth will govern the shape of the alveoli in the jaws, and this, in turn, shapes the contour of the dento-osseous portions facially.

The realization of these facts should have considerable influence in the diagnosis and prognosis of cases in Orthodontics. For instance, the premolars are succedaneous to the deciduous molars in identical sections of the maxillae and mandible. These sections are valuable combinations during development and after maturity. See "Dental Arch Formation," Chapter XVI. No other tooth combinations can serve as a substitute for the combined form of the premolars or the form of their osseous sections as completed around them. These beautiful and important teeth should not be sacrificed unless the patient's welfare demands it without question. The loss of any of the teeth brings about an atrophic reduction of valuable portions of the maxilla and mandible, a fact which adds disfigurement and psychological injury to the more obvious one of masticatory malfunction.

Chapter XV now includes new illustrations of the muscles of mastication, with illustrations of the muscles of facial expression.

The final chapter, Chapter XVI, on "Arrangement of the Teeth and Occlusion," has been carefully re-edited with figures placed in a manner which improves clarity and readability. Exercises have been suggested in chart tracing to be associated with simultaneous observation of three dimensional models or skulls.

The printed text on occlusion of the teeth is detailed. There is no "short cut" to the description of normal occlusal contacts during the various jaw movements. The student in dentistry must realize that normal occlusion of the teeth in his patients is the ultimate goal of the dental practitioner. All of his treatment plans, in dental development, in dental maintenance and in dental restoration, are to be devoted to that end.

The study of dental anatomy and physiology furnishes the *key* to that end; without it, there can be no real understanding of occlusion.

RUSSELL C. WHEELER

PREFACE TO THE FIRST EDITION

IN THE preparation of this book the author has attempted to simplify and coordinate the study of a fundamental subject in dentistry, namely, "Dental Anatomy and Physiology." Since *form* and *function* are so closely associated in the study of tooth design, "dental anatomy" and "dental physiology" must be considered and treated as one fundamental subject in the dental curriculum—hence the title of this book.

To date, a general lack of interest in this field, which is reflected in the meager literature and the dearth of research on the subject, makes it necessary for one textbook to attempt to cover the material. The author is very aware of this necessity, because his plan of separating the material on "Tooth Drawing and Carving" from that of the Textbook and placing the former in a laboratory manual has met with some criticism. Evidently there are those who think the subject too unimportant for enlargement, or for the allotment of sufficient time in the dental curriculum for proper assimilation. To the author this situation passes all understanding. No successful practitioner fails to recognize the importance of the fundamental form of the teeth, their alignment and their occlusion, as a basic subject serving as a background for *all phases* of dental practice.

This book is therefore humbly presented by one who fully realizes its brevity and its shortcomings. Criticism is to be expected and is requested. If the book has merit, constructive criticism will assist the author in improving any future editions. The material for this volume was not, however, accumulated overnight; twenty-one years of an active general practice in dentistry and sixteen years of association with dental school faculties have served as a "proving ground" for the text.

In general, the material on the following pages covers the macroscopic or gross anatomy of the individual teeth; their anatomy on cross section; the alignment of the teeth in the jaws; their occlusion during the various jaw relations, and the significance of the foregoing during function. Considerable space has been allotted to the bony foundations of the teeth, important maxillary and mandibular landmarks, and the temporomandibular articulation. A brief outline of the blood and nerve supply to the teeth has been added for reference purposes in order to complete the text. The drawing and carving of tooth forms, which is necessarily a laboratory course, is covered in a separate publication ("Tooth Form, Drawing and Carving, a Manual," W. B. Saunders Co., 1939).

Proper nomenclature often proves difficult, and is of course subject to change. Original terms are suggested only when those commonly used seemed to be inadequate. Most of the terms used are those generally recognized by dental teachers, although the consensus of opinion seems to be that the nomenclature covering landmarks on the teeth in particular is not entirely satisfactory.

Wherever feasible, the illustrations are cuts of actual photographs. Drawings are made directly from photographs or specimens. Any models of teeth that are shown are carved to definite specifications, which coincide with data arrived at through investigation and research.

Acknowledgment must be made of the positive influence exerted in this field upon the author by the works of Dr. G. V. Black, Dr. Martin Dewey and more recently, of Dr. Moses Diamond. Their books on dental anatomy in the author's library are much thumb marked and have been of invaluable assistance as reference works and inspirational sources.

It has been thirteen years since the first material was accumulated with the thought of future publication, therefore it would be impossible to list all those who have been instrumental in lending assistance. Four men who have inspired and guided the author from his earliest years in practice should be mentioned in particular. Through their idealism and exemplary professional standards they have wielded an influence they may not have realized. These four are Dr. Edgar H. Keys, Dr. Jesse D. White, Dr. Clarence O. Simpson and the late Dr. George B. W. Winter.

Special recognition must be given to Miss Catherine McKenzie, the author's efficient and most patient secretary. In addition to her difficult work as assistant in a busy dental practice, she has acted as editor, photographer, typist and copy reader.

Dean Thomas Purcell and individual faculty members of the St. Louis University School of Dentistry have been most cooperative at all times. Among these Dr. William Bauer and Dr. Ross Bleiker deserve special mention.

An effort has been made to give proper credit to all those who have granted permission so graciously to use illustrations from their published works. The hope is expressed that none of these has been overlooked.

Dr. Ruth Martin of Washington University, Dr. Geneve Riefling of St. Louis University, and Dr. Thomas Knox exhibited considerable interest in the chapter on deciduous teeth, and each one contributed valuable tooth specimens for the purpose of illustration.

Mr. Yandell Johnson, architect, deserves special mention for excellent illustrations and graphs in the textbook and manual. Mr. J. Wade McCarty executed the art work for Chapters VI to XII on the permanent teeth.

Lucille Wengler Wheeler has been personally interested and has been "literary critic" during the years the following material was being compiled; she has helped greatly in editing and correcting the manuscript.

Last, but far from least, the W. B. Saunders Company has done all a publisher could do to encourage and help the author.

RUSSELL C. WHEELER

CONTENTS

xiii

Chapter IX

Chapter X

Chapter XI

Chapter XII

Chapter XIII

Chapter XIV

A TEXTBOOK OF
Dental Anatomy
and Physiology

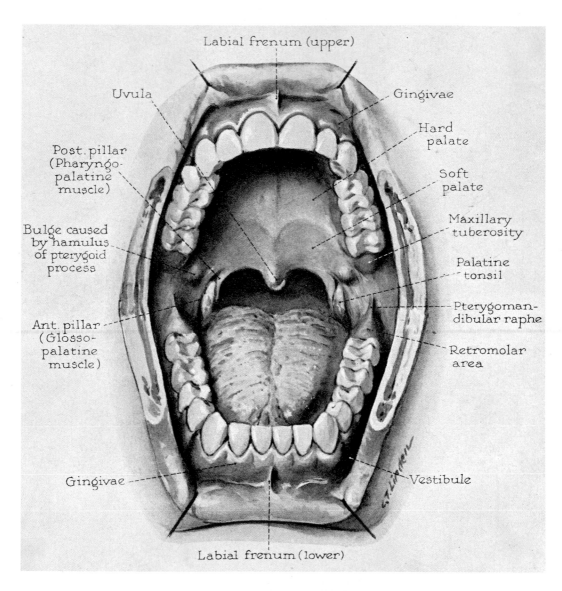

Labial frenum (upper)

Uvula

Gingivae

Post. pillar
(Pharyngo-
palatine
muscle)

Hard
palate

Soft
palate

Bulge caused
by hamulus
of pterygoid
process

Maxillary
tuberosity

Palatine
tonsil

Pterygoman-
dibular raphe

Ant. pillar
(Glosso-
palatine
muscle)

Retromolar
area

Gingivae

Vestibule

Labial frenum (lower)

THE ORAL CAVITY

(TAKEN FROM "ATLAS OF THE MOUTH," BY MASSLER AND SCHOUR.
AMERICAN DENTAL ASSOCIATION BUREAU OF PUBLIC RELATIONS.)

Chapter I

NOMENCLATURE AND
GENERAL CONSIDERATIONS

In ORDER to obtain a comprehensive view of any subject, one must learn the nomenclature and a general outline of what the subject includes. This can be done by reading an abstract or outline of the material which names and illustrates the terms. Chapters I, II, III, IV and V will cover such an outline. When a term is used for the first time it is emphasized in italics. If the definition is not clear at the time it is read in the text, further description may be found in proximate illustrations or elsewhere in the book. (Consult the index.)

NOMENCLATURE

The Deciduous Teeth

At birth, the individual has no functioning teeth in the mouth. Radiograms of the infant's jaws, however, show many teeth in various stages of the process of formation. The diet in early infancy is fluid or semifluid; therefore teeth are unnecessary until the reduction of solid food is required. Usually, at the age of two years or thereabout the *deciduous dentition* is complete.

The denomination and number of teeth for all Mammalia are expressed by formulae. The denomination of each tooth is represented by its initial letter, I for *incisor*, C for *canine*, P for *premolar*, M for *molar*; each letter is followed by a horizontal line, and the number of each type of tooth is placed above the line for the *maxilla*

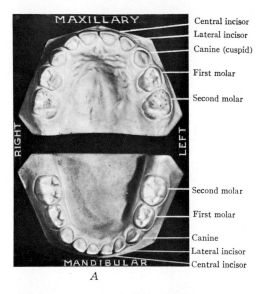

A

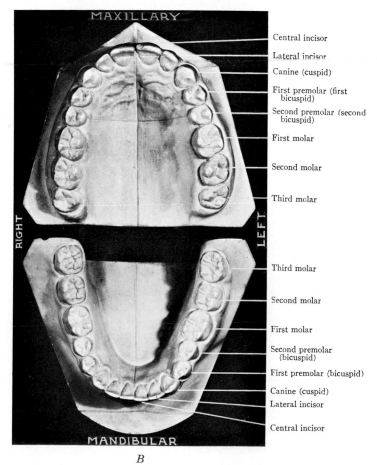

B

Figure 1. *A*, Plaster casts of deciduous or primary dentition. *B*, Casts of permanent dentition.

(upper jaw) and below the line for the *mandible* (lower jaw). The formula includes one side only:

The deciduous dental formula of man is:

$$I \frac{2}{2} \ C \ \frac{1}{1} \ M \ \frac{2}{2} = 10$$

This formula should be read thus: Incisors, two maxillary and two mandibular; canines, one maxillary and one mandibular; molars, two maxillary and two mandibular — or ten altogether on one side, right or left (Fig. 1, *A*).

The incisors are cutting teeth, the canines have a pointed cusp for tearing and incision, whereas the molars have broad occlusal surfaces with multiple cusps which break up food material as an aid in the digestive process.

The Permanent Teeth

By the time the child is about six years of age, the first permanent teeth (the first molars) appear in the maxilla and mandible, which have now become large enough to accommodate them. These teeth take their position *posterior* to the deciduous teeth. One by one the deciduous teeth are exfoliated, from the seventh year on, by a natural process brought about by *resorption* of their roots. *Succedaneous* permanent teeth take their places at the proper time. When the jaws have grown sufficiently, two additional molars are added posteriorly to the first molars.

The *permanent dental formula* of man is:

$$I \frac{2}{2} \ C \ \frac{1}{1} \ P \ \frac{2}{2} \ M \ \frac{3}{3} = 16$$

Premolars have now been added to the formula, two maxillary and two mandibular, and a third molar has been added, one maxillary and one mandibular (Fig. 1, *B*).

From the above we make the observation that the child has twenty deciduous teeth, and the adult thirty-two permanent teeth.

The Crown and Root

Each tooth has a *crown* and *root* portion. The crown is covered with *enamel*, and the root portion is covered with *cementum*. The crown and root join at the *cementoenamel* junction. This junction, also called the *cervical line* (Fig. 2), is plainly visible on a specimen tooth. The main bulk of the tooth is composed of *dentin*, which is clear in a cross section of the tooth. This cross section displays a *pulp chamber* and

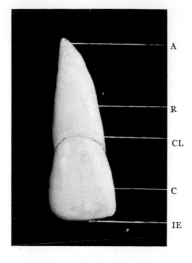

Figure 2. Maxillary central incisor (labial aspect). *A,* apex of root; *R,* root; *CL,* cervical line; *C,* crown; *IE,* incisal edge.

a *pulp canal* which normally contain the *pulp tissue.* The pulp chamber is in the crown portion mainly, and the pulp canal is in the root (Fig. 3). The spaces are continuous with each other and are spoken of collectively as the *pulp cavity.*

The four tooth tissues are *enamel, cementum, dentin* and *pulp.* The first three are known as *hard tissues,* the last as *soft tissue.* The pulp tissue furnishes the blood and nerve supply to the tooth.

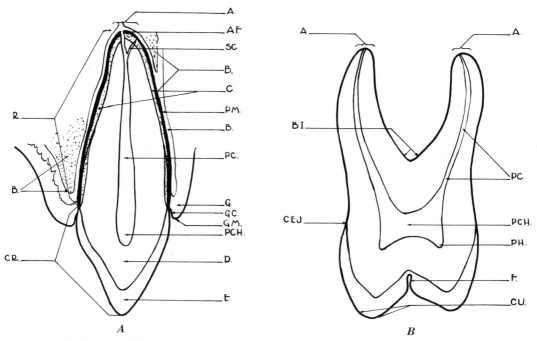

A   *B*

Figure 3. Schematic drawings of cross sections of an anterior and a posterior tooth.

A, Anterior tooth. *A,* apex; *AF,* apical foramen; *SC,* supplementary canal; *C,* cementum; *PM,* periodontal membrane; *B,* bone; *PC,* pulp canal; *G,* gingiva; *GC,* gingival crevice; *GM,* gingival margin; *PCH,* pulp chamber; *D,* dentin; *E,* enamel; *CR,* crown; *R,* root.

B, Posterior tooth. *A,* apices; *PC,* pulp canal; *PCH,* pulp chamber; *PH,* pulp horn; *F,* fissure; *CU,* cusp; *CEJ,* cementoenamel junction; *BI,* bifurcation of roots.

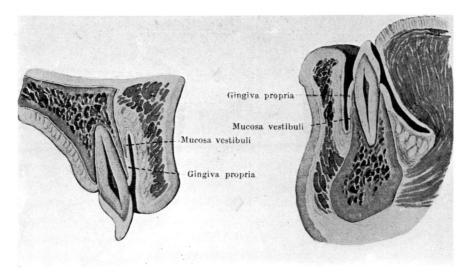

Figure 4. Sagittal sections through the central incisors and adjacent tissues (maxillary and mandibular). (Sicher, *Oral Anatomy,* The C. V. Mosby Company.)

The *crown* of an incisor tooth may have an incisal *ridge* or edge, as in the *central* and *lateral incisors;* a single *cusp,* as in the canines; or two or more cusps, as on premolars and molars. Incisal ridges and cusps form the cutting surfaces on tooth crowns.

The *root* portion of the tooth may be *single*, with one *apex* or terminal end, as usually found in *anterior* teeth and some of the premolars; or *multiple*, with a *bifurcation* or *trifurcation* dividing the root portion into two or more extensions or roots with their *apices* or terminal ends, as found on all molars and in some premolars.

The root portion of the tooth is firmly fixed in the bony process of the jaw, so that each tooth is held in its position relative to the others in the *dental arch*. That portion of the jaw which serves as a support for the tooth is called the *alveolar process*. The bone of the tooth socket is called the *alveolus* (plural, *alveoli*) (Fig. 6).

The crown portion is never covered by bone tissue after it is fully erupted, but it is partly covered at the *cervical third* in young adults by soft tissue of the mouth

Figure 5. Vertical section through the second maxillary molar and adjacent tissues. (Sicher, *Oral Anatomy,* The C. V. Mosby Company.)

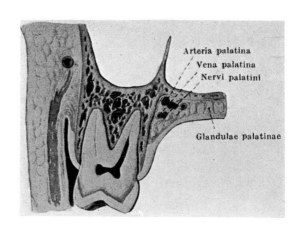

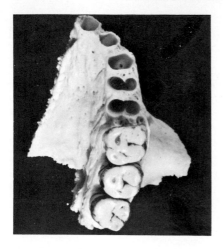

Figure 6. Left maxillary bone showing the alveolar process with three molars in place, and the alveoli of the central incisor, lateral incisor, canine, first and second premolars. Note the opening at the bottom of the canine alveolus, an opening which accommodates the nutrient blood and nerve supply to the tooth in life. Although they do not show in the photograph, the other alveoli present the same arrangement.

known as the *gingiva* or *gingival tissue*, or *gum tissue*. In older persons all of the enamel may be exposed in the oral cavity, and frequently some cervical cementum.

Surfaces and Ridges

The crowns of the incisors and canines have four surfaces and a ridge, and the crowns of the premolars and molars have five surfaces. The surfaces are named according to their positions and uses (Figs. 7 and 8). In the incisors and canines the surfaces toward the lips are called *labial surfaces*, and in the premolars and molars those facing the cheek are the *buccal surfaces*. When labial and buccal surfaces are spoken of collectively they are called *facial surfaces*. All surfaces facing toward the tongue are called *lingual surfaces*. The surfaces of the premolars and molars which come in contact with those in the opposite jaw during the act of closure (called *occlusion*) are called *occlusal surfaces*. In incisors and canines, those surfaces are called *incisal surfaces*.

The surfaces of the teeth facing toward adjoining teeth in the same dental arch are called *proximal* or *proximate surfaces*. The proximal surfaces may be called either *mesial* or *distal*. These terms have special reference to the position of the surface relative to the *median line* of the face. This line is drawn vertically through the center of the face, passing between the central incisors at their point of contact with each other in both the maxilla and the mandible. Those proximal surfaces which, following the curve of the arch, are faced toward the median line, are called *mesial surfaces*, and those most distant from the median line are called *distal surfaces*.

Four teeth have mesial surfaces which contact each other: the maxillary and mandibular central incisors. In all other instances the mesial surface of one tooth contacts the distal surface of its neighbor, except for the distal surfaces of third molars of permanent teeth and distal surfaces of second molars in deciduous teeth, which have no teeth distal to them. The area of the mesial or distal surface of a tooth which touches its neighbor in the arch is called the *contact area*.

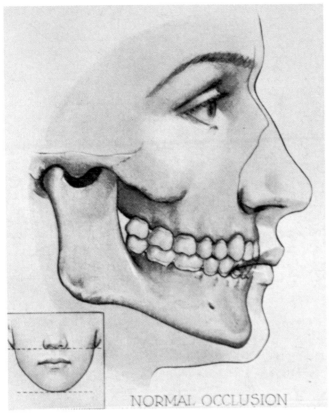

NORMAL OCCLUSION

Figure 7. Note the relation of the occlusal line to the profile of the face. (From Massler and Schour, *Atlas of the Mouth,* American Dental Association Bureau of Public Relations.)

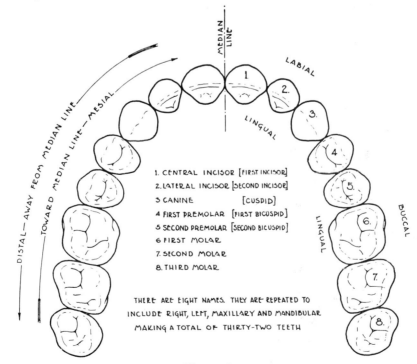

MEDIAN LINE

LABIAL

LINGUAL

DISTAL—AWAY FROM MEDIAN LINE

TOWARD MEDIAN LINE—MESIAL

LINGUAL

BUCCAL

1. CENTRAL INCISOR [FIRST INCISOR]
2. LATERAL INCISOR [SECOND INCISOR]
3. CANINE   [CUSPID]
4. FIRST PREMOLAR [FIRST BICUSPID]
5. SECOND PREMOLAR [SECOND BICUSPID]
6. FIRST MOLAR
7. SECOND MOLAR
8. THIRD MOLAR

THERE ARE EIGHT NAMES. THEY ARE REPEATED TO
INCLUDE RIGHT, LEFT, MAXILLARY AND MANDIBULAR
MAKING A TOTAL OF THIRTY-TWO TEETH

Figure 8.

Central and lateral incisors and canines as a group are called *anterior teeth;* premolars and molars as a group, *posterior teeth.*

Other Landmarks

In order to study an individual tooth intelligently one must be able to recognize all landmarks of importance by name. Therefore at this point it will be necessary to become familiar with additional terms such as:

cusp	triangular ridge	developmental groove
tubercle	transverse ridge	supplemental groove
cingulum	oblique ridge	pit
ridge	fossa	lobe
marginal ridge	sulcus	

A *cusp* is an elevation or mound on the crown portion of a tooth making up a divisional part of the occlusal surface (Figs. 3 and 9).

A *tubercle* is a smaller elevation on some portion of the crown produced by an extra formation of enamel (Fig. 100, Chapter IV). These are deviations from the typical form.

A *cingulum* is the lingual lobe of an anterior tooth. It makes up the bulk of the cervical third of the lingual surface. Its convexity mesiodistally resembles a girdle (cingulum is the Latin for girdle) encircling the lingual surface at the cervical third (Fig. 11 and Fig. 99, *A,* Chapter IV).

A *ridge* is any linear elevation on the surface of a tooth and is named according to its location: *buccal* ridge, *incisal* ridge, *marginal* ridge, etc.

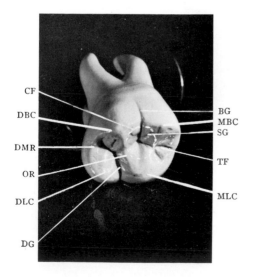

CF
DBC
DMR
OR
DLC
DG
BG
MBC
SG
TF
MLC

Figure 9. Some landmarks on the maxillary first molar. *BG,* buccal groove; *MBC,* mesiobuccal cusp; *SG,* supplemental groove; *TF,* triangular fossa; *MLC,* mesiolingual cusp; *DG,* developmental groove; *DLC,* distolingual cusp; *OR,* oblique ridge; *DMR,* distal marginal ridge; *DBC,* distobuccal cusp; *CF,* central fossa.

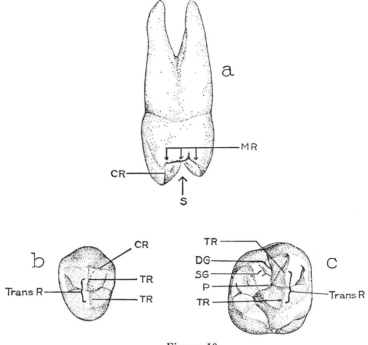

Figure 10.

a, Mesial view of a maxillary right first premolar. *S,* sulcus traversing occlusal surface; *MT,* marginal ridge; *CR,* cusp ridge.

b, Occlusal view of maxillary right first premolar. *CR,* cusp ridge; *TR,* triangular ridges; *Trans R,* transverse ridge, formed by two triangular ridges crossing the tooth transversely.

c, Occlusal view of a maxillary right first molar. *TR,* triangular ridge; *DG,* developmental groove; *SG,* supplemental groove; *P,* pit formed by junction of developmental grooves; *TR,* triangular ridge; *Trans R,* transverse ridge.

Marginal ridges are those rounded borders of the enamel which form the mesial and distal margins of the occlusal surfaces of premolars and molars and the mesial and distal margins of the lingual surfaces of the incisors and canines (Fig. 10, *a* and Fig. 11).

Triangular ridges are those ridges which descend from the tips of the cusps of molars and premolars toward the central part of the occlusal surfaces. They are so named because the slopes of each side of the ridge are inclined to resemble two sides of a triangle (Fig. 10, *b* and *c*, and Fig. 12). They are named after the cusps to which they belong—e.g., triangular ridge of the buccal cusp of the maxillary first premolar.

When a buccal and a lingual triangular ridge join, they form a *transverse ridge.* A transverse ridge is the union of two triangular ridges crossing transversely the surface of a posterior tooth (Fig. 10, *b* and *c*).

The *oblique ridge* is a variable ridge crossing obliquely the occlusal surfaces of maxillary molars. It, too, is formed by the union of two triangular ridges (Fig. 9).

A *fossa* is an irregular depression or concavity. *Lingual* fossae are on the lingual surface of incisors. *Central* fossae are on the occlusal surface of molars. They are formed by the converging of ridges terminating at a central point in the bottom of the depression, where there is a junction of grooves. *Triangular* fossae are found on molars and premolars on the occlusal surfaces mesial or distal to marginal ridges.

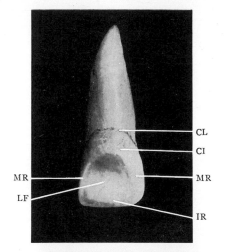

MR
LF
CL
CI
MR
IR

Figure 11.   Maxillary right central incisor (lingual aspect).* *CL*, cervical line; *CI*, cingulum; *MR*, marginal ridge; *IR*, incisal ridge; *LF*, lingual fossa.

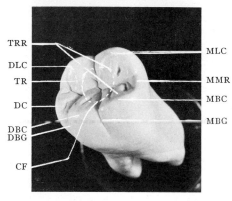

TRR
DLC
TR
DC
DBC
DBG
CF
MLC
MMR
MBC
MBG

Figure 12.   Mandibular right first molar.* *MLC*, mesiolingual cusp; *MMR*, mesial marginal ridge; *MBC*, mesiobuccal cusp; *MBG*, mesiobuccal groove; *CF*, central fossa; *DBG*, distobuccal groove; *DBC*, distobuccal cusp; *DC*, distal cusp; *TR*, triangular ridge; *DLC*, distolingual cusp; *TRR*, transverse ridge.

They are sometimes found on the lingual surfaces of maxillary incisors at the edge of the lingual fossae where the marginal ridges and the cingulum meet (Fig. 138, p. 132).

A *sulcus* is a long depression or valley in the surface of a tooth between ridges and cusps, the inclines of which meet at an angle. A sulcus has a developmental groove at the junction of its inclines. (The term "sulcus" must not be confused with the term *groove.*)

A *developmental groove* is a shallow groove or line between the primary parts of the crown or root. A *supplemental groove*, less distinct, is also a shallow linear depression on the surface of a tooth, but it is supplemental to a developmental groove and does not mark the junction of primary parts. *Buccal* and *lingual grooves* are developmental grooves found on the buccal and lingual surfaces of posterior teeth (Fig. 9; also Fig. 98, Chapter IV).

Pits are small pinpoint depressions located at the junction of developmental grooves or at terminals of those grooves. For instance, *central pit* is a term used to describe a landmark in the central fossa of molars where developmental grooves join (Fig. 10, *c*).

---

*For further graphic information on landmarks see Figs. 72, 133, 154, 175, 187, 199, 213, 223, 244 to 250 and 280 to 285.

A *lobe* is one of the primary sections of formation in the development of the crown. Cusps and mamelons are representative of lobes. A *mamelon* is any one of the three rounded protuberances found on the incisal ridges of newly erupted incisor teeth (Fig. 84, Chapter IV). (For further description of lobes see Figs. 98, 99 and 100, Chapter IV.)

The *roots* of the teeth may be single or multiple. Both maxillary and mandibular anterior teeth have only one root each. Mandibular first and second premolars and the maxillary second premolar are single-rooted, but the maxillary first premolar has two roots in most cases, one buccal and one lingual. Maxillary molars have three roots, one mesiobuccal, one distobuccal and one lingual. Mandibular molars have two roots, one mesial and one distal. It must be understood that description in anatomy can never follow a hard and fast rule. Variations frequently occur. This is especially true regarding tooth roots.

Division into Thirds, Line Angles and Point Angles

For purposes of description the crowns and roots of teeth have been divided into thirds, and junctions of the crown surfaces are described as *line angles* and *point angles*. Actually, there are no angles or points or plane surfaces on the teeth anywhere except those which appear from wear, or *abrasion*, or from accidental fracture. The terms "line angle" and "point angle" are used only as descriptive terms to indicate a location.

When the surfaces of the crown and root portions are divided into *thirds*, these thirds are named according to their location. Looking at the tooth from the *labial* or *buccal* aspect, one sees that the crown and root may be divided into thirds from the incisal or occlusal surface of the crown to the apex of the root (Fig. 13). The *crown* is divided into an incisal or occlusal third, a middle third and a cervical third. The *root* is divided into a cervical third, middle third and apical third.

The crown may be divided into thirds in three directions: inciso- or occlusocervically, mesiodistally, or labio- or buccolingually. Mesiodistally it is divided into the mesial, middle and distal thirds. Labio- or buccolingually it is divided into labial or buccal, middle and lingual thirds. Each of the five surfaces of a crown may be so divided. There will be one middle third and two other thirds, which are named according to their location as cervical, occlusal, mesial, lingual, etc.

A *line angle* is formed by the junction of two surfaces and derives its name from the combination of the two surfaces that join. For instance, on an anterior tooth, the junction of the mesial and labial surfaces is called the "mesiolabial line angle" (Fig. 14, *A*).

The *line angles* of the *anterior teeth* are:

mesiolabial	distolingual
distolabial	labioincisal
mesiolingual	linguoincisal

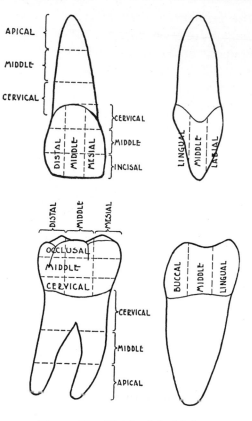

Figure 13.   Division into thirds.

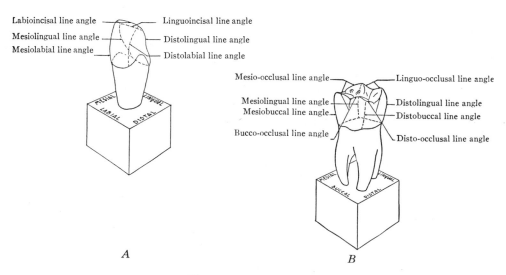

Figure 14.   Line angles.

Because the mesial and distal incisal angles of anterior teeth are rounded, *mesioincisal line angles* and *distoincisal line angles* are usually considered non-existent. They are spoken of as *mesial* and *distal incisal* angles only.

The *line angles* of the *posterior teeth* are:

mesiobuccal	distolingual	bucco-occlusal
distobuccal	mesio-occlusal	linguo-occlusal
mesiolingual	disto-occlusal	

A *point angle* is formed by the junction of three surfaces. The point angle also derives its name from the combination of the names of the surfaces forming it. For example, the junction of the mesial, buccal and occlusal surfaces of a molar is called the "mesiobucco-occlusal point angle." (Fig. 15, *B*.)

The *point angles* of the *anterior teeth* are:

mesiolabioincisal	mesiolinguoincisal
distolabioincisal	distolinguoincisal

The *point angles* of the *posterior teeth* are:

mesiobucco-occlusal	mesiolinguo-occlusal
distobucco-occlusal	distolinguo-occlusal

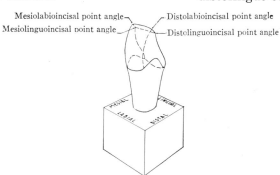

Mesiolabioincisal point angle Distolabioincisal point angle
Mesiolinguoincisal point angle Distolinguoincisal point angle

A. Anterior tooth.

Mesiolinguo-occlusal point angle Distolinguo-occlusal point angle
Mesiobucco-occlusal point angle Distobucco-occlusal point angle

B. Posterior tooth.
Figure 15. Point angles.

TOOTH FORM DRAWING AND CARVING

The subject of tooth drawing and carving is being introduced at this point because it has been found through experience that a laboratory course in tooth morphology (dissection, drawing and carving) must be carried on simultaneously with lectures and reference work on the subject of dental anatomy. Illustrations and instruction in tooth form drawing and carving will not, however, be included in this volume. A manual covering the subject is published in a separate binding (*An Atlas of Tooth Form*, W. B. Saunders Company).

Since form and function are allied so closely, the smallest details in dental anatomy are important. If restoration in operative dentistry is to be done scientifically, conscientious study through continuous close observation is required.

In an effort to establish more accuracy in restoration, an attempt was started some years ago to improve the teaching of tooth form by means of drawing to scale and carving to scale.

The author's plans and specifications for drawings and carvings of a complete model of dental arches began with the use of Dr. Greene Vardiman Black's table of average measurements for permanent teeth as a basis. (See tables, pages 427-428.) It was found, however, that teeth drawn or carved to those dimensions would not give what was wanted. Adjoining teeth in either of the dental arches were not always in good proportion, and opposing teeth in the opposite arch would not occlude properly when carvings were set up and occluded. Also, carving teeth natural size calibrated to tenths of a millimeter was found impracticable. Dr. Black's table being used as a starting point, therefore, deviation was made only when it seemed necessary to create the approach to the idealized norm. The only fractions listed in the model table are five-tenths of a millimeter and three-tenths of a millimeter, the latter in a few instances only. Fractions were avoided wherever possible in order to facilitate familiarity with the table and to avoid confusion.

Photographs of the five aspects of each tooth (mesial, distal, labial or buccal, lingual and incisal or occlusal) were taken with a lens capable of two diameter registrations. In short, the photographs show each tooth with its dimensions squared. These photographs were superimposed on squared millimeter cross section paper, obtainable from engineers' supply firms, which was a practical help in standardizing the relative positions of the tooth outlines on a given background. This procedure reduced the tooth outlines of each aspect to an accurate graph, so that it was possible to compare and record the contours (Figs. 16 and 17, also frontispiece).

Close observation of the outlines of the squared backgrounds shows the relationship of crown to root, extent of curvatures at various points, inclination of roots, relative widths of occlusal surfaces, height of marginal ridges, contact areas, etc. The *Atlas*, illustrating the methods of drawing and carving teeth, makes use of the scientific information discovered through these investigations.

Although there is no such thing as an established invariable norm in nature, in the study of anatomy it is necessary that there be a starting point; therefore we must

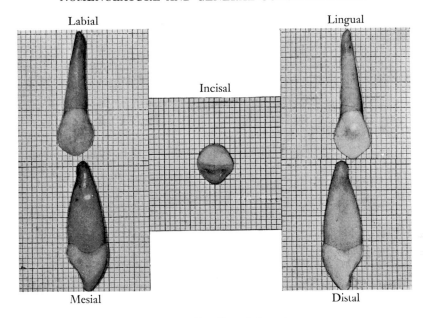

Figure 16.   Maxillary left canine.

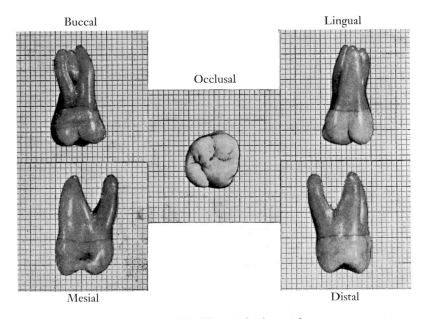

Figure 17.   Maxillary right first molar.

begin with an *arbitrary criterion*, accepted after experimentation and due consideration. Since restorative work in dentistry is a manual art which must approach the scientific as closely as manual dexterity will allow, models, plans, photographs and anatomic specimens should be given preference over the written text in this subject.

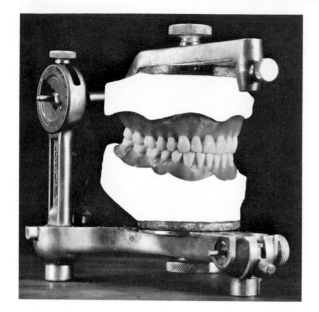

Figure 18. Carvings in Ivorine of individual teeth made according to the table of measurements on page 21. These models of teeth are set up into complete dental arches on an anatomic articulator. They have "balance" in lateral and protrusive movements as well as good centric relation.

Every curve and segment of a normal tooth has some functional basis, and it is important to reproduce them. *It is to be hoped that dental restoration will continue to develop as a science to restore function and not as a manual art to provide mere substitutes for lost tissue.*

Bulwer said, "Art and Science have their meeting point in method." With that statement in mind, these plans with a finished model are presented. The successful dental operator and restorative designer should be able to create mental pictures of various aspects of the teeth in his own mind. Complete pictures can be formed only

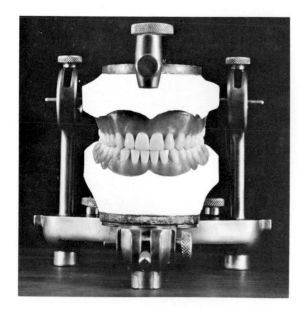

Figure 19. Another view of the models shown in Figure 18.

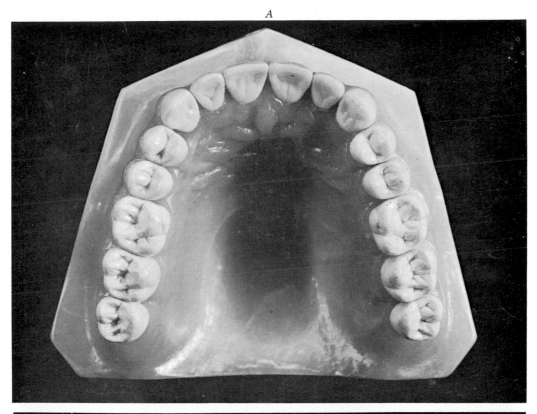

A

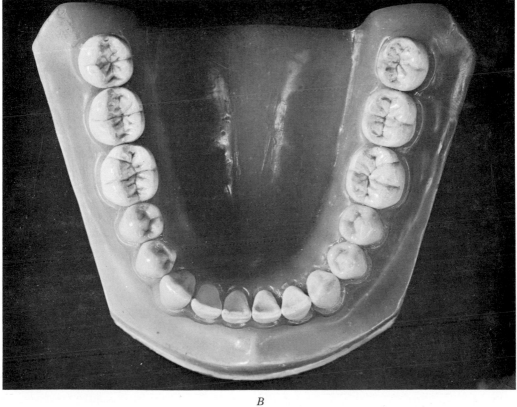

B

Figure 20. Occlusal view of the models shown in Figures 18 and 19.

when the individual is perfectly familiar with every detail — so familiar that it is possible for him to draw an outline of any aspect of any tooth in the human dental arches and draw it in good proportion without reference to a model drawing or carving. He should then be capable of carving any tooth in the mouth to correspond to his drawings.

Dental restoration must be approached from the engineer's viewpoint. Therefore the study of tooth reproduction must have a plan, and details of reconstruction should comply with the plan at all times. While it is impossible for the dentist to work with the precision of a mechanic operating a precision machine, and since the dentist's work must finally be the result of the coordination of hand and eye only, nevertheless, the engineer's viewpoint will give the operator an attitude of approach which will make him dissatisfied with anything less than logical sequence and good finish in technique.

Acute observation comes only after habitual study of detail. With the necessary application and interest, any dental operator can train himself to be an authority on the anatomy of the teeth — and that is the first step in becoming a master operator. To be a finished operator on human teeth, the intelligent student must absorb every detail of dental anatomy.

For excellence, a student must:

1. *Become so familiar with the table of measurements that it is possible to make instant comparisons mentally of the proportion of one tooth to another from any aspect.*
2. *Learn to draw accurate outlines of any aspect of any tooth.*
3. *Learn to carve with precision any design he can illustrate with line drawings.*

Although many individuals find the drawing and carving of teeth relatively easy, it is extremely difficult for others. It must also be remembered that a carving showing considerable skill and a beautiful finish often will fail to pass a rigid inspection with the caliper. Since this is a *scientific* course as well as an *art* course, *accuracy of outline* is paramount. Remember, *tooth contours affect function.*

When one is studying the *form* of anything, work will be facilitated by having a standard for comparative purposes. Since skulls and extracted teeth show so many variations and anomalies, an arbitrary norm for individual teeth had to be established for comparative study. Hence the thirty-two teeth were carved, natural size, in normal alignment and occlusion, and from the model a table of measurements was drafted. (Figs. 18, 19, 20.)

Although no claim is made that the table of measurements established by the carvings proves an average norm for tooth measurements which must be recognized as such, carvings and drawings made according to the measurements will illustrate teeth which will be accepted generally as close to the average in dimensions; close enough to prove observations on proportion in the study of form.

If the reader is not familiar with the *Boley gauge*, he should study its use before reading the following instructions on the use of the table of measurements on the opposite page.

Measurements of the Teeth—Millimeters: Specifications for Drawing and Carving Teeth of Average Size (This table was "proved" by carvings shown in Figures 18 and 19 and elsewhere in this book.)

Maxillary Teeth	Length of Crown	Length of Root	Mesio-distal Diameter of Crown*	Mesio-distal Diameter at Cervix	Labio- or Bucco-lingual Diameter	Labio- or Bucco-lingual Diameter at Cervix	Curvature of Cervical Line— Mesial	Curvature of Cervical Line— Distal
Central Incisor	10.5	13.0	8.5	7.0	7.0	6.0	3.5	2.5
Lateral Incisor	9.0	13.0	6.5	5.0	6.0	5.0	3.0	2.0
Canine	10.0	17.0	7.5	5.5	8.0	7.0	2.5	1.5
1st Premolar	8.5	14.0	7.0	5.0	9.0	8.0	1.0	0.0
2d Premolar	8.5	14.0	7.0	5.0	9.0	8.0	1.0	0.0
First Molar	7.5	b 12 l 13	10.0	8.0	11.0	10.0	1.0	0.0
Second Molar	7.0	b 11 l 12	9.0	7.0	11.0	10.0	1.0	0.0
Third Molar	6.5	11.0	8.5	6.5	10.0	9.5	1.0	0.0
Mandibular Teeth								
Central Incisor	9.0†	12.5	5.0	3.5	6.0	5.3	3.0	2.0
Lateral Incisor	9.5†	14.0	5.5	4.0	6.5	5.8	3.0	2.0
Canine	11.0	16.0	7.0	5.5	7.5	7.0	2.5	1.0
1st Premolar	8.5	14.0	7.0	5.0	7.5	6.5	1.0	0.0
2d Premolar	8.0	14.5	7.0	5.0	8.0	7.0	1.0	0.0
First Molar	7.5	14.0	11.0	9.0	10.5	9.0	1.0	0.0
Second Molar	7.0	13.0	10.5	8.0	10.0	9.0	1.0	0.0
Third Molar	7.0	11.0	10.0	7.5	9.5	9.0	1.0	0.0

* The sum of the mesiodistal diameters, both right and left, which gives the arch length, is: maxillary 128 mm., mandibular 126 mm.

† Lingual measurement approximately 0.5 mm. longer.

In order to understand the table, let us demonstrate the calibrations as recorded and the landmarks they encompass. There are *eight calibrations* of each tooth to be remembered. These measurements are shown in the accompanying example for the maxillary central incisor.

Measurements of the Teeth—Millimeters: Example

Maxillary Teeth	Length of Crown	Length of Root	Mesio-distal Diameter of Crown	Mesio-distal Diameter of Crown at Cervix	Labio- or Bucco-lingual Diameter of Crown	Labio- or Bucco-lingual Diameter at Cervix	Curvature of Cervical Line— Mesial	Curvature of Cervical Line— Distal
Central Incisor	10.5	13.0	8.5	7.0	7.0	6.0	3.5	2.5

The method of measuring an *anterior* tooth will be shown first, then a posterior one will be used for illustration.

Method of Measuring an Anterior Tooth

(Keep the long axis of the tooth vertical.)

1. LENGTH OF CROWN (LABIAL)*

Measurement $\Bigg\{$ Crest of curvature at cemento-enamel junction

Incisal edge

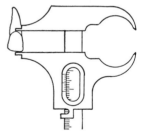

Figure 21. Length of crown.

2. LENGTH OF ROOT

Measurement $\Bigg\{$ Apex of root

Crest of curvature at crown cervix

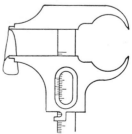

Figure 22. Length of root.

---

*Use the parallel beaks of the Boley gauge for measurements whenever feasible. The contrast of the various curvatures with the straight edges will help to make the close observer more familiar with tooth outlines.

3. MESIODISTAL DIAMETER OF CROWN

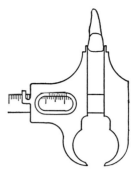

Measurement
{
Crest of curvature on the mesial surface (mesial contact area)

Crest of curvature on the distal surface (distal contact area)
}

Figure 23. Mesiodistal diameter of crown.

4. MESIODISTAL DIAMETER OF CROWN AT THE CERVIX

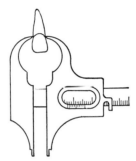

Measurement
{
Junction of crown and root on mesial surface

Junction of crown and root on distal surface (use caliper jaws of Boley gauge in this instance instead of parallel beaks)
}

Figure 24. Mesiodistal diameter of crown at cervix.

5. LABIOLINGUAL DIAMETER OF CROWN

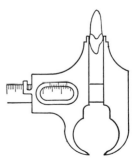

Measurement
{
Crest of curvature on the labial surface

Crest of curvature on the lingual surface
}

Figure 25. Labiolingual diameter of crown.

6. LABIOLINGUAL DIAMETER OF CROWN AT THE CERVIX

Measurement
{
Junction of crown and root on labial surface

Junction of crown and root on lingual surface (use caliper jaws in this instance also)

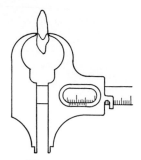

Figure 26. Labiolingual diameter of cervix.

7. CURVATURE OF CEMENTOENAMEL JUNCTION ON MESIAL*

Measurement
{
Crest of curvature of cemento-enamel junction, labial and lingual surface

Crest of curvature of cemento-enamel junction on the mesial surface

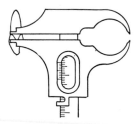

Figure 27. Curvature of cementoenamel junction on mesial.

8. CURVATURE OF CEMENTOENAMEL JUNCTION ON THE DISTAL

(Turn the tooth around and calibrate as in Fig. 27.)

Measurement
{
Crest of curvature of cemento-enamel junction on the labial and lingual surfaces

Crest of curvature of cemento-enamel junction on the distal surface

---

*This measurement is most important because, normally, it represents approximately the extent of curvature of the periodontal attachment when the tooth is in situ.

Method of Measuring a Posterior Tooth

(Keep the long axis of the tooth vertical.)

1. LENGTH OF CROWN (BUCCAL)

Measurement
{
Crest of buccal cusp or cusps

Crest of curvature at cementoenamel junction
}

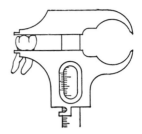

Figure 28. Length of crown.

2. LENGTH OF ROOT

Measurement
{
Crest of curvature at crown
cervix

Apex of root
}

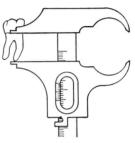

Figure 29. Length of root.

3. MESIODISTAL DIAMETER OF CROWN

Measurement
{
Crest of curvature on mesial
surface (mesial contact area)

Crest of curvature on distal surface (distal contact area)
}

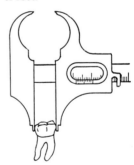

Figure 30. Mesio-distal diameter of crown.

4. MESIODISTAL DIAMETER OF CROWN AT THE CERVIX

Measurement
{
Junction of crown and root on
mesial surface

Junction of crown and root on
distal surface (use caliper jaws
of Boley gauge instead of
parallel beaks)
}

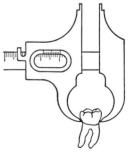

Figure 31. Mesio-distal diameter of crown at cervix.

5. BUCCOLINGUAL DIAMETER OF CROWN

Measurement
{
Crest of curvature on the buccal surface

Crest of curvature on the lingual surface
}

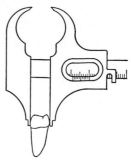

Figure 32. Buccolingual diameter of crown.

6. BUCCOLINGUAL DIAMETER OF CROWN AT THE CERVIX

Measurement
{
Junction of crown and root on buccal surface

Junction of crown and root on lingual surface (use caliper jaws)
}

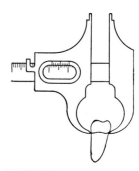

Figure 33. Buccolingual diameter of crown at cervix.

7. CURVATURE OF CEMENTOENAMEL JUNCTION ON MESIAL

Measurement
{
Crest of curvature of cementoenamel junction on the mesial surface

Crest of curvature of cementoenamel junction, buccal and lingual surfaces
}

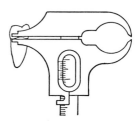

Figure 34. Curvature of cementoenamel junction on mesial.

8. CURVATURE OF CEMENTOENAMEL JUNCTION ON THE DISTAL

(Turn tooth around and measure as in Fig. 34.)

Measurement
{
Crest of curvature of cementoenamel junction on the distal surface

Crest of curvature of cementoenamel junction on the buccal and lingual surfaces
}

Chapter II

DEVELOPMENT OF THE TEETH, CALCIFICATION AND ERUPTION

THE CROWN and part of the root of a tooth are formed before emergence into the mouth. The crown is formed first; the root follows.

THE DECIDUOUS DENTITION

Calcification of the deciduous teeth begins about the fourth month of fetal life; near the end of the sixth month all of the deciduous teeth have begun to develop. Normally, at birth no teeth are visible in the mouth; occasionally, however, infants are born with erupted mandibular incisors. Such prematurely erupted teeth are usually lost soon after birth because of the incomplete development of the root attachment.

It must be emphasized at this point that all eruption schedules (and this includes calcification) must of necessity be approximate, because no two individuals are exactly alike in their development. Nevertheless, an approximation of averages in an eruption schedule can be a very valuable asset in diagnosis during the developmental years.

According to Schour, "It must be pointed out that the tooth is more than an organ of mastication. During the development of its enamel and dentin the tooth is also a biologic recorder of health and disease, especially of alterations in mineral metabolism. The incremental layer of enamel and dentin reflect metabolic fluctuations just as the growth rings of a tree reflect its life history (weather, nutrition, etc.)."

The deciduous *mandibular central incisors* appear in the mouth at the age of approximately six months. They are followed a month or so later by the *maxillary central incisors*. About two months elapse before the *maxillary lateral incisors* appear. The *mandibular lateral incisors* usually emerge a little earlier than maxillary laterals; in fact, to illustrate the variance in sequence in individuals, babies are often seen displaying four mandibular incisors and no maxillary teeth at all. However, the general rule to be kept in mind is that individual mandibular teeth usually precede the maxillary teeth in the process of eruption, and the teeth in both jaws erupt in *pairs*, one right and one left.

At the age of one year or a little later, the first deciduous molars erupt. The

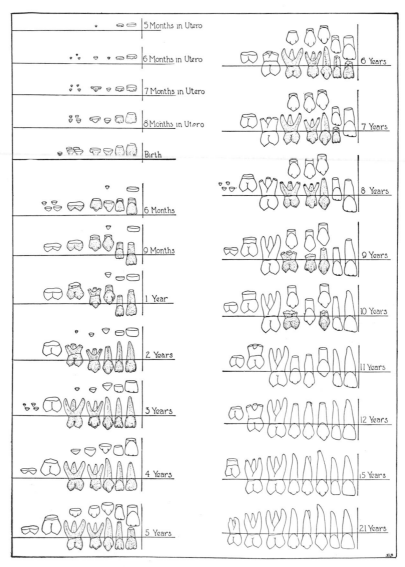

Figure 35. The chronology of the upper dentition. (Deciduous teeth stippled.) (From Noyes, Schour and Noyes, *Dental Histology and Embryology,* Lea & Febiger.) Refer also to Figures 36 and 37.

deciduous canines appear at about sixteen months. When the child is two or two and a half years of age, all of the deciduous teeth are expected to be in use. (Figs. 78 and 79, Chapter III.)

To repeat the usual order of appearance of the deciduous teeth in the mouth:

1. Central incisors
2. Lateral incisors
3. First molars
4. Canines
5. Second molars

Mandibular teeth usually precede the maxillary teeth in the order of appearance.

By the time the child is five years old or before, the jaw growth is made manifest by some separation of the deciduous teeth (Fig. 48, Chapter III).

A common impression, which is still widespread, is that the deciduous teeth are not to be taken seriously, since they will be lost at an early age in the process of making way for the permanent teeth. Many therefore think that since these deciduous teeth are to be replaced, any damage done them, or their premature loss, is not important. This is an erroneous view and one that has dire possibilities in the dental development of children. Possibly because they have been called "baby teeth" or "milk teeth," the laity at times regard the deciduous teeth as being temporary. That is not the case. All of the deciduous teeth are in use from the age of two until the age of seven years, or five years in all. Some of the deciduous teeth are in use from six months until twelve years of age, or eleven and a half years in all. The actual situation is, then, that these teeth are in use, contributing to the health and well-being of the individual, during his first years of greatest development, physically and mentally. With premature loss of deciduous teeth, normal jaw development may not take place. Unless the deciduous dental arches remain intact, therefore, the first permanent molars may not be guided into their normal position to act as "cornerstones" for the permanent dentition.

What is just as important to assure sufficient development for maturity, is normal function on both sides of the dental arches. Normal growth and development cannot take place without daily exercise and the use of both jaws. Without the comfortable activity of either side, one side will be favored to the detriment of normal formation.

PERMANENT DENTITION

The first teeth of the permanent dentition to emerge into the oral cavity are the *first molars*. They make their appearance immediately distal to the deciduous second molars at the age of approximately six years (Fig. 49, page 47). As a consequence, these teeth are often called the "six-year molars." They begin to calcify during the first month of life. They are much larger than any of the deciduous teeth and cannot make their entry until the jaw growth has progressed sufficiently to allow the space.

The second permanent tooth to take its place in the arch is the central incisor, which appears when the child is between six and seven years of age. As in the deciduous dentition, the mandibular permanent teeth tend to precede the maxillary teeth in the process of eruption. The mandibular central incisors usually show themselves some months previous to the maxillary central incisors. Often they erupt simultaneously with, or even previous to, the mandibular first molars and are often accompanied by the mandibular lateral incisors.

Before the permanent central incisor can come into position, the deciduous central incisor must be exfoliated. This is brought about by the phenomenon called *resorption* of the deciduous roots. The permanent tooth in its follicle attempts to force its way into the position held by its predecessor. The pressure brought to bear against the deciduous root evidently causes resorption of the root which continues until the deciduous crown has lost its anchorage, becomes loose and is finally exfoliated (Fig. 46). In the meantime, the permanent tooth has moved occlusally, so that when the deciduous tooth is lost, the permanent one is at the point of eruption and in proper position to succeed its predecessor.

Chronology of the Human Dentition

(LOGAN AND KRONFELD, slightly modified by SCHOUR)

		Tooth.	First evidence of calcification.	Crown completed.	Eruption.	Root completed
Deciduous dentition	Upper jaw	Central incisor	3–4 mos. *in utero*	4 mos.	7½ mos.	1½–2 yrs.
		Lateral incisor	4½ mos. *in utero*	5 mos.	8 mos.	1½–2 yrs.
		Canine	5¼ mos. *in utero*	9 mos.	16–20 mos.	2½–3 yrs.
		First molar	5 mos. *in utero*	6 mos.	12–16 mos.	2–2½ yrs
		Second molar	6 mos. *in utero*	10–12 mos.	20–30 mos.	3 yrs.
	Lower jaw	Central incisor	4½ mos. *in utero*	4 mos.	6½ mos.	1½–2 yrs
		Lateral incisor	4½ mos. *in utero*	4¼ mos.	7 mos.	1½–2 yrs
		Canine	5 mos. *in utero*	9 mos.	16–20 mos.	2½–3 yrs
		First molar	5 mos. *in utero*	6 mos.	12–16 mos.	2–2½ yrs
		Second molar	6 mos. *in utero*	10–12 mos.	20–30 mos.	3 yrs
Permanent dentition	Upper jaw	Central incisor	3–4 mos.	4– 5 yrs.	7– 8 yrs.	10 yrs
		Lateral incisor	10 mos.	4– 5 yrs.	8– 9 yrs.	11 yrs
		Canine	4–5 mos.	6– 7 yrs.	11–12 yrs.	13–15 yrs.
		First premolar	1½–1¾ yrs.	5– 6 yrs.	10–11 yrs.	12–13 yrs.
		Second premolar	2–2¼ yrs.	6– 7 yrs.	10–12 yrs.	12–14 yrs.
		First molar	At birth	2½– 3 yrs.	6– 7 yrs.	9–10 yrs.
		Second molar	2½–3 yrs.	7– 8 yrs.	12–13 yrs.	14–16 yrs.
		Third molar	7–9 yrs.	12–16 yrs.	17–21 yrs.	18–25 yrs.
	Lower jaw	Central incisor	3–4 mos.	4– 5 yrs.	6– 7 yrs.	9 yrs.
		Lateral incisor	3–4 mos.	4– 5 yrs.	7– 8 yrs.	10 yrs.
		Canine	4–5 mos.	6– 7 yrs.	9–10 yrs.	12–14 yrs.
		First premolar	1¾– 2 yrs.	5– 6 yrs.	10–12 yrs.	12–13 yrs.
		Second premolar	2¼–2½ yrs.	6– 7 yrs.	11–12 yrs.	13–14 yrs.
		First molar	At birth	2½– 3 yrs.	6– 7 yrs.	9–10 yrs.
		Second molar	2½– 3 yrs.	7– 8 yrs.	11–13 yrs.	14–15 yrs.
		Third molar	8–10 yrs.	12–16 yrs.	17–21 yrs.	18–25 yrs.

The *follicles* of the developing *incisors* and *canines* are in a position lingual to the deciduous roots (Fig. 42). The developing *premolars* which are to take the place of deciduous molars are within the bifurcation of deciduous molar roots (Figs. 43 and 44). The permanent incisors, canines and premolars are called *succedaneous teeth*, since they take the place of their deciduous predecessors.

Root resorption sometimes does not follow the routine procedure, with the result that the permanent tooth cannot emerge or else is kept out of its normal place. The failure of the deciduous root to resorb may bring about prolonged retention of the deciduous tooth (Figs. 44 and 45).

Mandibular lateral incisors erupt very soon after the central incisors, and often simultaneously. The *maxillary central incisors* erupt next in the chronological order, and the *maxillary lateral incisors* make their appearance about a year later (*cf.* "Chronology of Human Dentition," above and chart on page 33). The *first premolars* follow the maxillary laterals in sequence when the child is ten years old, approximately; the *mandibular canines* (cuspids) often appear at the same time. The *second premolars* follow during the next year and then the *maxillary canines*. Usually the second molars come in when the individual is about twelve; they are posterior to the first molars and are commonly called "twelve-year molars." The maxillary canines occasionally erupt along with the second molars, but in most instances of normal eruption the canines precede them somewhat.

The *third molars* do not come in until the age of seventeen years or later. Considerable jaw growth is required after the age of twelve to allow room for these teeth. Third molars are subject to many anomalies and variations of form. Insufficient jaw development for their accommodation complicates matters in the majority of cases. Individuals who have properly developed third molars in good alignment are very much in the minority. Third molar anomalies and variations with the complications brought about by malalignment and subnormal jaw development comprise a subject too vast to be covered here.

The usual order in which the permanent teeth appear is as follows:

1. First molars
2. Mandibular central and lateral incisors
3. Maxillary central incisors
4. Maxillary lateral incisors
5. Mandibular canines
6. First premolars
7. Second premolars
8. Maxillary canines
9. Second molars
10. Third molars

The "Chronology of the Human Dentition," which is a table of calcification and eruption of both deciduous and permanent teeth, was reported by Logan and Kronfeld in 1936 and modified later by McCall and Schour. The table has been recognized generally and has been utilized as an index of tooth development; in fact, this book uses the revised table as authority for all references to the chronology of tooth development.

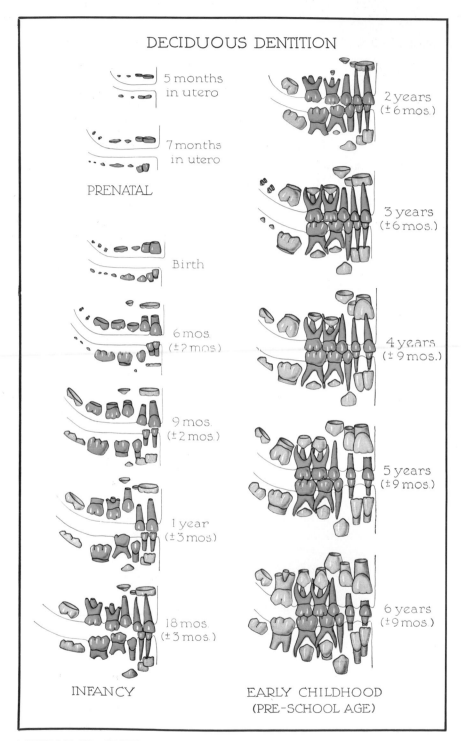

I. SCHOUR, D.D.S., Ph.D. and M. MASSLER, D.D.S., M.S., University of Illinois, College of Dentistry   2nd edition—1944

Figure 36.   Development of the human dentition to the sixth year. The deciduous or primary teeth are the darker ones in the illustration. (I. Schour and M. Massler, University of Illinois College of Dentistry.)

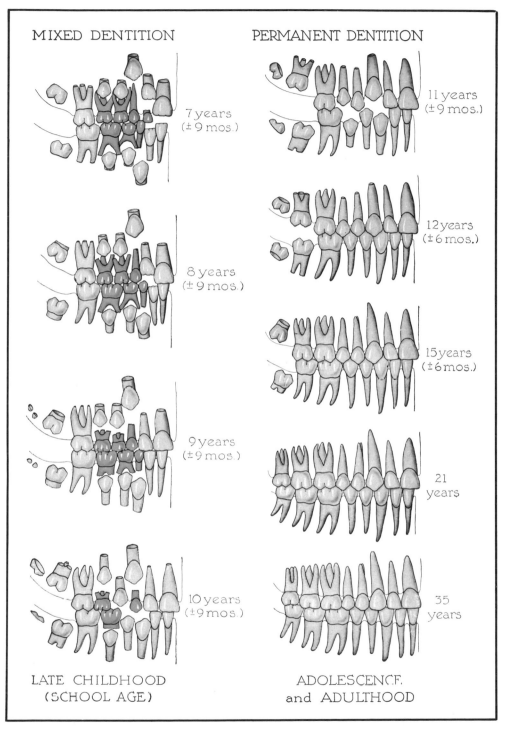

Figure 37. Development of the human dentition from the seventh year to maturity. Note the displacement of deciduous teeth by succedaneous permanent teeth. (I. Schour and M. Massler, University of Illinois College of Dentistry.)

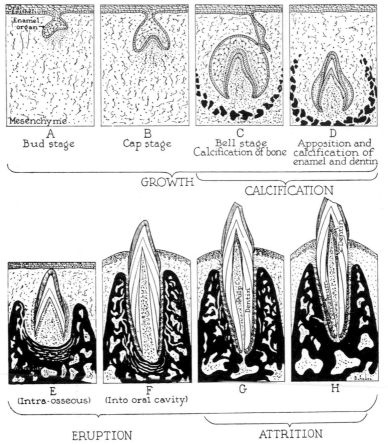

Figure 38. Diagram of life cycle of a human deciduous incisor. The normal resorption of the root is not indicated. Enamel and bone are drawn in black. (Slightly modified after Schour and Massler from Maximow and Bloom.) (Schour, *Oral Histology and Embryology,* Lea & Febiger, 8th ed.)

Dr. Carmen Nolla at the University of Michigan reported the results of new research in 1952. The report covered radiographic studies of tooth development, separating the records of boys and girls, at the Elementary School, University of Michigan. This work progressed over a long period under scientific procedure. The results are most interesting and promise to modify further the original work on this problem by Logan and Kronfeld. Dr. Carmen Nolla refers continually to their original table as modified and makes direct comparisons with it where her research seemed to differ in detail.

Some of the comments of Dr. Nolla, with illustrations and tables follow:

"A method for appraising the development of permanent teeth in terms of the amount of maturation was developed (radiographic records). The data obtained by this procedure are used to provide dental age values presented in the tables. The observational method used to appraise the development of each tooth in the maxillary and the mandibular arch is illustrated in Figures 39 and 40, titled calcification of maxillary and mandibular teeth, respectively.

"In order to obtain an appraisal of the development of a particular tooth, the radiograph is matched as closely as possible with the comparative figure. For

(Text continued on page 38.)

Teeth Mand.		Crown Completed (Nolla)		Root Completed (Nolla)		Logan and Kronfeld, 1944 (Modified by Schour and Massler) Root Completed
		Boys	Girls	Boys	Girls	
1	1	3 yrs. 8 mo.	3 yrs. 6 mo.	10 yrs.	8 yrs. 6 mo.	9 yrs.
2	2	4 yrs. 4 mo.	4 yrs.	10 yrs. 6 mo.	9 yrs. 8 mo.	10 yrs.
3	3	6 yrs.	5 yrs. 8 mo.	13 yrs. 6 mo.	12 yrs.	12–14 yrs.
4	4	7 yrs.	6 yrs. 6 mo.	14 yrs.	12 yrs. 6 mo.	12–13 yrs.
5	5	7 yrs. 8 mo.	7 yrs. 2 mo.	15 yrs.	14 yrs. 6 mo.	13–14 yrs.
6	6	4 yrs.	3 yrs. 10 mo.	11 yrs. 6 mo.	10 yrs.	9–10 yrs.
7	7	8 yrs. 2 mo.	7 yrs.	16 yrs. 6 mo.	15 yrs. 6 mo.	14–15 yrs.
Max.						
1	1	4½ yrs.	4½ yrs.	11 yrs.	10 yrs.	10 yrs.
2	2	5½ yrs.	5 yrs. 2 mo.	12 yrs.	11 yrs.	11 yrs.
3	3	6½ yrs.	5 yrs. 10 mo.	15 yrs.	12½ to 13 yrs.	13–15 yrs.
4	4	7 yrs. 4 mo.	6 yrs. 4 mo.	14½ yrs.	12 yrs. 9 mo.	12–13 yrs.
5	5	8 yrs. 5 mo.	7 yrs. 3 mo.	15½ yrs.	14 yrs.	13–14 yrs.
6	6	4½ yrs.	4 yrs. 2 mo.	11½ yrs.	9½ yrs.	9–10 yrs.
7	7	8 yrs. 2 mo.	7 yrs. 6 mo.	16½ yrs.	15 yrs. 6 mo.	14–16 yrs.

Norms for the Maturation of Permanent Teeth for Boys (NOLLA)

Dental Age (Yrs.)	Mandibular Teeth (Growth Stage)								Maxillary Teeth (Growth Stage)							
	1|1	2|2	3|3	4|4	5|5	6|6	7|7	8|8	1|1	2|2	3|3	4|4	5|5	6|6	7|7	8|8
3	5.2	4.5	3.2	2.6	1.1	5.0	.7		4.3	3.4	3.0	2.0	1.0	4.2	1.0	
4	6.5	5.7	4.2	3.5	2.2	6.2	2.0		5.4	4.5	3.9	3.0	2.0	5.3	2.0	
5	7.5	6.8	5.1	4.4	3.3	7.0	3.0		6.4	5.5	4.8	4.0	3.0	6.4	3.0	
6	8.2	7.7	5.9	5.2	4.3	7.7	4.0		7.3	6.4	5.6	4.9	4.0	7.4	4.0	
7	8.8	8.5	6.7	6.0	5.3	8.4	5.0	.8	8.2	7.2	6.3	5.7	4.9	8.2	5.0	
8	9.3	9.1	7.4	6.8	6.2	9.0	5.9	1.4	8.8	8.0	7.0	6.5	5.8	8.9	5.8	1.0
9	9.7	9.5	8.0	7.5	7.0	9.5	6.7	1.8	9.4	8.7	7.7	7.2	6.6	9.4	6.5	1.8
10	10.0	9.8	8.6	8.2	7.7	9.8	7.4	2.0	9.7	9.3	8.4	7.9	7.3	9.7	7.2	2.3
11			9.1	8.8	8.3	9.9	7.9	2.7	9.95	9.7	8.8	8.6	8.0	9.8	7.8	3.0
12			9.6	9.4	8.9		8.4	3.5		9.95	9.2	9.2	8.7		8.3	4.
13			9.8	9.7	9.4		8.9	4.5			9.6	9.6	9.3		8.8	4.9
14				10.0	9.7		9.3	5.3				9.8	9.8	9.6		9.3	5.9
15					10.0		9.7	6.2				9.9	9.9	9.9		9.6	6.6
16½							10.0	7.3								10.0	7.7
17								7.6									8.0

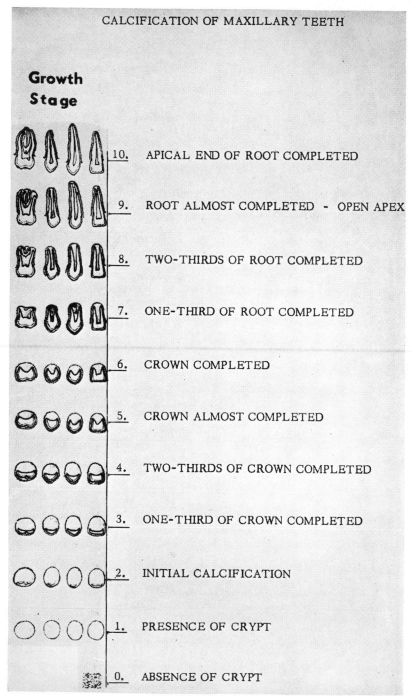

Figure 39. *(See legend on opposite page.)*

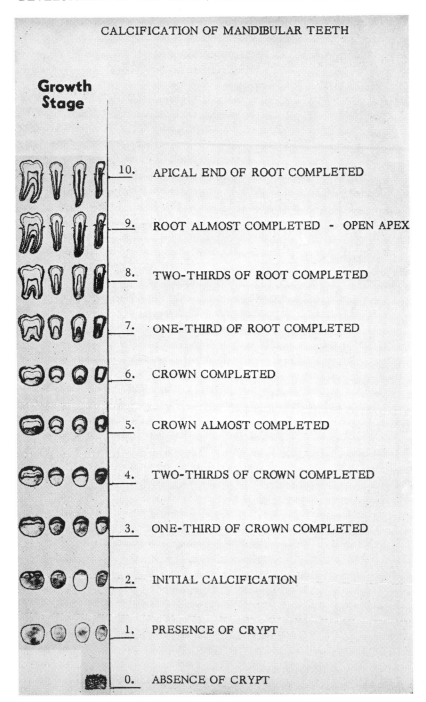

CALCIFICATION OF MANDIBULAR TEETH

Growth Stage

10. APICAL END OF ROOT COMPLETED

9. ROOT ALMOST COMPLETED - OPEN APEX

8. TWO-THIRDS OF ROOT COMPLETED

7. ONE-THIRD OF ROOT COMPLETED

6. CROWN COMPLETED

5. CROWN ALMOST COMPLETED

4. TWO-THIRDS OF CROWN COMPLETED

3. ONE-THIRD OF CROWN COMPLETED

2. INITIAL CALCIFICATION

1. PRESENCE OF CRYPT

0. ABSENCE OF CRYPT

Figure 40. (After Nolla)

Figures 39 and 40.   Under the column entitled growth stage is a set of drawings illustrating the ten stages of development of the teeth as observed radiographically. The first column (right) appraises the growth stage of the central and lateral incisors; the second the canine; the third the premolars and the fourth the molars. The drawings illustrate for each of the ten stages (1 to 10 inclusive) the appearance of the stage of tooth development as observed radiographically. (Child Development Laboratories, University of Michigan.)

Norms for the Maturation of Permanent Teeth for Girls (NOLLA)

Dental Age (Yrs.)	Mandibular Teeth (Growth Stage)								Maxillary Teeth (Growth Stage)							
	1͡1	2͡2	3͡3	4͡4	5͡5	6͡6	7͡7	8͡8	1͡1	2͡2	3͡3	4͡4	5͡5	6͡6	7͡7	8͡8
3	5.3	4.7	3.4	2.9	1.7	5.0	1.6		4.3	3.7	3.3	2.6	2.0	4.5	1.8	
4	6.6	6.0	4.4	3.9	2.8	6.2	2.8		5.4	4.8	4.3	3.6	3.0	5.7	2.8	
5	7.6	7.2	5.4	4.9	3.8	7.3	3.9		6.5	5.8	5.3	4.6	4.0	6.9	3.8	
6	8.5	8.1	6.3	5.8	4.8	8.1	5.0		7.4	6.7	6.2	5.6	4.9	7.9	4.7	
7	9.3	8.9	7.2	6.7	5.7	8.7	5.9	1.8	8.3	7.6	7.0	6.5	5.8	8.7	5.6	
8	9.8	9.5	8.0	7.5	6.6	9.3	6.7	2.1	9.0	8.4	7.8	7.3	6.6	9.3	6.5	2.1
9	10.0	9.9	8.7	8.3	7.4	9.7	7.4	2.3	9.6	9.1	8.5	8.1	7.4	9.7	7.2	2.4
10		10.0	9.2	8.9	8.1	10.0	8.1	3.2	10.0	9.6	9.1	8.7	8.1	10.0	7.9	3.2
11			9.7	9.4	8.6		8.6	3.7		10.0	9.5	9.3	8.7		8.5	4.3
12			10.0	9.7	9.1		9.1	4.7			9.8	9.7	9.3		9.0	5.4
13				10.0	9.4		9.5	5.8			10.0	10.0	9.7		9.5	6.2
14					9.7		9.7	6.5					10.0		9.7	6.8
15					10.0		9.8	6.9							9.8	7.3
16							10.0	7.5							10.0	8.0
17								8.0								8.7

(Continued from page 34.)

example, if one-third of the crown is completed, the observation is given the value 3; if one-third of the root is completed the observation is graded 7.0. When the radiographic reading lies between two grades, this appraisal is indicated as the value of 0.5. For example, if the X-ray reading is between one-third and two-thirds of the root completed, it is given the value of 7.5. When the X-ray shows a reading that is slightly greater than the illustrated grade, but not as much as halfway between that stage and the next, the value 0.2 is added. For example, if slightly more than two-thirds of the crown is completed, the grade will be 4.2, or if somewhat more than two-thirds of the root is completed it will be 7.2. If the development is slightly less than the grade indicated, the value 0.7 is added to the preceding grade. For example, if two-thirds of the crown is approximately completed, the grade will be 3.7, or if two-thirds of the root is almost completed, the grade will be 7.7.

"Thus, it is possible without too much difficulty to assign the observation value as seen on the growth level, above the growth level, halfway between the growth stage and close to the next level. Attempts to appraise radiographs more accurately than this do not seem feasible.

"In the succeeding annual radiographs, the quantitative increase in calcification easily is determined. The outline of the radiolucent pulp can be followed readily through the different stages of development. The completion of the apical end of the root is the final stage in the process of maturation to be observed radiographically.

"Maturation of teeth may, in this way, be used as a criterion of dental age and of the physiologic age of the patient. It provides an index of physiologic maturity of the permanent dentition."

In an article in the *Journal of Dentistry for Children*, Dr. Nolla stated:

"In the study of child growth and development it has been pointed out by various investigators that the development of the dentition has a close corelation to some other measures of growth. In the laboratory school of the University of Michigan, the nature of growth and development has been investigated by serial examination of the same children at yearly intervals, utilizing a set of objective measurements of various physical and mental attributes. It has been found by Olson and Hughes that there is an intimate relationship in the functioning of all the aspects of normal growth, as has been shown by the plotting of a number of measurements in the same graph. When this relationship is appreciated one thinks of the development of the teeth, not as an isolated process, but as one which relates to other developmental processes.

"So far, the only available measure of dental age has been secured by noting the eruption of teeth. Although the eruption of the teeth may differ greatly in the time of appearance in the mouths of different children, the majority of the children exhibit some pattern in the sequence of eruption. However, consideration of eruption alone makes one cognizant of only one phase of the development of the dentition. A measure of calcification (maturation) at different age levels will provide a more precise index for determining dental age and will contribute to the concept of the organism as a whole."

DEVELOPMENT OF THE TEETH

Apparently there are four or more *centers of formation* for each tooth. The formation of each center proceeds until there is a coalescence of all of them. Each of these centers (when one is speaking of the crown portion) is called a *lobe*.

Although no lines of demarcation are found in the dentin to show this development, there are signs to be found on the surfaces of the crowns and roots; these are called *developmental grooves* (Fig. 98).

After the *crown* of the tooth is formed, the *root portion* is begun. At the cervical border of the enamel, at the cervix of the crown, cementum starts to form as a root covering of the dentin. The *cementum* is hard tissue (similar in some ways to bone tissue) which covers the root of the tooth in a thin layer. The junction of enamel and cementum is called the *cementoenamel junction*. For descriptive purposes in dental anatomy this is spoken of as the *cervical line*, forming a line of demarcation between the crown and root.

The development of the crown and root takes place within a bony crypt in the jaw bone.*

Figures 42 to 46 are photographs of the skull of a child who was probably in his tenth year. The skull has been dissected to show the positions of the remaining deciduous teeth and their root resorption, as well as the positions and development of the permanent teeth.

After the crown and part of the root are formed, the tooth penetrates the mucous membrane and makes its entry into the mouth. Further formation of the root is supposed to be an active factor in pushing the crown toward its final position in the mouth. Eruption of the tooth is said to be completed when most of the crown is in evidence and when it has made contact with its antagonist or antagonists in the opposing jaw. Actually, eruption may and usually does continue after this; *i.e.,* more of the crown may become exposed, and the tooth may move farther occlusally to accommodate itself to new conditions.

Formation of root dentin and cementum continues after the tooth is in use. The *root* formation is about half finished when the tooth emerges. Ultimately the root is completed. Cementum covers the root. The pulp tissue continues to function with its blood and nerve supply after the tooth is formed. The pulp cavity within the tooth has by this time become small in comparison with the tooth size. Its outline is similar to the outline of the crown and root, and the opening of the pulp cavity at the apex is constricted. This opening is called the *apical foramen.* The pulp keeps its tissue-forming function, in that it may form *secondary dentin* on occasion as a protection to itself.

Formation of the tooth is said to be *completed* when the apex of the root is formed; as a matter of fact, however, this process continues slowly throughout the life of the tooth. The pulp cavity becomes smaller and more constricted with age. Sometimes the pulp chamber within the crown is entirely obliterated, and in rare instances the entire pulp cavity has been found filled with secondary deposit. This process is not so extensive in deciduous teeth, since the years of their usefulness are fewer; nevertheless, the same powers are inherent in the deciduous pulp. Deciduous teeth will show secondary dentin in their pulp chambers as a result of the irritation produced by caries or excessive wear.

The *dental pulp* is a connective-tissue organ containing a number of structures, among which are arteries, veins, a lymphatic system and nerves. Its primary function is to form the dentin structure of the tooth. When the tooth is newly erupted, the dental pulp is large; it becomes progressively smaller as the tooth is completed. The pulp is relatively large in deciduous teeth and also in young permanent teeth. For this reason the teeth of children and young people are more sensitive than teeth of older people to thermal change and dental operative procedure.

---

*Tooth development as treated here is necessarily incomplete. The aim is to give a short outline as an introduction to the *gross,* or *macroscopic,* anatomy of the teeth.

Microscopic anatomy of the teeth, or dental histology, must be studied for more complete information covering tooth tissues and their development.

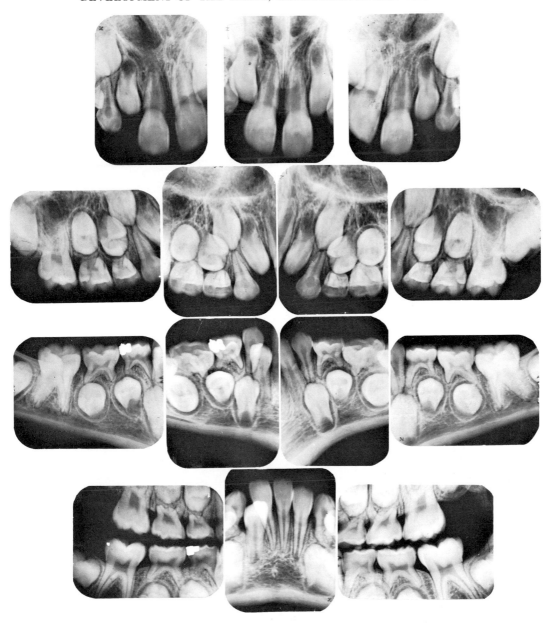

Figure 41. Radiographs of teeth of a child eight years old. Maxillary teeth have crowns pointed downward, whereas mandibular teeth have crowns pointed upward. Some of the permanent teeth have erupted, while others may be seen forming above or below deciduous predecessors. Note the resorption of the roots of deciduous teeth. (From the files of Dr. Clarence O. Simpson, St. Louis.)

At the time of its eruption, the enamel of the crown of the tooth is covered by the *enamel cuticle*. This is a thin horny material called *keratin*, which may be worn off in exposed areas, but which remains in places that are not subject to friction, such as the deepest portions of developmental grooves, interproximal areas and the cervix of the crown, where it is protected by the gingival tissue with its epithelial attachment. The enamel cuticle has been called *Nasmyth's membrane*.

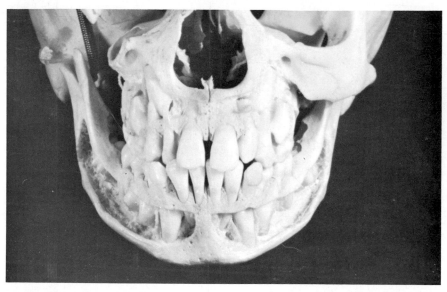

Figure 42. Front view of skull of child nine or ten years of age. Note the stages of development and eruption of the various teeth. The canines are lingual to the roots of predecessors. The relation and development of the teeth are normal except for the prolonged retention of the maxillary right lateral incisor, which is locked in a lingual relation to the mandibular teeth.

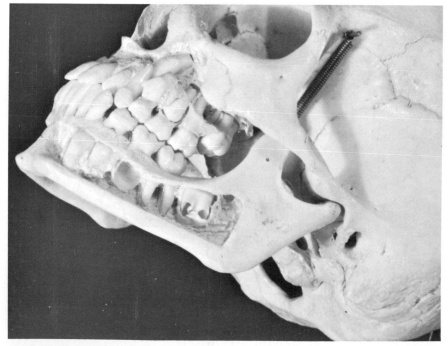

Figure 43. Left side of the skull shown in Figure 42. Note the placement of the permanent maxillary canine and the second premolar; also observe the position and stage of development of the maxillary second permanent molar.

The bony crypt of the mandibular second permanent premolar is in full view, since the developing tooth was lost from the specimen.

Observe the large openings in the developing roots of the mandibular second permanent molar.

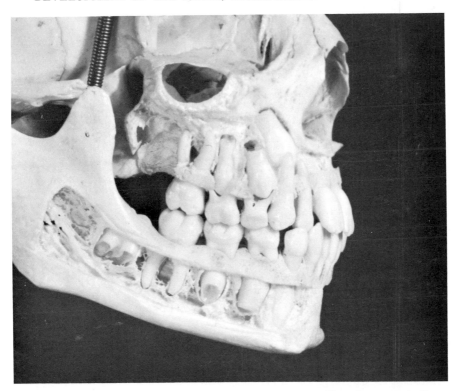

Figure 44. View of the right side of the skull shown in Fig. 42. Note the amount of resorption of the roots of the deciduous upper molars which has taken place and the relation of the developing premolars above them. The roots of the first permanent molars have been completed. Note the open pulp chambers and the pulp canals in the developing mandibular teeth. The lingual inclination of the lower second premolar is common. The developing upper second molar has been lost from the specimen.

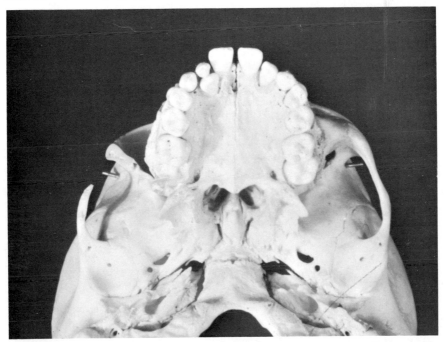

Figure 45. Occlusal view of the skull shown in the preceding illustrations. Both maxillary lateral incisors have erupted, but the right lateral has come in lingually to the deciduous tooth because of prolonged retention of the latter. (Compare with Fig. 42.) The deciduous canines and molars remain in position. The left maxillary second permanent molar is no longer covered by bone.

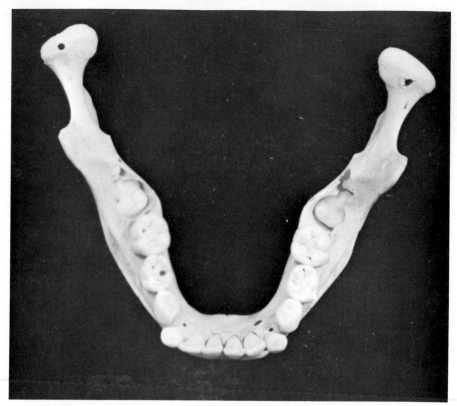

Figure 46. Occlusal view of the mandibular arch of the skull shown in Fig. 45. The development is typical, with a distal inclination of the lower lateral incisors (permanent) and a labial inclination of the canines (deciduous). Note the openings which have been started in the bone immediately lingual to the deciduous canines to facilitate the eruption of the permanent successors. Also note the developing second molars, typically located, and a tip of the developing third molar (right). The deciduous canines are approaching exfoliation. The deciduous molars remain in their normal positions with good contact relation.

BIBLIOGRAPHY

Broomell, I. N., and Fischelis, P.: Anatomy and Histology of the Mouth and Teeth. 6th ed., Philadelphia, Blakiston, 1923.

Finn, S. B.: Clinical Pedodontics. 2nd ed., Philadelphia, W. B. Saunders Co., 1962.

Logan, W. H. G., and Kronfeld, R.: Development of the human jaws and surrounding structures from birth to age fifteen. J.A.D.A., 20:379-424, 1935.

Massler, M., Schour, I., and Poncher, H. G.: Development pattern of the child as reflected in the calcification pattern of the teeth. American Journal of Dentistry for Children, July 1941.

McCall, J. O., and Wald, S. S.: Clinical Dental Roentgenology. 2nd ed., Philadelphia, W. B. Saunders Co., 1947.

Nolla, C. M.: Development of the permanent teeth. J. Den. Children, 27:254, 1960.

Nolla, C. M.: The Development of Permanent Teeth. Ann Arbor, Univ. of Michigan, 1962. Sixty page thesis.

Noyes, F. B., Schour, I., Noyes, H. J.: Dental Histology and Embryology, 5th ed., Philadelphia, Lea & Febiger, 1938.

Olson, W. C., and Hughes, B. O.: Growth of the Child as a Whole. In Barker, R. C., Kounin, J. S., and Wright, H. F.: Child Behavior and Development. New York, McGraw-Hill, 1943, pp. 199-208.

Schour, I., and Massler, M.: The development of the human dentition. J.A.D.A., 28:1153-60, 1941.

Schour, I., and McCall, J. O.: Chronology of the Human Dentition. In Orban, B.: Oral Histology and Embryology, St. Louis, C. V. Mosby, 1944, p. 240.

Schour, I., and Noyes, H. J.: Oral Histology and Embryology. 8th ed., Philadelphia, Lea & Febiger, 1960.

Watson, E. H., and Lowrey, G. H.: Growth and Development of Children. 2nd ed., Chicago, Year Book Publishers, 1954.

Chapter III

THE DECIDUOUS OR
PRIMARY TEETH

IMPORTANCE OF THE DECIDUOUS TEETH*

IN RECENT years, the dental profession has given the dental health of children increasing consideration. The medical profession is taking more interest also since no child health program is complete without the inclusion of a dental health division.

Since the deciduous teeth should be kept through some of the most important years of development of the human being, it is important that the one who has the responsibility of their care should learn all he can about them. He should know as much about their form, the significance of that form and the physiology of that form, as he does about the form of the permanent teeth. In this book, therefore, the deciduous teeth will be described in advance of the permanent teeth, so that they may be given their proper sequence in the study of dental anatomy, and this chapter will deal with the physiologic form of the various deciduous teeth, their alignment and their occlusion.

GENERAL DESCRIPTION OF THE DECIDUOUS TEETH

As the term "deciduous" implies, these teeth are shed in order to make way for their permanent successors. The process of exfoliation takes place between the seventh and the twelfth years. This does not, however, indicate the period at which

---

*The term "primary dentition" has been accepted as preferable to the term "deciduous dentition" by the Terminology Committee of the American Society of Dentistry for Children. However, the term "deciduous dentition" will have to be given preference in this text because it is more acceptable to all groups interested in dental anatomy, human or comparative.

the root resorption of the tooth begins. For in a year or two after the root is complete-ly formed and the apical foramen is established, resorption begins at the apical ex-tremity, and it continues in the direction of the crown until resorption of the entire root has taken place and the crown is lost from lack of support. Textbooks on dental histology should be consulted for complete information.

The deciduous teeth are *twenty* in number, ten in each jaw, and they are clas-sified as follows: four *incisors*, two *canines* and four *molars* in each jaw.

Beginning with the median line, the teeth are named in each jaw on each side of the mouth as follows: *central incisor, lateral incisor, canine, first molar, second molar.* These are replaced in the permanent dentition by the *central incisor, lateral incisor, canine, first premolar* and *second premolar*, respectively. The first permanent molar erupts immediately distal to the second premolar, and it is followed in turn by the second and third molars in the permanent dentition.

The deciduous teeth have been called "temporary," "milk," and "baby" teeth. These terms are improper because they foster the implication that these teeth are useful for a short period only. It should be emphasized again that they are needed for the child's welfare and comfort during early years of considerable physical develop-ment. Premature loss of deciduous teeth is to be avoided.

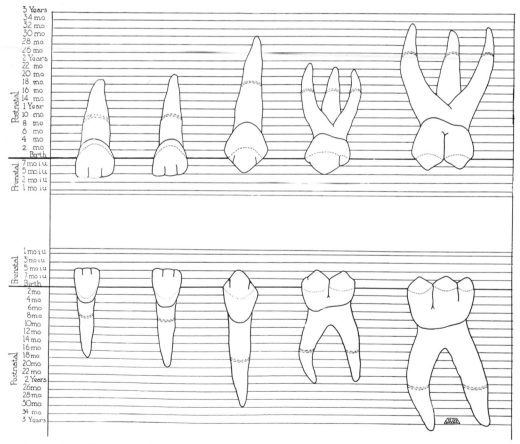

Figure 47. Diagrammatic representation of the chronology of the deciduous teeth. Eruption is completed at the approximate time indicated by the dotted area on the roots of the teeth. (Modified after McBeath, from Noyes, Schour and Noyes, *Dental Histology and Embryology,* Lea & Febiger.)

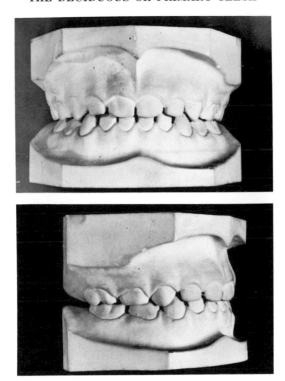

Figure 48. Casts of normally developed teeth of a child five years and six months old. Note the form and occlusion of the teeth and their even separation. *Top*, Labial aspect; *Bottom*, buccal aspect. Occlusal aspects of these casts are shown in Fig. 1, Chapter I. (Courtesy Columbia Dentoform Co., New York.)

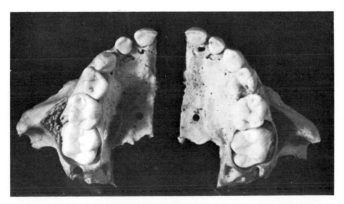

Figure 49. Occlusal aspect of maxillae of an individual approximately five and one-half years of age. The anterior teeth have separated considerably, and openings in the bone lingual to them have appeared in anticipation of the eruption of the permanent anterior teeth. The deciduous canines and molars remain in contact with each other. Well-formed permanent first molar crowns have lost their bone covering and are at the point of eruption distal to the second deciduous molars. The value of the deciduous second molar as a guide in influencing the future position of the permanent first molar is emphasized in this illustration.

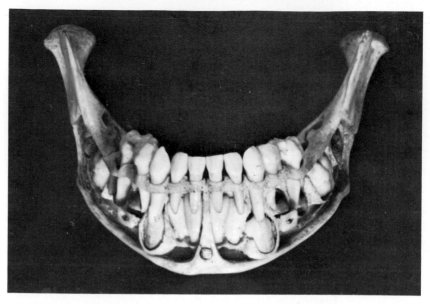

Figure 50. Anterior view of dissected mandible. From the same individual as specimens shown in Figs. 49, 51, 52, 53 and 77. The crown and root forms of the deciduous anterior teeth are well shown on this specimen. Note the positions and development of the permanent anterior teeth. The cervices of the canine crowns are near the lower border of the mandible. The crowns of the incisors are overlapped and placed much nearer the alveolar border, although root resorption of deciduous roots is not evident.

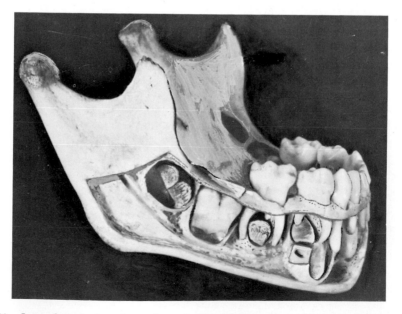

Figure 51. Lateral view of specimen shown in Fig. 50. Note the position and stages of development of the posterior permanent teeth. The root design of the deciduous molars is clear. The developing premolars are shown between the roots directly below each deciduous molar crown. The crown and part of the root of the permanent first molar have been completed. The crown of the permanent second molar is in the process of formation.

There has been considerable shrinkage and discoloration of partially formed crowns in this specimen.

Notice also the position of the mental foramen immediately below the deciduous first molar and the obtuse angle of the jaw where the ramus joins the body in the vicinity of the developing permanent second molar.

The first permanent molar, commonly called the *six-year molar,* makes its appearance in the mouth before any of the deciduous teeth are lost. It comes in immediately distal to the deciduous second molar.

The deciduous molars are replaced by *permanent premolars.* There are no premolars in the deciduous set, and there are no teeth in the deciduous set which resemble the permanent premolar. However, the crowns of the deciduous *maxillary* first molars resemble the crowns of the permanent premolars as much as they do any of the permanent molars. Nevertheless, they have three well-defined roots, which compare with the maxillary first permanent molar. The deciduous *mandibular* first molar also has a crown form unlike any permanent tooth. It has two well-defined roots, however, one mesial and one distal—an arrangement similar to that of a mandibular permanent molar. These two deciduous teeth, the maxillary and mandibular first molars, differ from any teeth in the permanent set when one compares the details of the outlines of the crowns with the outlines of the crowns of any of the permanent molars or premolars. The details of the form of the deciduous first molars will be described later.

SOME ESSENTIAL DIFFERENCES BETWEEN DECIDUOUS AND PERMANENT TEETH

A comparison of deciduous and permanent teeth will show the following *essential differences* in form:

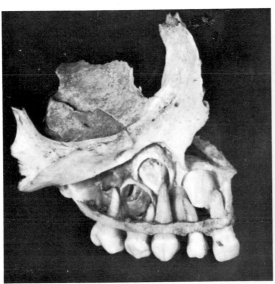 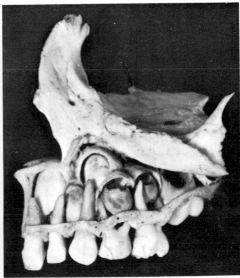

Figure 52.   Figure 53.

Figure 52. Right maxilla of child about five years of age. Note the lingual relation of the developing permanent anterior teeth and the separation of the anterior deciduous teeth which has taken place even at the age of five. The developing premolar crowns are between the roots of the deciduous molars and directly above them.

(The maxillae and mandible shown in Figs. 49, 50, 51, 52, 53 and 77 were loaned by Dr. Cornelia Morrison Thompson and were in the collection belonging to her grandfather, Dr. W. N. Morrison.)

Figure 53. Left maxilla of specimen shown in Fig. 52. Notice the developing premolars and the position of the permanent lateral incisor. Note the development of the first permanent molar.

(The developing first molar was lost from the right maxilla.) Compare the contact relation of the anterior deciduous teeth with that of the posterior teeth. Canines and molars usually remain in contact with each other, while the central and lateral incisors are separated.

1. The crowns of deciduous anterior teeth are wider mesiodistally in comparison with their crown length than are the permanent teeth.

2. The roots of deciduous anterior teeth are narrow and longer in comparison with crown length and width. Narrow roots with wide crowns present a design at the cervical third of crown and root which differs markedly from the permanent anterior teeth. From mesial and distal aspects the proportions are similar, except that the crown width is greatest at the cervical third, contrasting a wide crown with a narrow root.

3. The cervical ridge of enamel at the cervical third of the anterior crowns, labially and lingually, is much more prominent in the deciduous than in the permanent teeth. These prominent contours must be considered in operative procedures (Fig. 63).

4. The crowns and roots of deciduous molars are more slender mesiodistally at the cervical third than those of permanent molars.

5. The cervical ridges buccally on the deciduous molars is much more pronounced, especially on first molars, maxillary and mandibular (Figs. 73, 74, 75 and 76).

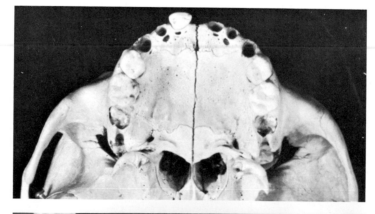

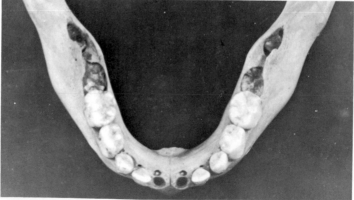

Figure 54.   Maxillae and mandible of a five-year-old child. Some of the anterior deciduous teeth have been lost from the specimen, which shows the empty alveoli. Note the relative position of the developing permanent second molar in the left maxilla. Tips of the mandibular central incisors are making their appearance lingual to the alveoli of the deciduous central incisors. The canines and first molars are still in contact with each other in this specimen.

6. The roots of the deciduous molars are relatively more slender and longer than the roots of the permanent teeth. They also flare out more apically, extending out beyond projected outlines of the crowns. This flare allows more room between the roots for the development of permanent tooth crowns before it is time for deciduous molars to lose their anchorage.

7. The buccal and lingual surfaces of deciduous molars are flatter above the cervical curvatures than those of permanent molars, thereby narrowing the occlusal surfaces with their taper occlusally.

8. The deciduous teeth are usually lighter in color than are the permanent teeth.

PULP CHAMBERS AND PULP CANALS
IN DECIDUOUS TEETH

Cross sections of deciduous teeth will emphasize morphological details which are important when considering the shape and relative size of pulp chambers and canals (Fig. 55).

1. Crown widths in all directions are large in comparison to root widths at the necks and cervices.

2. The enamel is relatively thin and has a consistent depth.

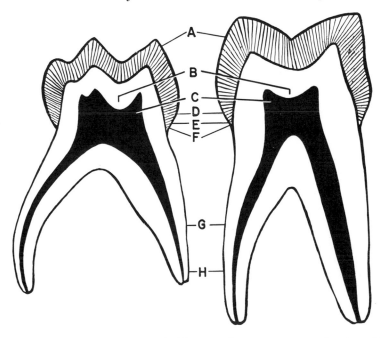

Figure 55. Comparison of maxillary, deciduous and permanent second molars, linguobuccal cross section. *A,* The enamel cap of deciduous molars is thinner and has a more consistent depth. *B,* There is a comparatively greater thickness of dentin over the pulpal wall at the occlusal fossa of deciduous molars. *C,* The pulpal horns are higher in deciduous molars, especially the mesial horns, and pulp chambers are proportionately larger. *D,* The cervical ridges are more pronounced, especially on the buccal aspect of the first deciduous molars. *E,* The enamel rods at the cervix slope occlusally instead of gingivally as in the permanent teeth. *F,* The deciduous molars have a markedly constricted neck compared to the permanent molars. *G,* The roots of the deciduous teeth are longer and more slender in comparison with crown size than those of the permanent teeth. *H,* The roots of the deciduous molars flare out nearer the cervix than do those of the permanent teeth. (From Finn, S. B.: *Clinical Pedodontics,* 2nd edition, W. B. Saunders Co.)

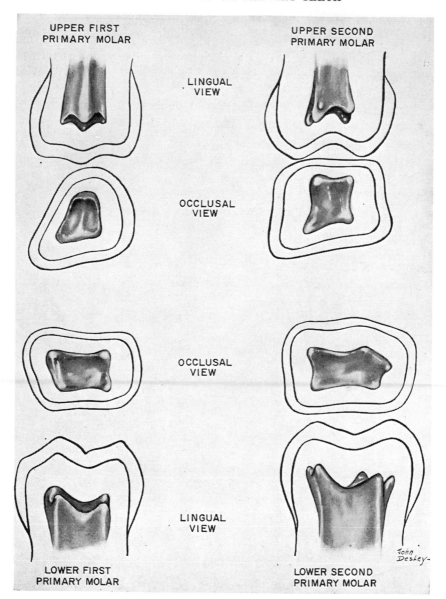

Figure 56. Pulp chambers in the primary molars. Note the contours of the pulp horns within them. (Finn, S. B.: *Clinical Pedodontics,* 2nd Edition.)

3. The dentin thickness between the pulp chambers and the enamel is limited, particularly in some areas (Fig. 56, lower second primary molar).

4. The pulpal horns are high and pulp chambers are large.

5. Deciduous roots are narrow and long when compared to crown width and length.

6. Molar roots of deciduous teeth flare markedly, and thin out rapidly as the apices are approached.

It is well, at all times, to study the comparisons between the deciduous and the permanent dentitions (Figs. 57 and 58). Further variations between the macroscopic

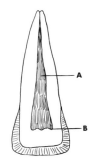
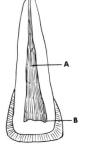

Figure 57.   Figure 58.

Figure 57. Permanent central incisor. This figure represents a sectioned permanent central incisor of a young person. Although the pulp canal is rather large, it is smaller than the pulp canal shown in Fig. 58 and it becomes more constricted apically. Note the dentin space between the pulp horns and the incisal edge of the crown. A, Pulp canal; B, pulp horn.

Figure 58. Deciduous central incisor. This figure represents a sectioned deciduous central incisor. It will be noted that the pulp chamber with its horns and the pulp canal are broader than those found in Fig. 57. The apical portion of the canal is much less constricted than that of the permanent tooth. Note the narrow dentin space incisally. A, Pulp canal; B, pulp horns.

form of the deciduous and the permanent teeth will follow with a detailed description of each deciduous tooth.

DETAILED DESCRIPTION OF EACH DECIDUOUS TOOTH

Maxillary Central Incisor

Labial Aspect (Fig. 59, *a*).   In the crown of the deciduous central incisor the mesiodistal diameter is greater than the cervicoincisal length. (The opposite is true of permanent central incisors.) The labial surface is very smooth and the incisal edge is nearly straight. Developmental lines are usually not seen. The root is cone-shaped with even, tapered sides. The root length is greater in comparison with the crown length than in the permanent central incisor. It will be well in studying the deciduous teeth, and also the permanent teeth later on, to make direct comparisons between the table of measurements of the deciduous teeth (page 58) and the table of measurements for the permanent teeth which was given in Chapter I (page 21).

Lingual Aspect (Fig. 61, *a*).   The lingual aspect of the crown shows definite well-developed marginal ridges and a highly developed cingulum. The cingulum extends up toward the incisal ridge far enough to make a partial division of the concavity on the lingual surface below the incisal edge, practically dividing it into a mesial and distal fossa.

The root narrows lingually and presents a ridge for its full length in comparison with a flatter surface labially. A cross section through the root where it joins the crown shows an outline which is somewhat triangular in shape, with the labial surface making one side of the triangle and mesial and distal surfaces making up the other two sides.

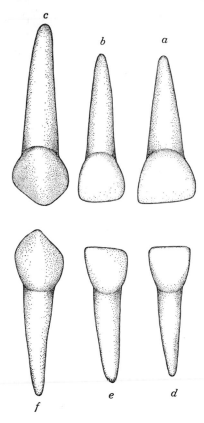

Figure 59. Deciduous right anterior teeth, labial aspect. *a*, Maxillary central incisor; *b*, maxillary lateral incisor; *c*, maxillary canine; *d*, mandibular central incisor; *e*, mandibular lateral incisor; *f*, mandibular canine.

Mesial and Distal Aspects (Fig. 63, *a*).　　The mesial and distal aspects of the deciduous maxillary central incisors are similar. The measurement of the crown at the cervical third shows the crown from this aspect to be wide in relation to its total length. The average measurement will be about 1 mm. less than the entire crown length cervicoincisally. Because of the short crown and its labiolingual measurement, the crown appears thick at the middle third and even down toward the incisal third. The curvature of cervical line, which represents the cementoenamel junction, is distinct, curving toward the incisal ridge. However, the curvature is not as great as that found on its permanent successor. The essential difference between the mesial aspect and the distal aspect of this tooth is that the cervical curvature *distally* is less than the cervical curvature *mesially*.

Although the root from this aspect appears more blunt than it did from the labial and lingual aspects, still it is of an even taper and is the shape of a cone. It is, however, blunt at the apex. Usually the mesial side of the root will have a developmental groove or concavity, whereas distally the surface is generally convex.

Note the development of the cervical ridges of enamel at the cervical third of the crown.

Incisal Aspect (Fig. 65, *a*).　　An important feature to note from the incisal aspect is the measurement mesiodistally as compared with the measurement labiolingually. The incisal edge is centered over the main bulk of the crown and is relatively straight. Looking down on the incisal edge, one sees that the labial surface is broader

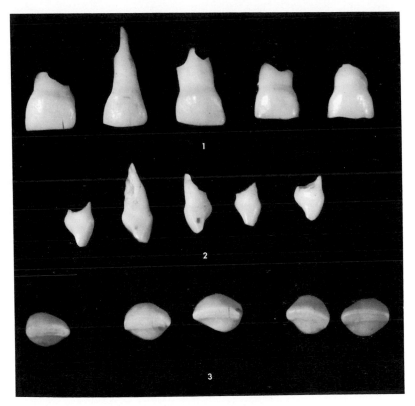

Figure 60. Deciduous maxillary central incisors (first incisors).

1. Labial aspect. Note the lack of character, or distinguishing mold form. Also pay attention to the large mesiodistal dimension compared to the cervicoincisal dimension.

2. Mesial aspect. The cervical ridges are quite prominent and the curvatures more extensive than those found on permanent incisors. This characteristic is common to all deciduous teeth. However, these curvatures are covered normally by gum tissue with its epithelial attachment. (See Chapter V, Physiologic Tooth Form Protecting the Periodontium.)

3. Incisal aspect.

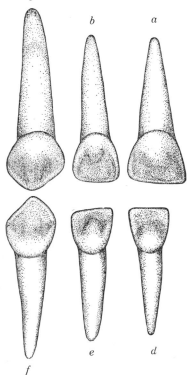

Figure 61. Deciduous right anterior teeth, lingual aspect. *a,* Maxillary central incisor; *b,* maxillary lateral incisor; *c,* maxillary canine; *d,* mandibular central incisor; *e,* mandibular lateral incisor; *f,* mandibular canine.

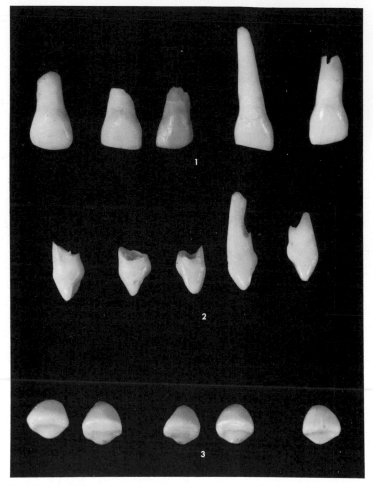

Figure 62.   Deciduous maxillary lateral incisors. (Second incisors.) 1, Labial aspect; 2, mesial aspect; 3, incisal aspect.

and smoother than the lingual surface. The lingual surface tapers toward the cingulum.

The mesial and the distal surfaces of this tooth are relatively broad. The mesial and distal surfaces toward the incisal ridge or at the incisal third are generous enough to make good contact areas with the adjoining teeth.

Maxillary Lateral Incisor (Figs. 59b, 61b, 63b, 65b)

The maxillary lateral incisor has an outline similar to the central incisor from all aspects, but its dimensions are different. Its crown is smaller in all dimensions. The cervicoincisal length of the crown is greater than its mesiodistal width. The distoincisal angles of the crown are more rounded. Although the root has a similar outline, it is much longer in proportion to its crown when one compares it with the central incisor.

Figure 63. Deciduous right anterior teeth, mesial aspect. *a,* Maxillary central incisor; *b,* maxillary lateral incisor; *c,* maxillary canine; *d,* mandibular central incisor; *e,* mandibular lateral incisor; *f,* mandibular canine.

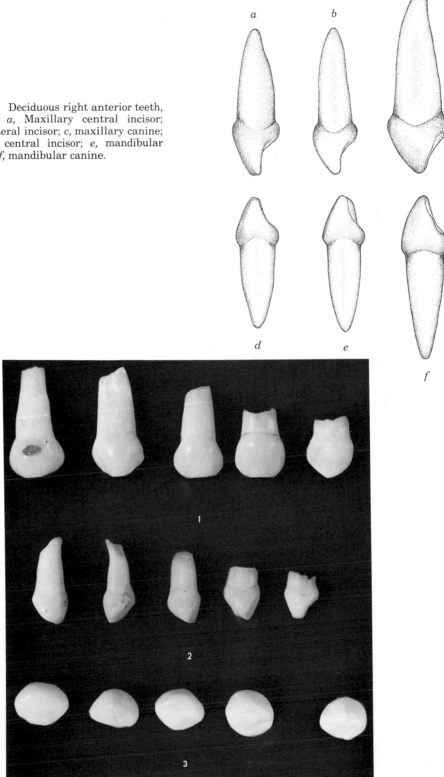

Figure 64. Deciduous maxillary canines. 1, Labial aspect; 2, mesial aspect; 3, incisal aspect.

57

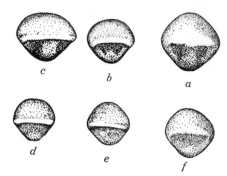

Figure 65. Deciduous right anterior teeth, incisal aspect. *a,* Maxillary central incisor; *b,* maxillary lateral incisor; *c,* maxillary canine; *d,* mandibular central incisor; *e,* mandibular lateral incisor; *f,* mandibular canine.

Table of Measurements of the Deciduous Teeth of Man (G. V. BLACK)
(Averages Only)

Upper Teeth	Length Over All	Length of Crown	Length of Root	Mesio-distal Diameter of Crown	Mesio-distal Diameter at Cervix	Labio-lingual Diameter of Crown	Labio-lingual Diameter at Cervix
Central Incisor	16.0*	6.0	10.0	6.5	4.5	5.0	4.0
Lateral Incisor	15.8	5.6	11.4	5.1	3.7	4.	3.7
Canine	19.0	6.5	13.5	7.0	5.1	7.0	5.5
First Molar	15.2	5.1	10.0	7.3	5.2	8.5	6.9
Second Molar	17.5	5.7	11.7	8.2	6.4	10.0	8.3
Lower Teeth							
Central Incisor	14.0	5.0	9.0	4.2	3.0	4.0	3.5
Lateral Incisor	15.0	5.2	10.0	4.1†	3.0	4.0	3.5
Canine	17.0	6.0	11.5	5.0	3.7	4.8	4.0
First Molar	15.8	6.0	9.8	7.7	6.5	7.0	5.3
Second Molar	18.8	5.5	11.3	9.9	7.2	8.7	6.4

* Millimeters.

Maxillary Canine

Labial Aspect (Fig. 59, c). Except for the root form, the labial aspect of the maxillary canine does not resemble either the central or the lateral incisors. The crown is more constricted at the cervix in relation to its mesiodistal width, and the mesial and distal surfaces are more convex. Instead of an incisal edge, which is relatively straight, it has a long, well-developed and sharp cusp.

Compared with that of the permanent maxillary canine, the cusp on the deciduous canine is much longer and sharper, and the crest of contour mesially is not so far down toward the incisal portion. A line drawn through the contact areas of the deciduous canine would bisect a line drawn from the cervix to the tip of the cusp. In the *permanent* canine the contact areas are not at the same level.

The root of the deciduous canine is long, slender and tapering and is more than twice the crown length.

Lingual Aspect (Fig. 61, c). The lingual aspect shows pronounced enamel ridges which merge with each other. They are the cingulum, mesial and distal marginal ridges, and incisal ridges, besides a tubercle at the cusp tip which is a continuation of the lingual ridge connecting the cingulum and the cusp tip. This lingual ridge divides the lingual surface into mesiolingual and distolingual fossae.

The root of this tooth tapers lingually. It is usually inclined distally above the middle third.

Mesial Aspect (Fig. 63, c). From the mesial aspect, the outline form is similar to that of the lateral and central incisors. However, there is a difference in proportion. The measurement labiolingually at the cervical third is much greater. This increase in crown dimension, in conjunction with the root length, permits resistance against forces the tooth must withstand during function. The function of this tooth is to punch, tear and apprehend food material.

Distal Aspect. The distal outline of this tooth is the reverse of the mesial aspect. No outstanding differences may be noted except that the curvature of the cervical line toward the cusp ridge is less than on the mesial surface.

Incisal Aspect (Fig. 65, c). From the incisal aspect one observes that the crown is essentially diamond-shaped. The angles which are found at the contact areas mesially and distally, at the cingulum on the lingual surface and at the cervical third, or enamel ridge, on the labial surface are more pronounced and less rounded in effect than are those found on the permanent canines. The tip of the cusp is distal to the center of the crown, and the mesial cusp slope is longer than the distal cusp slope. This allows for intercuspation with the lower, or mandibular, canine, which has its longest slope distally (Fig. 59).

Mandibular Central Incisor

Labial Aspect (Fig. 59, d). The labial aspect of this crown has a flat face with no developmental grooves. The mesial and distal sides of the crown are tapered evenly from the contact areas, the measurement being less at the cervix. This crown is wide in proportion to its length in comparison with that of its permanent successor.

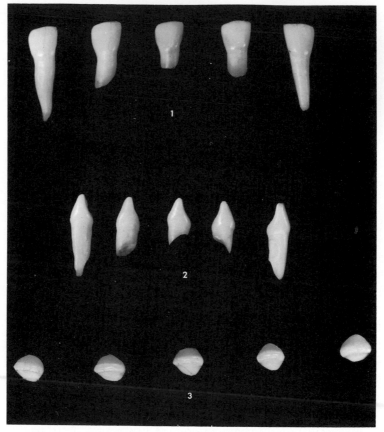

Figure 66. Deciduous mandibular central incisors. 1, Labial aspect; 2, mesial aspect; 3, incisal aspect.

The root of the deciduous central incisor is long, narrow and evenly tapered down to the apex, which is pointed. The root is almost twice the length of the crown.

Lingual Aspect (Fig. 61, d). On the lingual surface of the crown are seen the marginal ridges and the cingulum. The lingual surface of the crown at the middle third and the incisal third may have a flattened surface level with the marginal ridges, or it may present a slight concavity, called the *lingual fossa.* The lingual portion of the crown and root converges so that it is narrower toward the lingual than toward the labial surface.

Mesial Aspect (Fig. 63, d). The mesial aspect shows the typical outline of an incisor tooth even though the measurements are small. The incisal ridge is centered over the center of the root and between the crest of curvature of the crown, labially and lingually. The convexity of the cervical contours labially and lingually at the cervical third is just as pronounced as in any of the other deciduous incisors and more pronounced than the curvatures found at the same locations on a permanent mandibular central incisor.

Although this tooth is small, its labiolingual measurement is only a millimeter less than that of the deciduous maxillary central incisor.

The mesial surface of the root is nearly flat and is evenly tapered; the apex presents a more blunt appearance than is found when one observes the lingual or labial aspects.

Distal Aspect. The outline of this tooth from the distal aspect is the reverse of that found from the mesial aspect. There is little difference to be noted between these aspects except that the cervical line of the crown is less curved toward the incisal ridge than that found on the mesial surface. Often there is a developmental depression on the distal side of the root.

Incisal Aspect (Fig. 65, d). The incisal ridge is straight and bisects the crown labiolingually. The outline of the crown from the incisal aspect shows the crests of contour at the cervical third labially and lingually. There is a definite taper toward the cingulum on the lingual side.

The labial surface from this aspect presents a flat surface slightly convex, whereas the lingual surface presents a flattened surface slightly concave.

Mandibular Lateral Incisor (Figs. 59e, 61e, 63e, 65e)

The fundamental outlines of the deciduous mandibular lateral incisor are similar to those of the deciduous central incisor. These two teeth supplement each other in function. The lateral incisor is somewhat larger in all measurements except

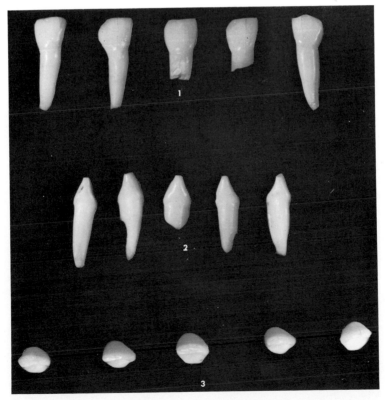

Figure 67. Deciduous mandibular lateral incisors. 1, Labial aspect; 2, mesial aspect; 3, incisal aspect.

the labiolingual, where the two teeth are practically identical. The cingulum of the lateral incisor may be a little more generous than that of the central incisor, and the lingual surface of the crown between the marginal ridges may be more concave. In addition, there is a tendency for the incisal ridge to slope downward distally. This design lowers the distal contact area apically in order that proper contact may be made with the mesial surface of the deciduous mandibular canine.

Mandibular Canine (Figs. 59f, 61f, 63f, 65f)

There is very little difference in functional form between this tooth and the maxillary canine. The difference is mainly in the dimensions. The crown is perhaps 0.5 mm. shorter, and the root is at least 2 mm. shorter. The outstanding variation in dimension is the labiolingual calibration. The deciduous maxillary canine is very much larger labiolingually.

The cervical ridges labially and lingually are not quite as pronounced as those found on the maxillary canine. The greatest variation in outline form when one compares the two teeth is seen from the labial and lingual aspects; the distal cusp slope is longer than the mesial slope. The opposite arrangement is true of the maxillary canine. This makes for proper intercuspation of these teeth during mastication.

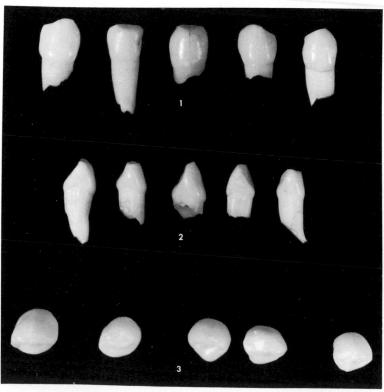

Figure 68.   Deciduous mandibular canines. l, Labial aspect; 2, mesial aspect; 3, incisal aspect.

Maxillary First Molar

Buccal Aspect (Fig 69, a).   The widest measurement of the crown of the maxillary first molar is at the contact areas mesially and distally. From these points the crown converges toward the cervix, the measurement at the cervix being fully 2 mm. less than the measurement at the contact areas. The occlusal line is slightly scalloped but with no definite cusp form. The buccal surface is smooth, and there is little evidence of developmental grooves.

The *roots* are slender and long, and they have a wide spread. All three roots may be seen from this aspect. The distal root is considerably shorter than the mesial one. The *bifurcation* of the roots begins immediately above the cervical line of the crown. The bifurcation buccally on permanent molars is located apical to the cervical line. Consequently, the permanent molars have a *root trunk* that shows greater development (Fig. 250).

Lingual Aspect (Fig. 70, a).   The general outline of the lingual aspect of the crown is similar to the buccal aspect. The crown converges considerably in a lingual direction.

The mesiolingual cusp is the most prominent cusp on this tooth. It is the longest and sharpest cusp. The distolingual cusp is poorly defined: it is small and rounded. From the lingual aspect the distobuccal cusp may be seen, since it is longer and better developed than the distolingual cusp. There is a type of deciduous maxillary first molar which is not uncommon and which presents one large lingual cusp with no developmental groove in evidence lingually. This type is apparently a three-cusped molar (Fig. 73, division 4, second from left).

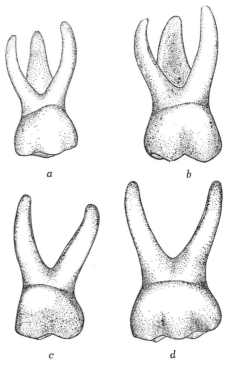

Figure 69. Deciduous right molars, buccal aspect. *a,* Maxillary first molar; *b,* maxillary second molar; *c,* mandibular first molar; *d,* mandibular second molar.

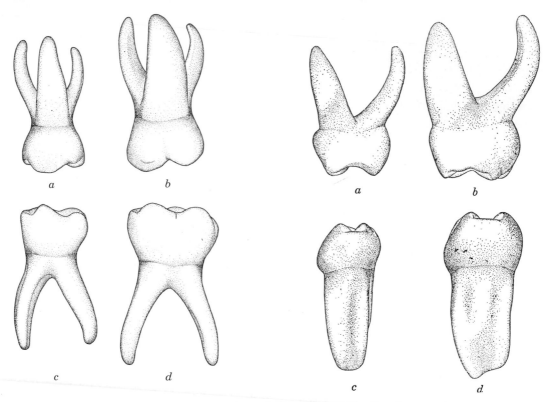

Figure 70. Deciduous right molars, lingual aspect. *a*, Maxillary first molar; *b*, maxillary second molar; *c*, mandibular first molar; *d*, mandibular second molar.

Figure 71. Deciduous right molars, mesial aspect. *a*, Maxillary first molar; *b*, maxillary second molar; *c*, mandibular first molar; *d*, mandibular second molar.

All three roots may be seen from this aspect also. The lingual root is larger than the others.

Mesial Aspect (Fig. 71, a).   From the mesial aspect the dimension at the cervical third is greater than the dimension at the occlusal third. This is true of all molar forms, but it is more pronounced on deciduous teeth than on permanent teeth. The mesiolingual cusp is longer and sharper than the mesiobuccal cusp. There is a pronounced convexity on the buccal outline in the cervical third. This convexity is an outstanding characteristic of this tooth. Actually, it gives the impression of over-development in this area when comparisons are made with any other tooth, deciduous or permanent. The cervical line mesially shows some curvature in the direction of the occlusal surface.

The mesiobuccal and lingual roots are visible when one looks at the mesial side of this tooth from a point directly opposite the contact area. The distobuccal root is hidden behind the mesiobuccal root. The lingual root from this aspect looks long and slender and extends lingually to a marked degree. It curves sharply in a buccal direction above the middle third.

Distal Aspect. From the distal aspect the crown is narrower distally than mesially. The distobuccal cusp is long and sharp, and the distolingual cusp is poorly developed. The prominence seen from the mesial aspect at the cervical third does not continue distally. The cervical line may curve occlusally, or it may extend straight across from the buccal surface to the lingual surface. All three roots may be seen from this angle, but the distobuccal root is superimposed on the mesiobuccal root so that only the buccal surface and the apex of the latter may be seen. The point of

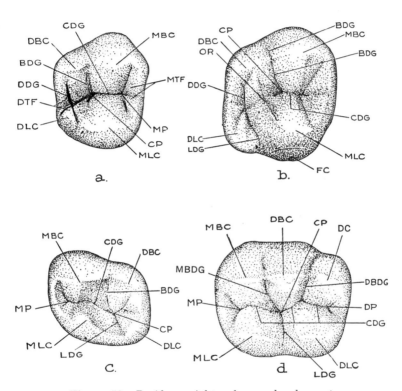

Figure 72. Deciduous right molars, occlusal aspect.

a, Maxillary first molar. *MBC,* mesiobuccal cusp; *MTF,* mesial triangular fossa; *MP,* mesial pit; *CP,* central pit; *MLC,* mesiolingual cusp; *DLC,* distolingual cusp; *DTF,* distal triangular fossa; *DDG,* distal developmental groove; *BDG,* buccal developmental groove; *DBC,* distobuccal cusp; *CDG,* central developmental groove.

b, Maxillary second molar. *BDG,* buccal developmental groove; *MBC,* mesiobuccal cusp; *CDG,* central developmental groove; *MLC,* mesiolingual cusp; *FC,* fifth cusp; *LDG,* lingual developmental groove; *DLC,* distolingual cusp; *DDG,* distal developmental groove; *OR,* oblique ridge; *DBC,* distobuccal cusp; *CP,* central pit.

c, Mandibular first molar. *CDG,* central developmental groove; *DBC,* distobuccal cusp; *BDG,* buccal developmental groove; *CP,* central pit; *DLC,* distolingual cusp; *LDG,* lingual developmental groove; *MLC,* mesiolingual cusp; *MP,* mesial pit; *MBC,* mesiobuccal cusp.

d, Mandibular second molar. *DBC,* distobuccal cusp; *CP,* central pit; *DC,* distal cusp; *DBDG,* distobuccal developmental groove; *DP,* distal pit; *CDG,* central developmental groove; *DLC,* distolingual cusp; *LDG,* lingual developmental groove; *MLC,* mesiolingual cusp; *MP,* mesial pit, *MBDG,* mesiobuccal developmental groove; *MBC,* mesiobuccal cusp.

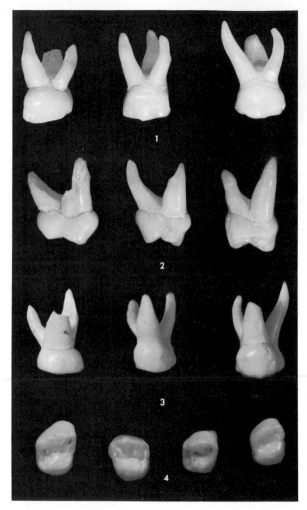

Figure 73. Deciduous maxillary first molars. 1, Buccal aspect; note the flare of roots. 2, Mesial aspect; the cervical ridge on the buccal surface is curved to the extreme. Also note the flat or concave buccal surface above this bulge as it approaches the occlusal surface. 3, Lingual aspect. 4, Occlusal aspect. This aspect emphasizes the extensive width of the mesial portion of deciduous first molars. The four specimens show size differentials even in deciduous teeth in individuals.

bifurcation of the distobuccal root and the lingual root is more apical to the cervical line at this point than the points of bifurcation described heretofore.

Occlusal Aspect (Fig. 72, a). The calibration of the distance between the mesiobuccal line angle and the distobuccal line angle is definitely greater than that found between the mesiolingual line angle and the distolingual line angle. Therefore, the crown outline converges lingually. Also, the calibration from the mesiobuccal line angle to the mesiolingual line angle is definitely greater than that found at the distal line angles. Therefore, the crown converges distally also. Nevertheless, the occlusal surface as outlined by the cusp tips and marginal ridges does not show this convergence. The occlusal surface is more nearly rectangular, with the shortest sides of the rectangle represented by the marginal ridges.

The occlusal surface has a *central fossa*. There is a *mesial triangular fossa,* just inside the mesial marginal ridge, with a mesial pit in this fossa and a sulcus with its *central groove* connecting the two fossae. There is also a well-defined *buccal developmental groove* dividing the mesiobuccal cusp and the distobuccal cusp occlusally. There are supplemental grooves radiating from the pit in the mesial triangular fossa. These grooves radiate as follows: one buccally, one lingually and one toward the marginal ridge, the last sometimes extending over the marginal ridge mesially.

Sometimes the deciduous maxillary first molar has a well-defined triangular ridge connecting the mesiolingual cusp with the distobuccal cusp. When well developed, it is called the *oblique ridge*. In some of these teeth the ridge will be very indefinite and the central developmental groove will extend from the mesial pit to the *distal developmental groove*. This disto-occlusal groove is always seen and may or may not extend through to the lingual surface, outlining a distolingual cusp. The distal marginal ridge is thin and poorly developed in comparison with the mesial marginal ridge.

Summary of the Occlusal Aspect of This Tooth.　　The form of the maxillary first deciduous molar varies from that of any tooth in the permanent dentition. Although there are no premolars in the deciduous set, in some respects the crown of this deciduous molar resembles a permanent maxillary premolar. Nevertheless, the divisions of the occlusal surface and the root form with its efficient anchorage make it a molar, both in type and function.

Maxillary Second Molar

Buccal Aspect (Fig. 69, b).　　The deciduous maxillary second molar resembles the *permanent* maxillary first molar except in size (Fig. 251).

The buccal view of this tooth shows two well-defined buccal cusps with a buccal developmental groove between them. Characteristically, the crown is narrow at the cervix in comparison with its mesiodistal measurement at the contact areas. This crown is considerably larger than that of the first deciduous molar. Although the roots, from this aspect, appear slender, they are much longer and heavier than those found on the deciduous maxillary first molar. The point of bifurcation between the buccal roots is close to the cervical line of the crown. The two buccal cusps are more nearly equal in size and development than those of the deciduous maxillary first molar.

Lingual Aspect (Fig. 70, b).　　Lingually, the crown shows three cusps: (1) the mesiolingual cusp, which is large and well developed; (2) the distolingual cusp, which is well developed (more so than that of the deciduous first molar), and (3) a third supplemental cusp, which is apical to the mesiolingual cusp and which is sometimes called the *tubercle of Carabelli* or the fifth cusp. This cusp is poorly developed and merely acts as a buttress or supplement to the bulk of the mesiolingual cusp. A well-defined developmental groove separates the mesiolingual cusp from the distolingual cusp and connects with the developmental groove which outlines the fifth cusp.

All three roots are visible from this aspect; the lingual root is large and thick in comparison with the other two roots. It is approximately the same length as the mesiobuccal root.

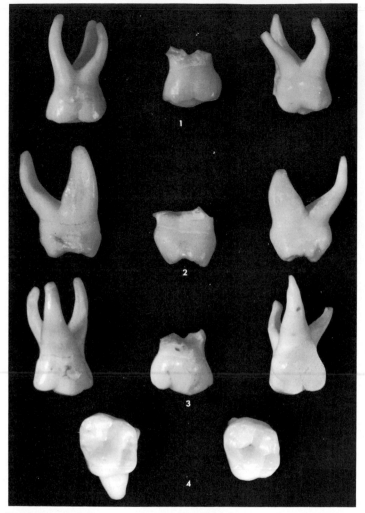

Figure 74.   Deciduous maxillary second molars. 1, Buccal aspect; 2, mesial aspect; 3, lingual aspect; 4, occlusal aspect.

Mesial Aspect (Fig. 71, b).   From the mesial aspect the crown has a typical molar outline and resembles that of the permanent molars. The crown appears short because of its width buccolingually in comparison with its length. The crown of this tooth is usually only about 0.5 mm. longer than the crown of the first deciduous molar, but the buccolingual measurement is 1.5 to 2 mm. greater. In addition, the roots are 1.5 to 2 mm. longer. The mesiolingual cusp of the crown with its supplementary fifth cusp appears large in comparison with the mesiobuccal cusp. The mesiobuccal cusp from this angle is relatively short and sharp. There is very little curvature to the cervical line. Usually it is almost straight across from buccal surface to lingual surface.

The mesiobuccal root from this aspect appears broad and flat. The lingual root has somewhat the same curvature as the lingual root of the maxillary first deciduous molar. It extends lingually far out beyond the crown outline. The point of bifurcation between the mesiobuccal root and the lingual root is 2 or 3 mm. apical to the cervical line of the crown and approximately two thirds the distance from buccal surface to lingual surface. The mesiolingual cusp is directly below this point. Although the curvature lingually on the crown from this aspect is great at the cervical portion, as on most deciduous teeth, the crest of curvature buccally at the cervical third is slight and resembles the curvature found at this point on the permanent maxillary first molar. In this it differs entirely from the accented curvature found on the deciduous maxillary first molars at the cervical third buccally.

Distal Aspect. From the distal aspect it is apparent that the distal measurement of the crown is less than the mesial measurement, but not to the degree found on the deciduous maxillary first molar. From both the distal and the mesial aspects the outline of the crown lingually appears almost semicircular, whereas a line describing the buccal surface is almost straight from the crest of curvature to the occlusal surface. The distobuccal cusp and the distolingual cusp are about the same in length. The cervical line is approximately straight, as was found mesially.

All three roots are seen from this aspect, although only a part of the outline of the mesiobuccal root may be seen, since the distobuccal root is superimposed over it. The distobuccal root is shorter and narrower than the other roots. The point of bifurcation between the distobuccal root and the lingual root is more apical in position than any of the other points of bifurcation. The point of bifurcation between these two roots on the distal is more nearly centered above the crown than that on the mesial between the mesiobuccal and lingual roots.

Occlusal Aspect (Fig. 72, b). From the occlusal aspect this tooth resembles the permanent first molar. It is somewhat rhomboidal and has four well-developed cusps and one supplemental cusp: mesiobuccal, distobuccal, mesiolingual, distolingual and fifth cusps. The buccal surface is rather flat, with the developmental groove between the cusps less marked than that found on the first permanent molar. Developmental grooves, pits, oblique ridge, etc., are almost identical.

The occlusal surface has a *central fossa* with a *central pit*, a well-defined *mesial triangular fossa*, just distal to the *mesial marginal ridge*, with a mesial pit at its center. There is, too, a well-defined developmental groove called the *central groove* at the bottom of a sulcus connecting the mesial triangular fossa with the central fossa. The *buccal developmental groove* extends buccally from the central pit, separating the triangular ridges which are occlusal continuations of the mesio- and distobuccal cusps. Supplemental grooves often radiate from these developmental grooves.

The *oblique ridge* is prominent and connects the mesiolingual cusp with the distobuccal cusp. Distal to the oblique ridge one finds the *distal fossa*, which harbors the *distal developmental groove*. The distal groove has branches of supplemental grooves within the *distal triangular fossa* which is rather indefinitely outlined just mesial to the distal marginal ridge.

The distal groove acts as a line of demarcation between the mesiolingual and distolingual cusps and continues on to the lingual surface as the *lingual developmental groove*. The *distal marginal ridge* is well developed as the *mesial marginal ridge*. It will be remembered that the marginal ridges are not developed equally on the deciduous maxillary first molar.

Mandibular First Molar

This tooth does not resemble any of the other teeth, deciduous or permanent. Because it varies so much from all others, it appears strange and primitive.

Buccal Aspect (Fig. 69, c). From the buccal aspect the mesial outline of the crown of the deciduous mandibular first molar is almost straight from the contact area to the cervix, constricting the crown very little at the cervix. The outline describing the distal portion, however, converges toward the cervix more than usual, making the contact area extend distally to a marked degree.

The distal portion of the crown is shorter than the mesial portion, the cervical line dipping apically where it joins the mesial root.

The two buccal cusps are rather distinct, although there is no developmental groove between them. The mesial cusp is larger than the distal cusp. There is a

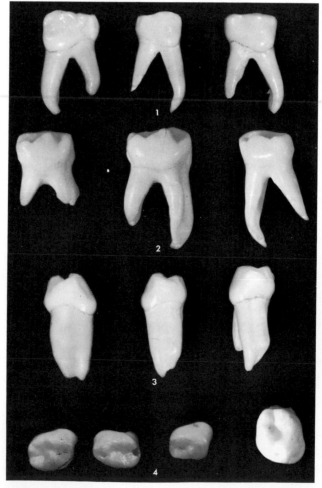

Figure 75. Deciduous mandibular first molars. This tooth has characteristics in detail unlike any other tooth in the mouth, deciduous or permanent. See text. 1, Buccal aspect; 2, lingual aspect; 3, mesial aspect; 4, occlusal aspect.

developmental depression dividing them, which extends over to the buccal surface.

The roots are long and slender, and they spread greatly at the apical third beyond the outline of the crown.

As is characteristic of all deciduous molars, the point of bifurcation between the roots is very close to the cervical line of the crown.

Lingual Aspect (Fig. 70, c).   The crown and root converge lingually to a marked degree on the mesial surface. Distally the opposite arrangement is true of both crown and root; the crown is rhomboidal in outline. The distolingual cusp is rounded and well developed and suggests a developmental groove between this cusp and the mesiolingual cusp. The mesiolingual cusp is long and sharp at the tip, more so than any of the other cusps. It will be noted that the mesial marginal ridge is so well developed that it might almost be considered another small cusp lingually. Part of the two buccal cusps may be seen from this angle.

From the lingual aspect the crown length mesially and distally is more uniform than it is from the buccal aspect. The cervical line is straighter.

Mesial Aspect (Fig. 71, c).   The most noticeable detail from the mesial aspect is the extreme curvature buccally at the cervical third. Except for this detail, the crown outline of this tooth from this aspect is similar to the mesial aspect of the deciduous second molar and the permanent mandibular molars. In comparison, the buccal cusps are placed over the root base, and the lingual outline of the crown extends out lingually beyond the confines of the root base.

Both the mesiobuccal cusp and the mesiolingual cusp are in view from this aspect, as is the well-developed mesial marginal ridge. Since the mesiobuccal crown length is greater than the mesiolingual crown length, the cervical line slants upward buccolingually. Note the flat appearance of the buccal outline of the crown from the crest of curvature of the buccal surface at the cervical third to the tip of the mesiobuccal cusp. All of the deciduous molars have flattened buccal surfaces above this crest.

The outline of the mesial root from the mesial aspect does not resemble the outline of any other deciduous tooth root. The buccal and lingual outlines of the root drop straight down from the crown and are approximately parallel for over half their length, tapering only slightly at the apical third. The root end is flat and almost square. A developmental depression usually extends almost the full length of the root.

Distal Aspect.   The distal aspect of the mandibular first molar differs from the mesial aspect in the following points: There is less curvature at the cervical third buccally. The length of crown buccally and lingually is more uniform, and the cervical line extends almost straight across buccolingually. The distobuccal cusp and the distolingual cusp are not as long or as sharp as the two mesial cusps. The distal marginal ridge is not as straight and well-defined as the mesial marginal ridge. The distal root is rounder and shorter and tapers more apically.

Occlusal Aspect (Fig. 72, c).   The general outline of this tooth from the occlusal aspect is rhomboidal. The prominence mesiobuccally is noticeable from this aspect also, a fact which accents the mesiobuccal line angle of the crown in comparison with the distobuccal line angle.

The mesiolingual cusp may be seen as the largest and the best developed of all the cusps, and it has a broad flattened surface lingually. The *buccal developmental groove* of the occlusal surface divides the two buccal cusps evenly. This developmental groove is short, extending from between the buccal cusp ridges to a point approximately in the center of the crown outline at a *central pit*. The *central developmental groove* joins it at this point and extends mesially, separating the mesiobuccal cusp and the mesiolingual cusp. The central groove ends in a *mesial pit* in the *mesial triangular fossa* which is immediately distal to the *mesial marginal ridge*. Two supplemental grooves join the developmental groove in the center of the mesial triangular fossa; one supplemental groove extends buccally and the other extends lingually.

The mesiobuccal cusp exhibits a well-defined triangular ridge on the occlusal surface which terminates in the center of the occlusal surface buccolingually at the *central developmental groove*. The *lingual developmental groove* extends lingually from ths point, separating the mesiolingual cusp and the distolingual cusp. Usually the lingual developmental groove does not extend through to the lingual surface but stops at the junction of lingual cusp ridges. There are some supplemental grooves immediately mesial to the *distal marginal ridge* in the *distal triangular fossa* which join with the central developmental groove.

Mandibular Second Molar

The deciduous mandibular second molar resembles the permanent mandibular first molar except in its dimensions.

Buccal Aspect (Fig. 69, d).   From the buccal aspect, the deciduous mandibular second molar has a mesiodistal measurement at the cervix much less in proportion to its mesiodistal measurement at the contact areas than that measurement on mandibular first permanent molars. A mesiobuccal and a distobuccal developmental groove divide the buccal surface occlusally into three cusps which are almost equal in size.

The roots of the deciduous second molar from this angle are slender and long. They have a characteristic flair mesiodistally at the middle and apical thirds. The roots of this tooth are usually twice as long as the crown, if not longer.

The point of bifurcation of the roots starts immediately below the cervical line of the crown buccally.

Lingual Aspect (Fig. 70, d).   From the lingual aspect one sees two cusps of almost equal dimensions. Between them is a short lingual groove. The two lingual cusps are not quite as wide as the three buccal cusps; this arrangement narrows the crown lingually. The cervical line is relatively straight, and the crown extends out over the root more distally than it does mesially. A portion of each of the three buccal cusps may be seen from this aspect.

The roots from this aspect give somewhat the same appearance as from the buccal aspect. Note the length of the roots.

Mesial Aspect (Fig. 71, d).   From the mesial aspect the outline of the crown resembles the permanent mandibular first molar. The variations are: The crest of contour buccally is more prominent on the deciduous molar, and the tooth seems to

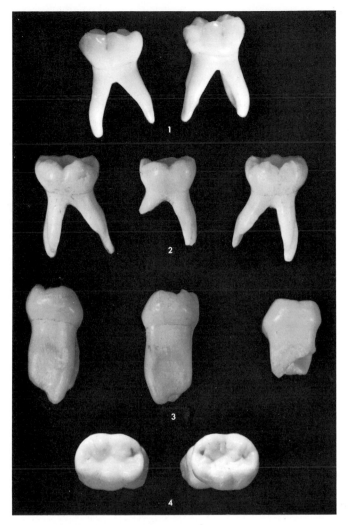

Figure 76. Deciduous mandibular second molars. 1, Buccal aspect; 2, lingual aspect; 3, mesial aspect; 4, occlusal aspect.

be more constricted occlusally because of the flattened buccal surface above the crest of contour.

The crown has the characteristic position over the root of all mandibular posteriors with its buccal cusp over the root and the lingual outline of the crown extending out beyond the root outline. The marginal ridge is high, a characteristic which makes the mesiobuccal cusp and the mesiolingual cusp appear rather short. The lingual cusp is longer, or extends higher at any rate, than the buccal cusp. The cervical line is regular, although it extends upward buccolingually, making up for the difference in length between the buccal and lingual cusps.

The mesial root is broad and flat with a blunt apex.

Distal Aspect. The crown is not so wide distally as it is mesially; therefore it is possible to see the mesiobuccal cusp as well as the distobuccal cusp from the distal aspect. The distolingual cusp appears well developed, and the triangular ridge from the tip of this cusp extending down into the occlusal surface is seen over the distal marginal ridge.

The distal marginal ridge dips down more sharply and is shorter buccolingually than the mesial marginal ridge. The cervical line of the crown is regular, although it has the same upward incline buccolingually on the distal as on the mesial.

The distal root is almost as broad as the mesial root, and it is flattened on the distal surface. The distal root tapers more at the apical end than does the mesial root.

Occlusal Aspect (Fig. 72, d). The occlusal aspect of the deciduous mandibular second molar is somewhat rectangular. The three buccal cusps are similar in size. The two lingual cusps are also equally matched. However, the total mesiodistal width of the lingual cusps is less than the total mesiodistal width of the three buccal cusps.

There are well-defined triangular ridges extending occlusally from each one of these cusp tips. The triangular ridges end in the center of the crown buccolingually in a *central developmental groove* which follows a staggered course from the *mesial triangular fossa,* just inside the *mesial marginal ridge,* to the *distal triangular fossa,* just mesial to the *distal marginal ridge.* The distal triangular fossa is not so well defined as the mesial triangular fossa. Developmental grooves branch off from the central groove both buccally and lingually, dividing the cusps. The two *buccal*

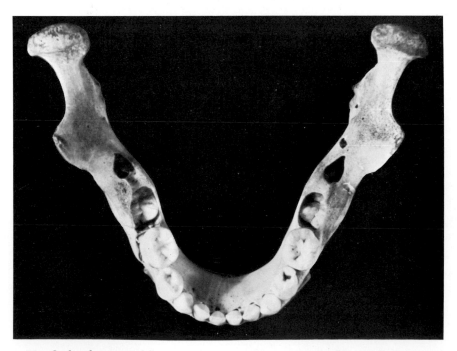

Figure 77. Occlusal aspect of the mandible of specimen shown in Fig. 50. Permanent first molar crowns are well developed, and openings in the bone have appeared over the developing permanent second molars. Note the extent of development of the mandible between the distal surface of the second deciduous molar and the anterior border of the ramus.

grooves are confluent with the buccal developmental grooves of the buccal surface, one *mesial* and one *distal*, and the single *lingual developmental groove* is confluent with the *lingual groove* on the lingual surface of the crown.

Scattered over the occlusal surface are supplemental grooves on the slopes of triangular ridges and in the mesial and distal triangular fossae. The mesial marginal ridge is better developed and more pronounced than the distal marginal ridge. The outline of the crown converges distally. An outline following the tips of the cusps and the marginal ridges conforms to the outline of a rectangle more closely than does the gross outline of the crown in its entirety.

A comparison between the deciduous mandibular second molar and the permanent mandibular first molar brings out the following points of difference: The deciduous molar has its mesiobuccal, distobuccal and distal cusps almost equal in size and development. The distal cusp of the permanent molar is smaller than the other two. Because of the small buccal cusps, the deciduous tooth crown is narrower buccolingually in comparison with its mesiodistal measurement, than is the permanent tooth.

THE OCCLUSION OF THE DECIDUOUS TEETH

The deciduous teeth are arranged in the jaws in the form of two arches: a maxillary and a mandibular. An outline following the labial and buccal surfaces of the maxillary teeth describes the segment of an ellipse, an outline which is larger than the segment following the same surfaces on the mandibular teeth (see Fig. 1, *A,* Chapter I).

The relation between the maxillary and mandibular deciduous teeth when in occlusion is such that each tooth, with the exception of the mandibular central incisor and the maxillary second molar, occludes with two teeth of the opposite jaw. The deciduous teeth should be in normal alignment and occlusion shortly after the age of two, with all the roots fully formed by the time the child is three years old. A year or so after the teeth have fully erupted and have assumed their respective positions in the arches, the rapid development of the jaws is sufficient to create a slight space, or *diastema,* between some of them.

The anterior teeth separate and usually show greater separation as time goes on — a process which is caused by the growth of the jaws and the approach of the permanent teeth from the lingual side. This separation usually begins between the ages of four and five years. The canines and molars are supposed to keep their positive contact relation during all the jaw growth. However, some shifting and separation is often seen. Since the teeth do not hold their relative positions for long, they are worn off rapidly on incisal ridges and occlusal surfaces. As an example, when a deciduous canine is lost eight years or more after its eruption, its long, sharp cusp has in most instances been worn flat. If the deciduous teeth are in good alignment, the occlusion is most efficient during the time that these teeth are in their original positions (see Figs. 78 and 79).

After normal jaw growth has resulted in considerable separation, the occlusion is supported and made more efficient by the eruption and occlusion of the first per-

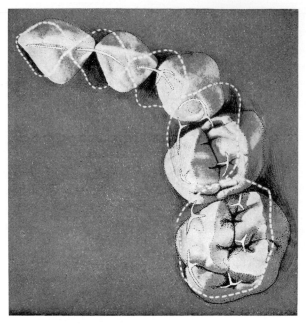

Figure 78. Occlusal surfaces of the maxillary deciduous teeth, with the outlines of the opposing teeth superposed in occlusion. (Freil, Internat. J. Orthodontia and Oral Surgery.)

manent molars immediately distal to the deciduous second molars. The child is now approximately six years of age, and he will use some of his deciduous teeth for six more years.

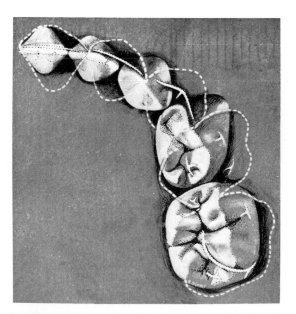

Figure 79. Occlusal surface of the mandibular deciduous teeth, with the outlines of the opposing teeth superposed in occlusion. Three years of age. (Freil, Internat. J. Orthodontia and Oral Surgery.)

Details of Occlusion (Figs. 78 and 79)

The occlusion of deciduous teeth, in a three-year-old child, may be described. After separation has begun, the migration of the teeth changes the occlusion. Nevertheless, if development is normal, the spacing of the teeth is rather uniform (Fig. 48).

Normal occlusion of deciduous teeth at the age of three years is as follows:

1. Mesial surfaces of maxillary and mandibular central incisors are in line with each other at the median line.

2. The maxillary central incisor occludes with the mandibular central incisor and the mesial third of the mandibular lateral incisor. The mandibular anterior teeth strike the maxillary anterior teeth lingually above the level of the incisal ridges.

3. The maxillary lateral incisor occludes with the distal two-thirds of the mandibular lateral incisor and that portion of the mandibular canine which is mesial to the point of its cusp.

4. The maxillary canine occludes with that portion of the mandibular canine distal to its cusp tip and the mesial third of the mandibular first molar (that portion mesial to the tip of the mesiobuccal cusp).

5. The maxillary first molar occludes with the distal two-thirds of the mandibular first molar and the mesial portion of the mandibular second molar, which portion is represented by the mesial marginal ridge and the mesial triangular fossa.

6. The maxillary second molar occludes with the remainder of the mandibular second molar, the distal surface of the maxillary molar projecting slightly over the distal portion of the mandibular second molar.

The interrelation of cusps and incisal ridges of the opposing arches of deciduous teeth may be studied in the illustrations by Sheldon Freil. The relation in size of deciduous and permanent arches is also illustrated by him in Figure 80. (See also Fig. 1, Chapter I.)

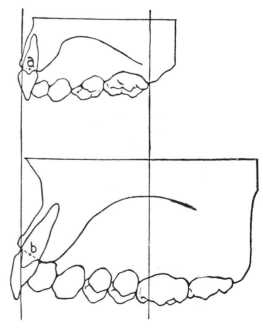

Figure 80. Drawing of a sagittal section through the permanent and deciduous maxillary incisors. The labial surface at the cervical margin is oriented in the same plane. Note that the midalveolar point of the permanent incisors, *b*, is more lingual than the midalveolar point of the deciduous incisors, *a*, but that the incisal edge of the permanent incisors is more labial than that of the deciduous incisors. (Freil, Internat. J. Orthodontia and Oral Surgery.)

Chapter IV

GENERAL CONSIDERATIONS
IN THE PHYSIOLOGY
OF THE PERMANENT DENTITION

FORM AND FUNCTION

THE TEETH must be regarded as instruments—instruments to be used for the cutting and *comminution* of food during the process of mastication. Since they need to be kept sound and firmly attached in the jaws for a lifetime, it is necessary that the supporting tissues be kept in good condition also. Normal tooth form, plus proper alignment, assures efficiency in masticating food. This form also helps to insure the life of the tooth and its position in the jaw by protecting vulnerable tissues with protective and efficient contours.

Since the design of the individual teeth protects their investing tissues, in addition to serving for the mastication of food, we come to the familiar term "Form and Function." To illustrate: Surgical instruments, carpenters' tools, and the like, are designed for definite purposes. The better each tool or instrument obeys fundamental physical laws in design, the more efficient it will be in application. Its form governs its function, and its function in turn requires a definite design.

Human teeth are no exception to this rule: Their anatomy is such that they are enabled to perform two major functions during life: (1) *they incise and reduce food material during mastication,* and (2) *they help sustain themselves in the dental arches by assisting in the development and protection of the tissues that support them.*

Protection of the investing tissues and stabilization of alignment are provided by the normal form of the individual teeth, by their proper alignment with others in the

78

same jaw, by normal development of the jaws, and by the proper relation of one jaw to the other during functional movements.

The relation of one jaw to the other has an effect upon the forces brought to bear on the teeth. A normal jaw relation applies the forces equally in directions which the teeth, in normal alignment, are designed to withstand.

The function of the dental apparatus is primarily the mastication of food. It has other important values however.

Good teeth make one physically more attractive. Socially good diction is an asset and correct speech is assisted by the normal development of teeth and jaws.

Psychologically, physical and mental concentration are aided by clenching the teeth firmly together during almost any activity. Strong teeth with good occlusion add in this manner to one's assets and capabilities.

Alignment, Contacts and Occlusion

When the teeth in the mandibular arch come into contact with those in the maxillary arch in any *functional relation*, they are said to be *in occlusion*. There is therefore a central relation of one arch to the other, which is called *centric* or *central occlusion* When the occlusion of the teeth of one jaw with those in the opposing jaw is abnormal, the teeth are said to be in *malocclusion.*

In proper alignment the teeth are arranged in arches in each jaw and placed in strong contact with their neighbors (Fig. 81). If, in addition, each tooth in the arch is placed at its most advantageous angle to withstand forces brought to bear upon it, each tooth is more efficient and the arches are stabilized by the collective action of the teeth in supporting each other (Figs. 82 and 83). Compare the plaster casts in Figure 84, for example, with those in Figure 85. It is readily seen that irregularly arranged teeth subject to jaw forces are less likely to stabilize themselves or to help in stabilizing the others.

Contact of each tooth with its fellows in the arch protects the *gingiva* between them in the *interproximal spaces*. Figures 86 and 87 are given as examples. The gingiva is the soft tissue in the mouth which covers the alveolar bone and surrounds the teeth.

Interproximal Form

The interproximal space between the teeth is a triangular region, normally filled with gingival tissue, which is bounded by two proximal surfaces of contacting teeth and alveolar bone.

The gingiva within this space is called the *gingival or interdental papilla* (Fig. 126). Normally, the gingiva covers part of the cervical third of the tooth crowns and fills the interproximal spaces (Figs. 86 and 121). The *gingival line* follows the curvature, but not necessarily, the level of the cervical line. The cervical line has been

A

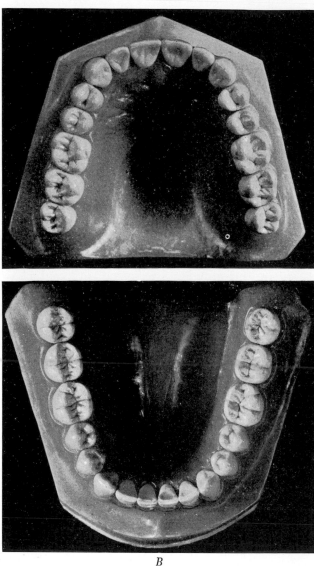

B

Figure 81. Model teeth placed in "ideal" alignment and contact relation. *A,* Maxillary arch; *B,* mandibular arch.

defined previously as the "cementoenamel junction of crown and root." The gingival line and the cervical line must not be confused; although they normally follow a similar curvature, they are seldom at the same level on the tooth. The cervical line is a stable anatomic demarcation, whereas the gingival line merely represents the gingival level on the tooth at any one period in the individual's life, and this level is variable. Malalignment of the teeth will change the gingival line—a fact which is not conducive to the health of the tissue (Fig. 88).

Even though the teeth are in good alignment, unless the proper relation is kept between the *width* of the tooth *at the cervix* and the width *at the point of contact,* the

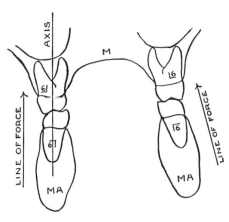
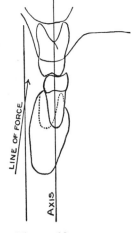

Figure 82   **Figure 83**

Figure 82. Outline of a cross section through the maxilla and mandible at the site of the first molars. The line of force exerted when the teeth come into contact should be parallel to the long axis of the teeth. If the teeth are in the proper position to withstand this force their positions will be stable.

Figure 83. A drawing showing the first mandibular molar out of normal position. Its axis is not parallel with the line of force, and consequently the act of mastication would tend to change the position and angulation of the teeth, making them unstable.

A

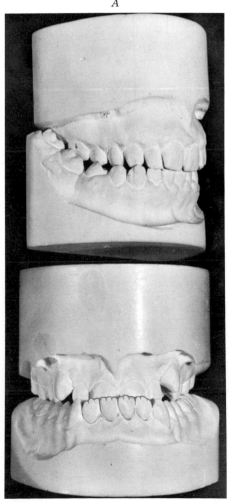

Figure 84. Plaster casts of two sets of jaws, each demonstrating malocclusion. *A,* Fair occlusion of maxillary central and lateral incisors with those of the mandible, but gross malocclusion of the right canines and posterior teeth. *B,* Extensive malocclusion with improper relationship of the maxillary and mandibular arches. Note the *mamelons,* which are still intact on the incisal portion of the mandibular central and lateral incisors. (Courtesy of Dr. Henry Westhoff.)

B

81

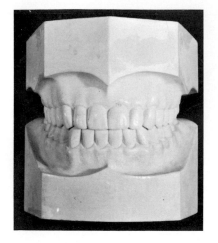

Figure 85. This cast demonstrates normal occlusion. The teeth in each arch are in proper alignment, the jaw relationship is normal, and therefore the relationship of each mandibular tooth to its antagonist in the maxilla is normal. These teeth will support each other in keeping normal arch relationship.

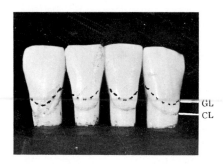

Figure 86. The mandibular centrals and laterals contact each other at the incisal third. The form of each tooth, plus the location of the contact areas, creates narrow pointed spaces between the teeth which differ from other interproximal spaces in other segments of the arches. *CL,* cervical line as established by the cementoenamel junction. *GL,* the variable gingival line which represents the gingival level.

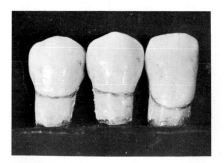

Figure 87. Contact design and interproximal (sometimes called interdental) spaces illustrated by the mandibular canine and first and second premolars. Note the variation in contact areas in relation to crown length.

spacing interdentally will be changed. This is an important point to observe in drawing and carving and in tooth restoration.

When considering the tooth form from the *mesial* and *distal aspects,* we find curvature on the crowns at the cervical third above the cervical line, labially or buccally and lingually—a factor which must be treated with respect. This curvature holds the gingiva under proper tension and serves to protect the investing tissues of the teeth during mastication; it is often called the "cervicoenamel ridge" (Figs. 16 and 17, Chapter I).

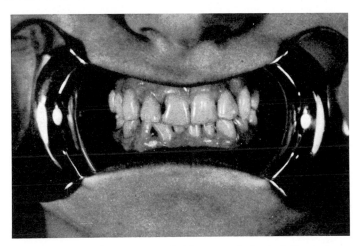

Figure 88. The maxillary teeth are surrounded by normal gingival tissue, because these teeth are in good alignment. Observe the irregular outline of the gingiva around the mandibular teeth and the destruction apparent in this young individual between the right lateral incisor and canine. The alignment is especially bad at this point, and therefore the contact and interproximal spacing are abnormal.

Important Physiologic Relations

The *length* and *shape of the root* (or roots) of each tooth must be considered. The canine, for instance, because of its position and the work it performs, would be torn out of its socket, or at least displaced, by forces brought to bear upon it, if it were not for the fact that the root is of extra size and length (Fig. 89). Fracture would be

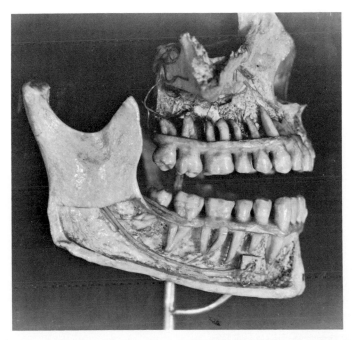

Figure 89. A view of a specimen from a point opposite the first molar. Note that the teeth are placed at different angulations. The position of the tooth in the jaw and the relation between its axis and the lines of force brought to bear upon it are very important.

imminent if the root were not larger than that of other single-root teeth. The root form therefore is associated with the *size* of the tooth and the *work* it has to do.

The *angle* at which the incisal and occlusal surfaces of the tooth crowns are placed with respect to the root bases is also important. The mesial view of an anterior tooth will show that the incisal ridge or cusp is centered over the root (Fig. 16, Chapter I). The mesial view of an upper first molar will show the occlusal surface of the crown contacting the opposing teeth to be well within the confines of the root base. (Note the flare of the roots for stabilization—Fig 17, Chapter I.) The measurement from cusp to cusp buccolingually is definitely less than the buccolingual diameter of the root where it joins the crown.

Compensating Occlusal Curvature

Close observation shows that the occlusal and incisal surfaces of all the crowns taken together in either arch would not contact a flat plane. Looking at the teeth from a point opposite the first molars buccally, one sees that a line following the occlusal and incisal surfaces describes a curve.

This arrangement was described originally in the German literature in 1890 by F. Graf von Spee, and it is called the *Curve of Spee* (Fig. 90). The occlusal curvature of tooth alignment was described as conforming to arcs of circles. Today we prefer to think of the composite arrangement of the occlusal surfaces of all of the teeth in each dental arch and of their approximate conformation to a segment of a sphere, which gives the curvature three-dimensional quality (Figs. 91 and 398). This curvature is called the *compensating occlusal curvature*. We say that the compensating occlusal curvature of the mandibular teeth is *concave* and that of the maxillary teeth *convex* (Fig. 91). Also, the compensating occlusal curvature of all the teeth is reflected in the design of each tooth. The occlusal surface of the maxillary first molar, for instance, shows a definite *acute* angulation *mesially* with the long axis of the roots (Fig. 92).

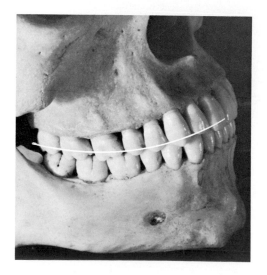

Figure 90. Centric occlusion. The occlusion of natural teeth is seldom if ever "ideal." This illustration shows normal occlusion. Note the "Curve of Spee." Also note the margin of the alveolar bone in its relation to the cervical line of the teeth. (Observe fourth mandibular molar, an anomaly.)

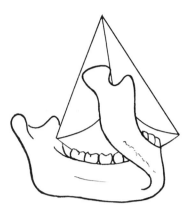

Figure 91. A segment of a sphere placed on the occluding surfaces of the mandibular teeth, showing their compensating occlusal curvature.

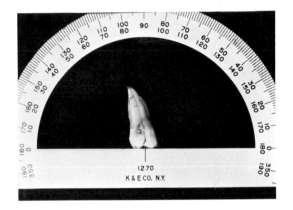

Figure 92. Individual tooth placed within a protractor to show axial inclinations.

The length and shape of the roots, the angle at which the incisal and occlusal surfaces are placed with respect to the roots, sufficient dimensions for strength, and efficient design for thorough work with resistance against lines of force; all these play a part in a magnificent scheme to stabilize the dental arches and to resist physiologic change.

Comparative Dental Anatomy

The fundamentals of tooth form in the human subject can be better understood by making comparisons with the dentition of the lower animals. The physiologic significance of important landmarks on the teeth will be realized only after a study of development and its relation to function; detailed descriptions of the form of individual teeth will then have more meaning.

Paleontologists tell us that the *primordial form* of tooth was a single cone. From this primitive form, which is found in lower animal organisms today, other more highly developed forms have been derived by multiplication of the single cone or lobe, until we come finally to the human teeth, each of which is made up of four or more

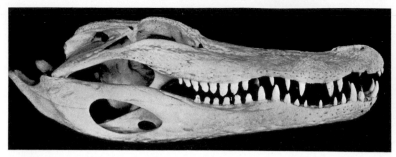

Figure 93. The Mississippi alligator. (Kronfeld, *Dental Histology and Comparative Dental Anatomy*, Lea & Febiger.)

lobes. An example of the single-lobe form may be found in the teeth of the Mississippi alligator (Fig. 93).

Jaw movements are always related to tooth forms. Single-pointed cones will lock together when the jaws are closed, and therefore the jaw movement for these simple conical teeth resolves itself into the simple hinge action, or up-and-down movement.

A major change which takes place among the higher forms of animal life is the development of the *tritubercular form* of tooth, which presents a fusion of three lobes or cusps. A common example of this is in the dog (Fig. 94). The jaw movement is still limited to the simple hinge action because of the interlocking cusps.

An animal which has jaw movements which begin to approach those of the human being is the bear (Fig. 95). The bear has a dentition similar in some respects to that of the dog, except that the premolars and molars are adapted to a more mixed diet. The dog is carnivorous (by nature), the bear omnivorous. The premolars and molars of the bear have acquired occlusal surfaces which are more regular in outline; the cusps have an intercusping relation and the design is more efficient in reducing vegetable food than in the dog. The incisors and canines are still of the true carnivorous type. The

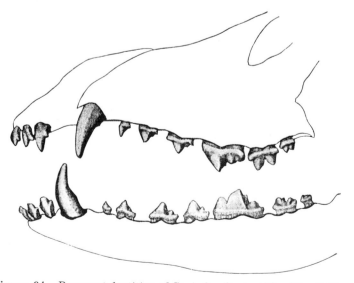

Figure 94. Permanet dentition of Canis familiaris. (After Marett Tims.)

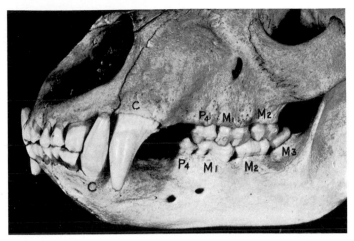

Figure 95. The bear. (Kronfeld, *Dental Histology and Comparative Dental Anatomy*, Lea & Febiger.)

temporomandibular joint permits some lateral excursion to correspond with the tooth design posteriorly.

The animal that has a dental mechanism most nearly like that of man is the anthropoid ape (Fig. 96). His dentition has the same formula as that of man. There is considerable difference, however, in the size and in the development of individual teeth, in the dental arch form, and the range of lateral movement. The jaw movements are limited by the interlocking of the canines in centric relation, which is typical of "carnivorous" development.

The reader would do well to make a further study of the subject of comparative dental anatomy. It will serve to orientate his thinking on the functional form of the teeth, while he pursues a fascinating and important area in anthropology.

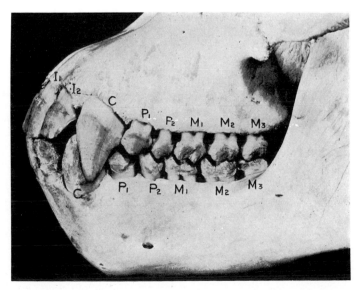

Figure 96. The ape. (Kronfeld, *Dental Histology and Comparative Dental Anatomy,* Lea & Febiger.)

From the foregoing we draw the conclusion that tooth forms and jaw movements are closely related.

Lobe Form

Lobe formation in human teeth is apparent on observation of the development and the functional form of the teeth. Representative instances follow:

The multiplication and fusion of lobes during tooth development are demonstrated graphically when teeth are viewed from the mesial or distal aspects. Anterior teeth, which are used for incising or apprehending food, reflect the single cone; whereas the posterior or multicusp teeth, which are used for grinding food in addition to a shearing action, appear to be two or more cones fused (Fig. 97). Although the functional form of the teeth from the mesial and distal aspects is that of a single cone, or the fusion of two or three cones, observation of all aspects proves the development of each tooth crown to be a combination of *four lobes* or more. Each lobe represents a primary center of formation.

All anterior teeth show traces of four lobes, three labially and one lingually, the lingual lobe being represented by the cingulum. Each labial lobe of the incisor terminates incisally in rounded eminences known as *mamelons*. These mamelons are prominent in newly erupted incisors (Fig. 84). Soon after eruption they are worn down by use unless through malalignment they escape incisal wear. Maxillary central incisors often show traces of the fusion of three lobes on the labial face by visible markings in the enamel called *labial grooves* (Fig. 98, *a*).

In the anterior teeth the four lobes are called the *mesial, labial, distal* and *lingual lobes* In *premolars* they are called *mesial buccal distal* and *lingual lobes;* or, as in

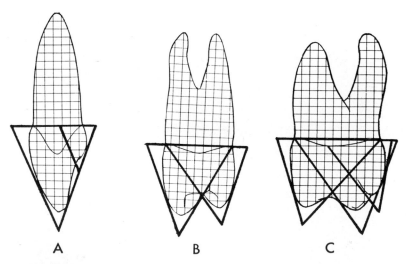

A   B   C

Figure 97. The functional form of the teeth when outlined schematically from the mesial or distal aspects is that of the fusion of two or three cones. *a*, Maxillary incisor; *b*, maxillary premolar; *c*, maxillary first molar. Note that the major portion of the incisor in view is made up of one cone or lobe.

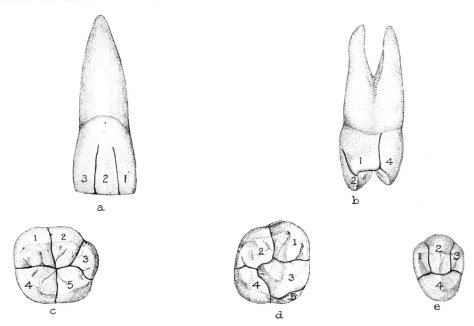

Figure 98. This illustration shows the general outlines of some of the lobes.

a, Labial aspect of maxillary central incisor, showing the labial grooves marking the division of the lobes. 1, Mesial lobe; 2, labial lobe; 3, distal lobe. (Lingual lobe or cingulum not in view.) (See Fig. 99, *A*-4.)

b and *e*, Mesial and occlusal aspects of maxillary first premolar. 1, Mesial lobe; 2, buccal lobe; 3, distal lobe, 4, lingual lobe.

c, Occlusal aspect of mandibular first molar. 1, Mesiobuccal lobe; 2, distobuccal lobe; 3, distal lobe; 4, mesiolingual lobe; 5, distolingual lobe. (Lobes on molars are named the same as cusps.)

d, Occlusal aspect of maxillary first molar. 1, Mesiobuccal lobe; 2, distobuccal lobe; 3, mesiolingual lobe; 4, distolingual lobe; 5, fifth lobe (fifth cusp).

Figure 99. *A*, Lingual aspect of maxillary canine, which shows the primary centers of formation. 1, Mesial lobe; 2, central lobe (cusp); 3, distal lobe; 4, lingual lobe (cingulum).

B, Incomplete formation demonstrated by a developmental groove distolingually on a maxillary lateral incisor. This groove will sometimes harbor fissures at various points along its length, especially in the coronal portion. A tooth with this handicap is more subject to caries as well as gum infections around it.

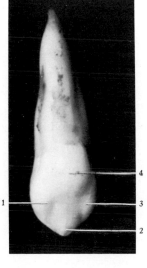

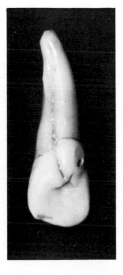

A

B

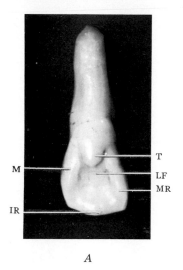
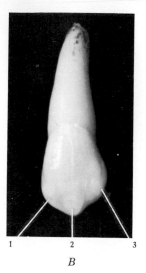

A   *B*

Figure 100. *A,* Maxillary lateral incisor which shows prominences at the centers of calcification. *T,* Tubercle, prominence equal to a small cusp at the cingulum; *LF,* lingual fossa; *MR,* marginal ridges; *IR,* incisal ridge with a prominent enamel rise.

B, Maxillary canine showing evidences of lobe formation. 1, Mesial lobe; 2, labial lobe; 3, distal lobe.

the case of the mandibular second premolar, which often has two lingual cusps, the *mesial, buccal, distal, mesiolingual* and *distolingual lobes,* making five in all (Fig. 239).

The *molar lobes* are named the same as the cusps: *mesiobuccal lobe,* etc. The tip of each cusp represents the primary center of formation of each lobe.*

It is possible, of course, to find a variation in the number of lobes in molars. Tubercles of enamel may be found in addition to the primary lobes. When present, they are usually smaller than, and supplementary to, the major lobes.

A GEOMETRIC CONCEPT OF CROWN OUTLINES

In a general way, all aspects of each tooth crown except the incisal or occlusal aspects may be outlined within three geometric figures: a *triangle,* a *trapezoid* and a *rhomboid.* To one unfamiliar with dental anatomy it may seem an exaggeration to say that curved outlines of tooth crowns can be included within geometric figures. Nevertheless, to one who realizes the problems involved in crown design it seems very plausible to consider fundamental outlines schematically to assist in visualization.

In freehand drawing, the outlines of a subject are sketched roughly at first in order to get proportion and outline form. In sculpture the subject is "blocked in," a method which follows the same plan as sketching in drawing except that three

---

*Tables of development of the teeth will be given under the complete description of each tooth. The description of the formation of the teeth histologically, however, will not be included. For this refer to a textbook on dental histology.

dimensions are involved. Therefore, since it is possible to reduce the fundamental outline of tooth crowns to three generalizations (except, as has been pointed out, for the incisal or occlusal aspects), this method of approach will be used.

Facial and Lingual Aspects of All Teeth

The outlines of the facial and lingual aspects of all the teeth may be represented by *trapezoids* of various dimensions. The shortest of the uneven sides represent the bases of the crowns at the crevices, and the longest of the uneven sides represent the working surfaces, or the incisal and occlusal surfaces, through the points of contact of neighboring teeth in the same arch (Fig. 101). Disregarding the overlap of anterior teeth and the cusp forms of the cusped teeth in the schematic drawing, one can easily see the fundamental plan governing the form and arrangement of the teeth from this aspect.

The occlusal line which forms the longest uneven side of each of the trapezoids represents the approximate point at which the opposing teeth come together when the jaw is closed. The student must not become confused at this point and think that the teeth actually occlude at their points of contact. The illustration is made to help the student visualize the fundamental outline of the teeth from the labial and buccal aspects. (See Fig. 102.)

This arrangement brings out the following *fundamentals* of form:

1. Interproximal spaces accommodate interproximal gingival tissue.

2. Spacing between the roots of one tooth and those of another allows sufficient bone tissue for a foundation or investment for the teeth and a supporting structure required to hold up gingival tissue to a normal level. Sufficient circulation of blood to the parts would be impossible without this necessary spacing.

3. Each tooth crown in the dental arches must be in contact at some point with

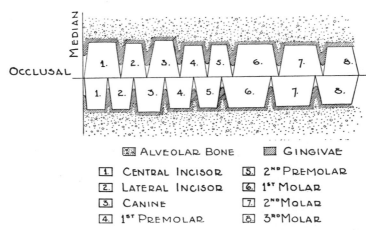

Figure 101. Schematic drawing of facial (labial and buccal) aspects of the teeth only, illustrating the teeth as trapezoids of various dimensions. Note the relations of each tooth to its opposing tooth or teeth in the opposite arch. Each tooth has two antagonists except number 1 below and number 8 above.

its neighbor, or neighbors, to protect the interproximal gingival tissue from trauma during mastication. The contact of one tooth with another in the arch tends to insure their relative positions by mutual support.

4. Each tooth in each dental arch has two antagonists in the opposing arch, excepting the mandibular central incisor and the maxillary third molar. In the event of loss of any tooth, this arrangement tends to prevent elongation of antagonists and helps stabilize the remaining teeth over a longer period than would be likely if each tooth had a single antagonist.

Mesial and Distal Aspects of the Anterior Teeth

The mesial and distal aspects of the anterior teeth, central incisors, lateral incisors and canines, maxillary and mandibular, may be included within *triangles*. The base of the triangle is represented by the cervical portion of the crown, and the apex by the incisal ridge (Fig. 102, *a*).

The fundamentals portrayed here are:

1. A wide base to the crown for strength.

2. A tapered outline labially and lingually, narrowing down to a relatively thin ridge which facilitates biting through food material.

Mesial and Distal Aspects of Maxillary Posterior Teeth

The outlines of the mesial and distal aspects of all maxillary posterior teeth (premolars and molars) can be included within *trapezoidal* figures. Naturally, the uneven sides of the premolar figures are shorter than those of the molars (Fig. 102, *e* and *f*). Notice that in this instance the trapezoidal figures show the longest uneven side representing the base of the crown instead of the occlusal line, as was the case in showing the same teeth from the buccal or lingual view. In other words, the schematic outline used to represent the buccal aspect of premolars or molars is turned upside down to represent the mesial or distal aspects of the same teeth. (In Fig. 102, compare maxillary figures *c* and *d* with *e* and *f*.)

The fundamentals of the mesial aspects are:

1. Because the occlusal surface is constricted the tooth can be forced into food material more easily.

2. If the occlusal surface were as wide as the base of the crown the additional chewing surface would multiply the forces of mastication; then, too, the tooth would be less "self cleansing" during the process.

It has been found necessary to emphasize the fundamental outlines of these aspects through the medium of schematic drawings because the correct anatomy is overlooked so often.

The tendency is to take for granted that the tooth crowns are narrowest at the cervix *from all angles,* which is not true.

The measurement of the cervical portion of a posterior tooth is smaller than that of the occlusal portion from buccal or lingual aspects only; when observed from the

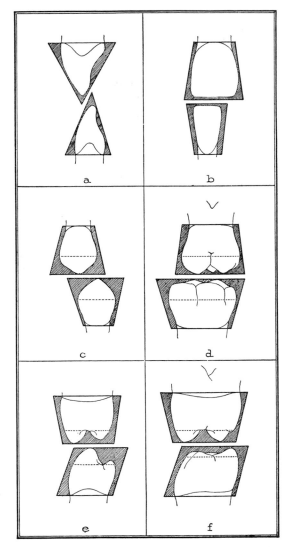

Figure 102. Outlines of crown forms within geometric outlines — triangles, trapezoids and rhomboids. The upper figure in each square represents a maxillary tooth, the lower figure a mandibular tooth. Note that the trapezoid outline will not include the cusp form of posteriors actually. It does include the crowns from cervix to contact point or cervix to marginal ridge, however. Remember that this is a schematic drawing to emphasize certain fundamentals. *a,* Anterior teeth, mesial or distal; *b,* anterior teeth, labial or lingual; *c,* premolars, buccal or lingual; *d,* molars, buccal or lingual; *e,* premolars, mesial or distal; *f,* molars, mesial or distal.

mesial or distal aspects, the comparison is just the reverse, the occlusal surface tapering from the wide root base. (Compare *e* and *f,* Fig. 102, with *c* and *d*.)

Mesial and Distal Aspects of Mandibular Posterior Teeth

Finally, the mandibular posterior teeth, when approached from the mesial or distal aspects, are somewhat *rhomboidal* in outline (Fig. 102, *e* and *f*). The occlusal surfaces are constricted in comparison with the bases—similar to the maxillary posterior teeth. The rhomboidal outline inclines the crowns lingual to the root bases, bringing the cusps into proper occlusion with the cusps of their maxillary opponents. At the same time, the axes of crowns and roots of the teeth of both jaws are kept parallel (Figs. 82 and 83). If the mandibular posterior crowns were to be set on the roots with the same relation of crown to root as the maxillary crowns exhibit, the cusps would clash with each other during mastication instead of allowing the proper intercusp relations.

SUMMARY OF SCHEMATIC OUTLINES

Outlines of the tooth crowns, when viewed from the labial or buccal, lingual, mesial and distal aspects, are described in a general way by triangles, trapezoids or rhomboids (Fig. 102, *a* to *f*).

Triangles
    Six anterior teeth, maxillary and mandibular
        1. Mesial aspect
        2. Distal aspect
Trapezoids
    A. Trapezoid with longest uneven side toward occlusal or incisal surface
        1. *All anterior teeth,* maxillary and mandibular
            a. Labial aspect
            b. Lingual aspect
        2. *All posterior teeth*
            a. Buccal aspect
            b. Lingual aspect
    B. Trapezoid with shortest uneven side toward occlusal surface
        1. *All maxillary posterior teeth*
            a. Mesial aspect
            b. Distal aspect
Rhomboids
    All mandibular posterior teeth
        1. Mesial aspect
        2. Distal aspect

Chapter V

PHYSIOLOGIC TOOTH FORM PROTECTING THE PERIODONTIUM

FUNDAMENTAL CURVATURES

THE TEETH possess certain fundamental curvatures that serve to give the proper degree of protection to the *periodontium*. Some of these protective curvatures are so finely drawn that an increase or decrease in dimensions at vulnerable areas would affect seriously the future of a tooth. In short, these protective contours are physiologic.

Research on the physiologic significance of tooth forms has been very limited. Authorities are, nevertheless, agreed on this; that certain fundamental outlines of the individual teeth have functional significance which is important to them singly and collectively in improving or decreasing their efficiency. The term efficiency implies, of course, that each tooth must help insure its own position, thereby doing its share toward the stability of the entire dental arch. It does this by contributing toward the protection of investing tissues in addition to its efficiency in mastication. This chapter will concern itself with the subject of *tooth form and dental maintenance*.

Without sound tissues supporting it, a tooth cannot last long. Teeth are subject to *abnormal development* and *anomalies of form,* as are other parts of the body. Undoubtedly many teeth are lost prematurely because certain functional outlines fail to develop properly or because malalignment of well-formed teeth in the dental arches made the important protective contours inoperative. Naturally, a good diagnosis for subsequent dental treatment of any sort must take into serious consideration all that is known of physiologic tooth form, alignment and occlusion.

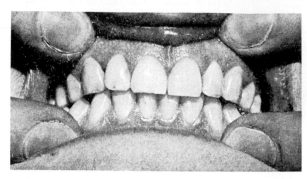

Figure 103. Normal, healthy gums, showing the interdental tissue papillae reaching well up into the embrasures. (Courtesy of Dr. Russell W. Bunting. From Hill, *Textbook of Oral Pathology,* Lea & Febiger.)

Briefly, the study of the protective functional form of the tooth crowns must include, among other things, the following:

1. Proximal contact areas.
2. Interproximal spaces (formed by proximal surfaces in contact).
3. Embrasures (spillways).
4. Labial and buccal contours at the cervical thirds (cervical ridges) and lingual contours at the middle thirds of crowns. (Both are protective contours.)
5. Curvatures of the cervical lines on mesial and distal surfaces (cementoenamel junction).

The above headings include the form which has a direct or primary bearing on the protection of the periodontium. Many other details of tooth form have an indirect bearing on the stability of the teeth through their contribution to the maintenance of efficiency during function. Some of these details are cusp forms, the proportions of various measurements of the crowns and roots, root form and anchorage and angles at which teeth are set in the jaws.

Further observation of the details of tooth form soon establishes another important fact: from all aspects, when well formed teeth are in normal alignment with normal gingival attachment (Fig. 103) they are remarkably "self cleansing." The smooth rounded form of the teeth contributes toward proper *dental hygiene* when assisted by the brushing activity of tongue and cheeks, the flushing action of saliva and the intake of fluids, plus the friction of food material during the functional activity of mastication. Needless to say, this form contributes to the efficient use of the tooth brush during home care of the teeth.

1. PROXIMAL CONTACT AREAS

Soon after the alignment of all of the teeth in their respective positions in the jaws takes place, there should be a positive contact relation mesially and distally of one tooth with another in each arch. Excepting the last molars (third molars, if

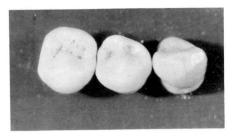

Figure 104. This is a photograph of three mandibular teeth removed from the same individual. This person was evidently well past middle age, but it so happened that the canine had never been in contact with the first premolar. The premolars had been in strong contact relation, as evidenced by their adaptation to each other at the contact areas.

The teeth were set up in their proper alignment to show the contrast between the "marble" contact of the canine and first premolar, a contrast which represents the contact design in extreme youth, since there had been no wear at the contact areas in this case, and the adaptation of one premolar to the other at the point of contact after many years of functional use.

present), each tooth has *two* contacting members adjoining it. The last molar is in contact only with the tooth mesial to it. Although the areas of contact are still very circumscribed, especially on anterior teeth, these are *areas* and not mere *points* of contact. Actually the term "contact point," which term is often used to designate the contact of teeth in the same arch, is a misnomer. When the individual is quite young and the teeth are newly erupted, some of the teeth come close to having point contacts only when the contacting surfaces are nearly perfect curvatures (Fig. 104). Examples of the few contacts made by such rounded surfaces are located distally on canines and mesially on first premolars maxillary and mandibular.

The proper contact relation between neighboring teeth in each arch is important for the following reasons: (1) it serves to keep food from packing between the teeth, and (2) it helps to stabilize the dental arches by the combined anchorage of all the teeth in either arch in positive contact with each other. Excepting the third molars, each tooth in the arch is supported in part by its contact with two neighboring teeth, one mesial and one distal. The third molars (and the second molars also if there is no third molar) are prevented from drifting distally where there is no contacting tooth by the angulation of their occlusal surfaces with their roots and by the direction of the occlusal forces which are in their favor. This will be explained at length later.

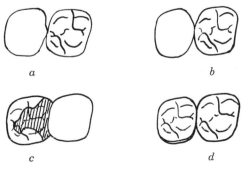

Figure 105. *a,* The projection of a point contact, as in a faulty restoration. This arrangement would not reproduce normal contact form or embrasure form. *b,* The contact is better than in *a,* but the supplementary embrasure form is faulty. *c,* Contact area is too great, with insufficient embrasure opening, buccal and lingual. *d,* Normal contact and embrasure form.

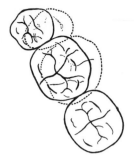

Figure 106. Outline drawings from the occlusal aspect of the mandibular second premolar, first molar and second molar. Shadow drawings of occluding teeth show the adaptation of the contact and embrasure design to the occlusal relation.

If for any reason food is allowed to escape between the teeth past the contact areas, the result may be pathologic. The gingival tissue which normally fills the interdental spaces may become inflamed so that *gingivitis* ensues. This inflammation may be followed by further degenerative processes unless it is checked. The final result may be a complete breakdown of the tissues, including destruction of the alveolar bone and the possible loss of one or more teeth. Separation of the teeth through loss of contact causes a change in tooth alignment, which in turn brings about a shifting of the forces brought to bear upon the tooth or teeth in question during mastication.

When a tooth is subjected to occlusal forces at an angle that it is not designed to withstand, or if it must absorb more than its share of those forces through lack of support by its neighbors, it suffers from *occlusal trauma*. Prolonged occlusal trauma may also cause destruction of the supporting tissues.

Contact areas must be observed from *two aspects* in order to obtain the proper perspective for locating them: (1) the labial or buccal aspect, and (2) the incisal or occlusal aspect.

The *labial* or *buccal* view will demonstrate the relative positions of the contact areas cervicoincisally and cervico-occlusally. The center of the area from this aspect can be gauged in its relation to the length of the crown (Figs. 109 and 110).

The *incisal* or *occlusal* view will show the relative position of the contact areas labiolingually or buccolingually. In this instance the center of the area may be located in its relation to the labiolingual or buccolingual diameter of the crown (Figs. 113 and 114). The point at which the area is bisected will also depend upon the outline of the form of the crown from the incisal or occlusal aspect. This outline is governed by the *alignment* of the tooth in the arch and also by the *occlusal relation* with its antagonists in the opposing arch. The mandibular first molar is an excellent example (Fig. 106). The contact and embrasure design for this tooth will be explained later when the incisal and occlusal aspects of the teeth are considered.

2. INTERPROXIMAL SPACES (FORMED BY PROXIMAL SURFACES IN CONTACT)

The interproximal spaces between the teeth are triangularly shaped spaces normally filled by *gingival tissue (gingival papillae)*. The base of the triangle is the alveolar process; the sides of the triangle are the proximal surfaces of the contacting

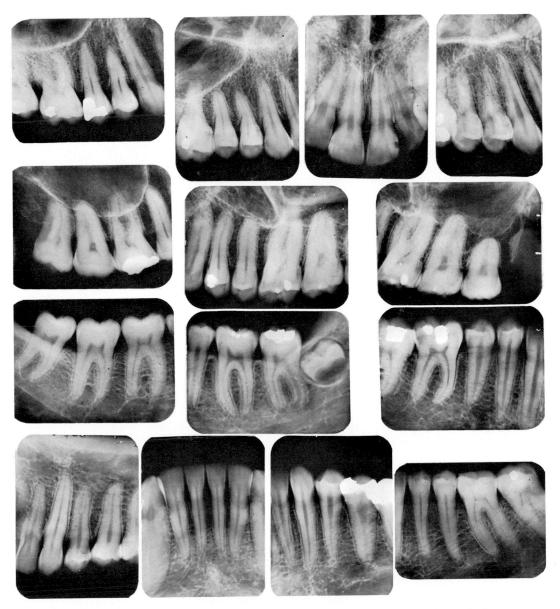

Figure 107. Radiographs of various groups of the permanent dentition. The radiographs demonstrate contact areas, occlusal embrasures, interproximal spacing, root forms, pulp cavities, root spacing, bone levels between the teeth, a developing unerupted tooth (right lower third molar), etc. (Courtesy of Dr. Clarence O. Simpson, St. Louis.)

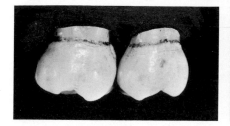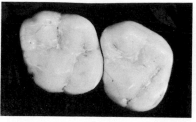

Figure 108. Photographs of maxillary first and second molars, taken from an elderly individual, showing considerable wear at their contact areas.

teeth, and the apex of the triangle is in the area of contact. The form of the inter-proximal space will vary with the form of the teeth in contact and will depend also upon the relative position of the contact areas (compare Figs. 109, *A* and *D*).

Proper contact and alignment of adjoining teeth allow proper spacing between them for the necessary gingival tissue that is attached to the bone and teeth. This gingival tissue, which is a continuation of the gingiva covering all of the alveolar process, is a valuable aid in mouth hygiene. Assisted by the saliva and the friction of food during mastication, and aided somewhat by the fluid intake, the gingiva serves to prevent the stasis of food about the teeth by its elasticity and smoothness.

Since the teeth are narrower at the cervix mesiodistally than they are toward the occlusal surfaces and the outline of the root continues to taper from that point to the apices of the roots, considerable spacing is created between the roots of one tooth and those of the adjoining teeth. This arrangement allows sufficient bone tissue between one tooth and another, anchoring the teeth securely in the jaws. It also simplifies the problem of the blood and nerve supply to the surrounding alveolar process and the other investing tissues of the teeth (Fig. 107).

The *type of tooth* in the individual case also has a bearing upon the interproximal space. Some individuals have teeth which are wide at the cervices, constricting the space at the base. Others have teeth which are more slender at the cervices than usual; this type of tooth widens the space. Teeth which are oversize or unusually small will likewise affect the interproximal spacing. Nevertheless, this spacing will conform to a plan which is fairly uniform, provided the anatomic form for the teeth is normal and the teeth are in good alignment.

3. EMBRASURES (SPILLWAYS)

When two teeth in the same arch are in contact, their curvatures adjacent to the contact areas form spillway spaces called *embrasures*. The spaces that widen out from the area of contact labially or buccally and lingually are called *labial* or *buccal* and *lingual interproximal embrasures*. These embrasures are continuous with the in-terproximal spaces between the teeth (Fig. 113). Above the contact areas incisally and occlusally, the spaces, which are bounded by the marginal ridges as they join the cusps and incisal ridges, are called the *incisal* or *occlusal embrasures*. These embra-sures, and the labial or buccal and lingual embrasures, are continuous (Figs. 109 and

111). The curved proximal surfaces of the contacting teeth roll away from the contact area at all points, occlusally, labially or buccally, and lingually and cervically, and the embrasures and interproximal spaces are continuous, as they surround the areas of contact.

This embrasure form *serves two purposes:* (1) it makes a spillway for the escape of food during mastication, a physiologic form which reduces forces brought to bear upon the teeth during the reduction of any material which offers resistance; and (2) it makes the teeth more self cleansing because the rounded smooth surfaces of the enamel of the crowns are more exposed to the cleansing action of foods, fluids and the friction of the tongue, lips and cheeks. If the spaces did not widen out so freely, or if the surfaces of the teeth presented angles or corners for the lodgment of food, the situation would not be conductive to proper dental hygiene.

The embrasure and contact form, when normal, protects the gingival tissue from undue frictional trauma, and paradoxically it allows proper stimulation by permitting the proper degree of frictional massage during mastication. Proper form provides *protection* or *stimulation* as needed, whereas improper contact and embrasure form will encourage pathologic change in supporting tissues.

The design of contact areas, interproximal spaces and embrasures varies with the form and alignment of the various teeth in each mouth. They will be described individually from the labial and buccal aspects, and following that, from the incisal and occlusal aspects.

Contact Areas and Incisal and Occlusal Embrasures from the Labial and Buccal Aspects

It is advisable to refer continually to the illustrations of contacts and embrasures during the reading of the following descriptions.

Figures 109 and 111 are close-ups of the labial and buccal surfaces of the teeth taken from several angles for the purpose of showing normal contacts and incisal or occlusal embrasures. Some of the interproximal spacing may be seen also. Outline drawings of the tooth crowns in contact supplement the photographs (Figs. 110, 112, 114 and 116). These outlines emphasize the crests of curvature on the crowns which locate the contact areas. Dotted lines have been used to show the approximate points at which the contact areas may be bisected.

Locate the individual illustration of interest (i.e., Fig. 110, *a*) while reading the details concerning contact area levels in the following text.

Maxillary Teeth

Central Incisors. The contact areas mesially on both central incisors are located at the incisal third of the crowns. Since the mesioincisal third of these teeth approaches a right angle, the incisal embrasure is very slight.

Central and Lateral Incisors. The distal outline of the central incisor crown is rounded. The lateral incisor has a shorter crown and has a more rounded mesioincisal angle. The form of these two teeth coming into contact with each other therefore

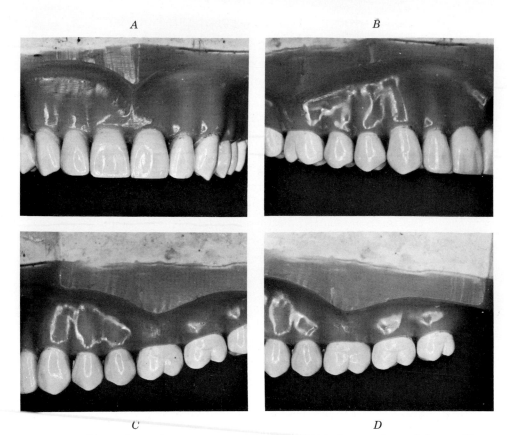

Figure 109. These photos demonstrate normal contact and embrasure form of the maxillary teeth from the labial and buccal aspects. (See Fig. 81.) Some of the interproximal spacing is visible. The interproximal, or interdental, space is normally filled by gingival tissue. *A*, Central and lateral incisors. *B*, Lateral incisor, canine and first premolar. *C*, Canine, first and second premolars and first molar. *D*, Second premolar, first, second and third molars.

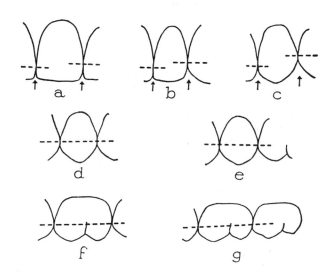

Figure 110. Outline drawings of the maxillary teeth in contact, with dotted lines bisecting the contact areas at the various levels as found normally. Arrows point to embrasure spaces. *a*, Central and lateral incisors. *b*, Central and lateral incisors and canine. *c*, Lateral incisor, canine and first premolar. *d*, Canine, first and second premolars. *e*, First and second premolars and first molar. *f*, Second premolar, first molar and second molar. *g*, First, second and third molars.

places the contact areas differently from the mesial contact areas of the central incisors. A line bisecting the contact areas approaches the junction of the middle and incisal thirds of each crown.

The rounded distoincisal angle of the central incisor and the rounded mesioincisal angle of the lateral incisor open up a distinct incisal embrasure.

Lateral Incisor and Canine.   The distal contact area on the lateral incisor is approximately at the middle third. The mesial contact area on the canine is at the junction of the incisal and middle thirds. The form of these teeth creates an embrasure which is more open than the two previously described.

Canine and First Premolar.   The canine has a long distal slope to its cusp, which puts the distal crest of curvature at the center of the middle third of the crown. The contact area is, therefore, at the point.

The first premolar has a long cusp form also, which puts its mesial contact area rather high up on the crown. Usually it is just cervical to the junction of the occlusal and middle thirds. The embrasure between these teeth has a wide angle.

First and Second Premolars.   The contact areas of these teeth are in a similar relative position—usually a little cervical to the junction of the occlusal and middle thirds of the crowns. The form of these teeth creates a wide occlusal embrasure.

It should be noted that the design of the interproximal spaces changes with the form and dimensions of the teeth in contact.

Second Premolar and First Molar.   The position of the contact areas cervicoocclusally is about the same as that found between the premolars.

The embrasure form changes somewhat because the mesiobuccal cusp of the molar is shorter than the cusp of the second premolar.

First and Second and Second and Third Molars.   These two contact and embrasure forms may be described together, since they are similar. The distal outline of the first molar is round—a fact that puts the contact area approximately at the center of the middle third of the crown.

The mesial contact area of the second molar also approaches the middle third of the crown. The occlusal embrasure is distinct as a consequence, even though the cusps are not long.

The contact and embrasure design of the second and third molars is similar to those of the first and second molars. The molars become progressively shorter from the first to the third. Naturally, the dimensions of the tooth crowns influence the contact and embrasure design.

Mandibular Teeth

Central Incisors.   The mesial contact areas on the mandibular central incisors are located at the incisal third of the crowns. At the time of the eruption of these teeth, the mesial and distal incisal angles are slightly rounded and the mamelons are noticeable on the incisal ridges. Soon, however, incisal wear reduces the incisal ridge to a straight surface, and the mesial and distal angles approach right angles in sharpness. This is due partly to wear at the contact areas (Fig. 111, *A*). In many instances the contact areas extend to the mesioincisal angle. There will therefore be a small incisal embrasure mesially between the mandibular central incisors until wear through usage obliterates it.

A   *B*

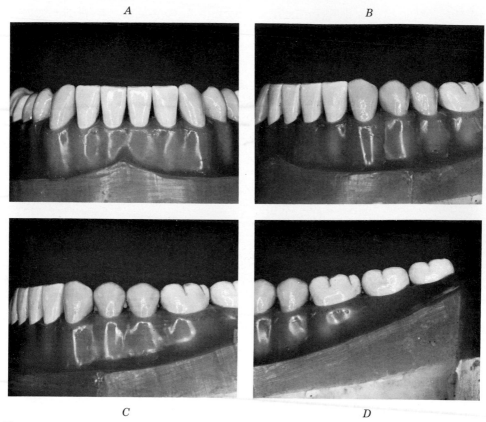

C   *D*

Figure 111. Normal contact and embrasure form of the mandibular teeth from the labial and buccal aspects. *A,* Central and lateral incisors. *B,* Lateral incisor, canine and first premolar. *C,* Canine, first and second premolars and first molar. *D,* Second premolar, first, second and third molars.

Central and Lateral Incisors.   The distal contact areas and the incisal embrasures on the central incisors and the mesial contact areas and incisal embrasures on the lateral incisors are similar to those just described. Since the mandibular central and lateral incisors are small mesiodistally and supplement each other in function, the design of their crowns brings about similar contact and embrasure forms.

Note the slender gothic arches which circumscribe the interproximal spaces between them.

Lateral Incisor and Canine.   The positions of the contact areas distally on the lateral incisor and mesially on the canine are approximately the same, cervicoincisally, as the other two just described. The teeth are in contact at the incisal third close to the incisal ridges. However, the mesioincisal angle of the canine is more rounded than the others, which form opens up a small incisal embrasure at this point.

The interproximal spacing is very similar in outline to the two interproximal spaces mesial to it.

Canine and First Premolar.   The distal slope of the cusp of the mandibular canine is pronounced, a formation which places the distal contact area on this tooth somewhat cervical to the junction of the incisal and middle thirds.

The first premolar has a long buccal cusp, and although its crown is shorter than the canine, the mesial contact area has about the same relation cervico-occlusally as that found distally on the canine—just cervical to the junction of the occlusal and middle thirds.

The occlusal embrasure is quite wide and pronounced because of the cusp forms of the two teeth. The interproximal space has been reduced by the lowering of the contact areas cervically.

First and Second Premolars.   From the buccal aspect the crowns of these two teeth are similar. The buccal cusp of the second premolar is not quite as long as that of the first premolar. The contact of these teeth is nearly level with that of the canine and first premolar. The slope of the cusps creates a large occlusal embrasure. The interproximal space is smaller than that between the canine and first premolar.

Second Premolar and First Molar.   The contact and embrasure design for these teeth is similar to that just described for the premolars. The mesiobuccal cusp of the first molar is shorter and more rounded than the cusp of the second premolar, which varies the embrasure somewhat, and since the crown of the molar is a little shorter, it reduces the interproximal space to some extent as well.

First and Second and Second and Third Molars.   These two contact and embrasure designs may be described together, since they are similar.

The proximal surfaces of the teeth listed below are quite round: distal surface of the first molar, mesial surface of the second molar, distal surface of the second molar, and mesial surface of the third molar. The occlusal embrasures are, therefore, distinct above the points of contact even though the cusps are short and rounded.

Because the molars become progressively shorter from the first to the third, the centers of the contact areas drop cervically also. A line bisecting the contact areas of

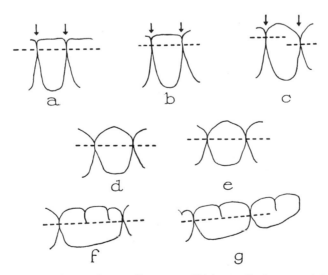

Figure 112.   Contact levels found normally on mandibular teeth. Arrows point to embrasure spaces. *a,* Central and lateral incisors. *b,* Central and lateral incisors and canine. *c,* Lateral incisor, canine and first premolar. *d,* Canine, first and second premolars. *e,* First and second premolars and first molar. *f,* Second premolar, first and second molars. *g,* First, second and third molars.

the second and third molars is located approximately at the center of the middle thirds of those crowns.

The interproximal spaces have been reduced considerably in comparison with those mesial to them.

Contact Areas, and Labial, Buccal and Lingual Embrasures, from the Incisal and Occlusal Aspects*

The contact areas of all of the teeth tend to approach a line bisecting the crowns labiolingually and buccolingually. In order to get the proper perspective in locating the contact areas buccolingually and labiolingually, each tooth must be observed on a line parallel to its own axis. The eye must be directly above the tooth, and the position of the contact area must be related to the labiolingual or buccolingual diameter. This point of view will give a better perspective in making comparisons of the embrasure designs labially, buccally and lingually. It will be noted that the labial and buccal embrasures are pronounced when the contact areas are properly located in their relation to labiolingual and buccolingual outlines and to the long axes of the teeth.

A general rule which may be followed in locating contact areas in their labiolingual and buccolingual relation is: *Anterior teeth will have their contact areas centered labiolingually, whereas posterior teeth will have their contact areas slightly buccal to lines bisecting the crowns buccolingually.* The buccal inclination of contact areas on posterior teeth must not be overemphasized however.

Excepting the maxillary first molar, all of the crowns converge more lingually from the contact areas than they do labially or buccally. This design widens the embrasures lingually in comparison. The lingual embrasures of the maxillary central and lateral incisors serve as good examples.

Maxillary Teeth

Central Incisors.   The contact areas of these teeth are centered labiolingually. The labial embrasure is a V-shaped space created by the labial form of these crowns. The lingual embrasure widens out more than the labial embrasure because of the lingual convergence of the crowns (Fig. 113, *A*). Note the centering of the labioincisal edge in respect to the crown outline of these teeth, and the narrowness of the lingual surfaces in comparison with the broad labial faces.

Central and Lateral Incisors.   The contact areas of these teeth are centered labiolingually also.

Lateral Incisor and Canine.   The contact area is centered labiolingually on both canine and lateral incisors. The lingual embrasure is similar to that of the central and lateral incisors, but the labial embrasure is changed somewhat by a definite convexity at the mesiolabial line angle of the canine.

---

*Refer to Figs. 113, 114, 115 and 116.

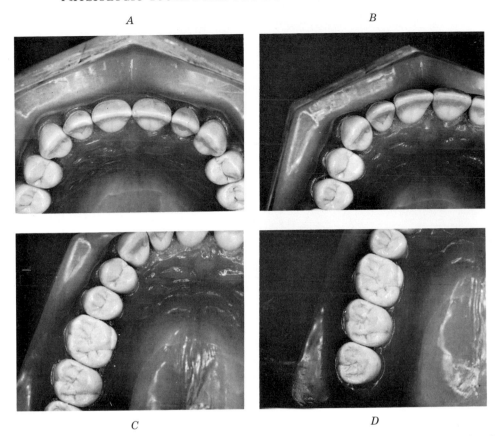

A *B*

C *D*

Figure 113. Normal contact and embrasure form of the maxillary teeth from incisal and occlusal aspects. *A,* Central and lateral incisors. *B,* Lateral incisor, canine and first premolar. *C,* Canine, first and second premolars and first molar. *D,* First, second and third molars.

Canine and First Premolar.   The contact area is centered on the distal surface of the canine, but is a little buccal to center on the mesial surface of the first premolar. The embrasure design lingually is marked by a concavity in the region of the distolingual line angle of the canine and by a developmental groove crossing the mesial marginal ridge of the first premolar.

First and Second Premolars.   The contact areas are nearly centered buccolingually. The embrasures buccally and lingually are regular in outline.

The prominence of the mesio- and distobuccal line angles of the premolars is in direct contrast to the even taper of these teeth lingually, as viewed from the occlusal aspect. This form will demonstrate a variation between buccal and lingual embrasures.

Second Premolar and First Molar.   As usual, a line bisecting the contact areas of these teeth will be nearly centered in its relation to the crowns buccolingually. The area on the mesial surface of the first molar will be located farther buccally than is usual for the other contact areas on the maxillary posterior teeth. The contact areas are wider because of the greater diameter buccolingually of the first molar.

The buccal embrasure between these teeth and the location of the mesial contact

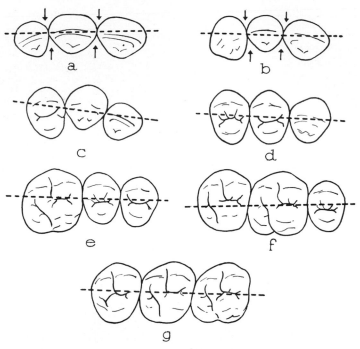

Figure 114. Outline drawings of the maxillary teeth from the incisal and occlusal aspects with broken lines bisecting the contact areas. These illustrations show the relative positions of the contact areas labiolingually and buccolingually. Arrows point to embrasure spaces. *a,* Central incisors and lateral incisor. *b,* Central and lateral incisor and canine. *c,* Lateral incisor, canine and first premolar. *d,* Canine, first premolar and second premolar. *e,* First premolar, second premolar and first molar. *f,* Second premolar, first molar and second molar. *g,* First, second and third molars.

area of the first molar are influenced by the prominence of the mesiobuccal line angle of the *maxillary* first molar. The lingual embrasure is not unusual, although the distal outline of it may be changed somewhat — a change dependent upon the development of the fifth cusp of the first molar. Sometimes this cusp (cusp of Carabelli) is large and well developed, but usually it is small or absent.

The mesiolingual lobe of this tooth is always large, however, causing the tooth to be wider lingually from its mesiolingual line angle to its distolingual line angle than it is from the mesiobuccal line angle to the distobuccal line angle. If it were not for this fact, the rhomboid form of the first molar in contact with the tapered form of the second premolar would open up a lingual embrasure of extremely large proportions. The large mesiolingual lobe makes up for the change in occlusal outline from premolar form to molar form, keeping the conformity of the lingual embrasures (Fig. 114, *e*).

First and Second and Second and Third Molars.   These contact and embrasure forms may be described together, since they are similar.

Although the mesiobuccal line angles of the second and third molars are not as sharp as that of the first molar, they are prominent nevertheless.

The distobuccal line angles of all the maxillary molars are indistinct and rounded, so that the buccal embrasure forms are shaped and characterized mainly by the prominent mesiobuccal line angle.

The mesiolingual line angles of the second and third molars are rounded and in conjunction with the rounded distolingual line angles; the lingual embrasures between first, second and third molars present a regular and open form (Fig. 114, *f* and *g*).

The contact areas are broad and centered buccolingually. The embrasures are uniform. Note the generous proportions of the buccal embrasures.

Mandibular Teeth

Central Incisors and Central and Lateral Incisors.   These contact areas and embrasures may be described together, since they are similar.

Although these teeth are narrow mesiodistally, their labiolingual measurements are not very different from those of the maxillary central and lateral incisors. The mandibular central incisors will come within a millimeter or so of having the same labiolingual diameter as that of the maxillary central incisors; the *mandibular* lateral incisors will have a labiolingual diameter as great if not greater than that of the *maxillary* lateral incisors.

The contact areas are centered labiolingually and the embrasures are uniform. Although the mesiodistal dimensions are less, the outline form of the incisal aspects of the mandibular central and lateral incisors is similar to that of the maxillary

A

B

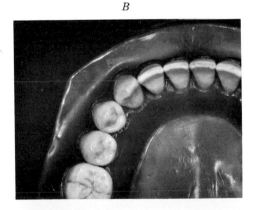

Figure 115. Normal contact and embrasure form of the mandibular teeth from the incisal and occlusal aspects. *A,* Central and lateral incisors. *B,* Lateral incisor, canine and first and second premolars. *C,* Second premolar, first, second and third molars.

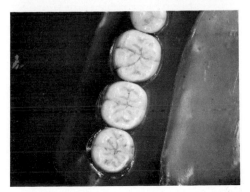

C

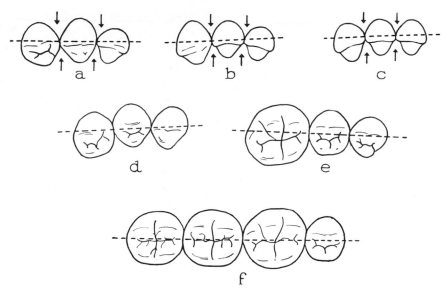

Figure 116. Contact relation of mandibular teeth labiolingually and buccolingually when surveyed from the incisal and occlusal aspects. Arrows point to embrasure spaces. *a,* Central incisors and lateral incisor. *b,* Central and lateral incisor and canine. *c,* Lateral incisor, canine and first premolar. *d,* Canine, first premolar and second premolar. *e,* First premolar, second premolar and first molar. *f,* Second premolar, first, second and third molars.

central and lateral incisors in that the lingual outlines have a rounded taper in comparison with broad, flattened labial faces.

Lateral Incisor and Canine. The contact areas are centered, and the lingual embrasure is similar to those just described. The labial embrasure is influenced by the prominence of the mesiolabial line angle of the canine. It will be remembered that the maxillary canine presents the same characteristic.

Canine and First Premolar. The contact areas are approximately centered, and the buccal embrasure is smooth and uniform in outline. The lingual embrasure is opened up somewhat by a slight concavity on the canine distolingually and by a characteristic developmental groove across the marginal ridge of the first premolar mesiolingually.

First and Second Premolars. The contact areas are nearly centered buccolingually, but are broader than those found mesial to them because the distal curvature of the first premolar describes a larger arc than the mesial curvature, and the mesial contacting surface of the second premolar is relatively broad and describes an even greater arc than that of the distal surface of the first premolar.

Because of the lingual convergence of the first premolar and the narrow lingual cusp form, the lingual embrasure is as wide as the one mesial to it.

Second Premolar and First Molar. The contact areas are wide and almost centered. The extent of the contact areas is sometimes increased by a slight concavity in the outline of the mesial surface of the first molar below the marginal ridge. The mesial contact area of the first molar is located farther buccally than any of the other contact areas on mandibular posterior teeth.

The prominence of the first molar at the mesiobuccal line angle is readily apparent. The mesial outline of the crown tapers to the lingual, forming a generous lingual embrasure in conjunction with the smooth curvature of the second premolar distolingually.

First and Second Molar. The contact areas are nearly centered buccolingually, although they are not so broad as the contact just described. This variation is brought about by the design of the first molar distally. The distal contact area of the first molar is confined to the distal cusp, which does not present the broad surface for contact with the second molar that was found mesially in contact with the second premolar. This form, along with the rounded outline at the distobuccal line angle, opens up both embrasures wider than those found immediately mesial.

The outline of the first molar crown just lingual to the distal contact area presents a straight line and occasionally a concavity.

The second molar outline buccally and lingually on both sides of the mesial contact area is uniformly rounded.

Second and Third Molars. The contact areas are broad, and they are nearly centered buccolingually. When the third molar is normally developed, it is similar in outline to the second molar from the occlusal aspect.

The buccal and lingual embrasures between these teeth are almost alike in form and extent.

A straight line may be drawn through the contact areas of the second premolar and the three molars, and it will come very near to bisecting all of the contact areas. These four mandibular teeth are set in a line that is almost straight.

4. LABIAL AND BUCCAL CONTOURS AT THE CERVICAL THIRDS (CERVICAL RIDGES) AND LINGUAL CONTOURS AT THE MIDDLE THIRDS OF CROWNS*

It will be found that the tooth crowns, when viewed from mesial or distal aspects, have rather uniform curvatures at the cervical thirds and at the middle thirds labially or buccally and lingually, depending upon the teeth under consideration (Fig. 117, *d* and *e*). These contours must be recognized as having considerable physiologic importance. Apparently, the curvatures hold the gingiva under definite tension and also protect the gingival margins by deflecting food material away from the margins during mastication (Fig. 117, *a*). The proper degree of curvature will deflect food over the gingival margin, thereby preventing undue frinctional irritation. Proper curvature will allow some stimulation of soft tissue.

If the curvature is absent or too slight, the gingival tissue will be driven apically, and this will result in a recession of gum tissue and possible pathologic changes Fig. 117, *b*). If the curvature is too great, another complication may arise: The gingiva is protected too much and loses tissue "tone." Food material and debris pack around the gingival area under this exaggerated contour and a veritable "back-

---

*Both are protective contours. See page 16, line 30, also Figs. 121 through 125.

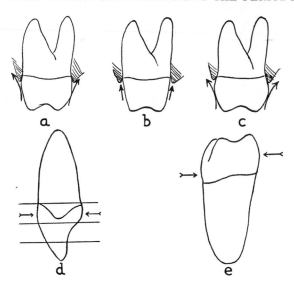

Figure 117. Schematic drawings of curvatures labially, buccally and lingually. *a,* Normal curvatures as found on maxillary molar. Arrow shows path of food material as it is avalanched over these curvatures during mastication. *b,* Molar with little or no curvature. The gingiva is apt to be stripped or pushed apically through lack of protection and consequent overstimulation. *c,* Molar with curvature in excess of the normal. The gingiva will be protected too much and will suffer from lack of proper stimulation. Food material and bacterial cultures may lodge under these curvatures, promoting pathologic disturbance. *d,* Normal cervical curvatures as found on maxillary incisors. The crests of curvature are opposite each other labiolingually. *e,* Curvatures as found on mandibular posterior teeth. The protective curvature is located at the cervical third to the buccal and at the middle third to the lingual.

water" results; this is accompanied by stagnation of foreign material and chronic inflammation of the gingiva (Fig. 117, *c*).

A very important observation at this point has to do with the soft tissue attachment to the teeth. The *epithelial attachment* of soft tissue to the teeth, soon to be described more fully, is entirely within the area of the cervical third of the crown, the area involved in the cervical curvatures.

An attempt will be made to describe what seems to be the *average cervical contour* labially or buccally and lingually for each group of teeth in the maxillary and mandibular arches. This phase of tooth form has not been emphasized in dental literature, although it is most valuable in preserving the gingival line and investment tissues about the teeth. The contour under consideration is the curvature possessed by all tooth crowns above the cementoenamel junction, labially or buccally and lingually, which is usually found at the cervical third or at the middle third when one observes the teeth from the mesial and distal aspects.

The curvatures above the cementoenamel junction seem to describe rather constant arcs, depending upon the locality in the mouth, *i.e.,* maxillary anterior teeth, maxillary posteriors, mandibular anteriors and mandibular posteriors. Each group exhibits an arc of curvature that is characteristic of that group, both as to location of the curvatures and as to the extent of the curvatures.

Variations are always possible, and therefore no invariable rule can be made. But one may strike an *average* for that particular feature. Values that are "averages" or "norms" must be established in order properly to judge requirements in diagnosis or in restoration. Variations from the average are then better understood. Cervical contours may vary in individuals. If curvatures in any given case are found to be greater or less than average, it has been the author's observation that the variation will be uniform in that individual. Since there are variations, therefore, and since it is extremely difficult to restore the curvature once it is removed during operative procedures, these curvatures or "cervical ridges" should be treated with respect and should be allowed to remain as they are whenever practicable.

In young people, most of the curvature lies beneath the gingival crest (Fig. 121).

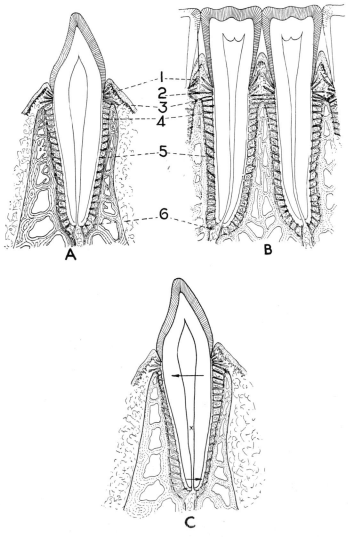

Figure 118. Diagrammatic representation of the arrangement of the principal fibers of the periodontal ligament. **A**, Labiolingual, and **B**, mesiodistal sections through a lower central incisor. 1, Free gingival group; 2, transseptal group; 3, alveolar crest group; 4, horizontal group; 5, oblique group; 6, apical group. **C**, shows the tipping of the tooth lingually and the changes in the periodontal membrane under incisal stress. X indicates approximate fulcrum point. The periodontal ligament is shown disproportionately wide for clarity. (From Schour, I.: Noyes' *Oral Histology and Embryology,* 8th Edition, 1960, Lea and Febiger.)

In older persons, the cementoenamel line may be visible or may be just under the gingival crest, with most of the prominent curvature exposed.

Gradual recession of the gingivae throughout life may be a normal procedure, with no pathologic change in evidence. This process varies in different persons. If the recession occurs early with no apparent pathologic evidence, it may be found that the individual has "flat-faced" tooth crowns with little or no curvature, labially or lingually or buccally, to act as a protector of the gingiva. At least, such teeth are not favored by normal cervical curvature. By the same token, teeth having an excess of curvature over the average may be predestined to premature loss through their contribution to unhygienic conditions about the gingival sulci of their own periodontium.

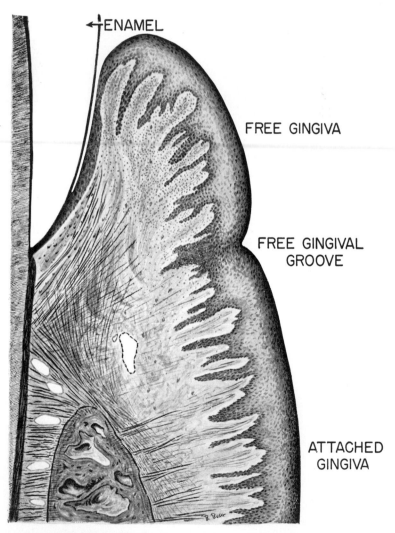

Figure 119.   Drawing of longitudinal section of the free and attached gingiva separated by the free gingival groove. Note the free gingiva, the alveolar crest, and the horizontal fibers. (From Schour, I.: Noyes' *Oral Histology and Embryology,* 8th Edition, 1960, Lea and Febiger.)

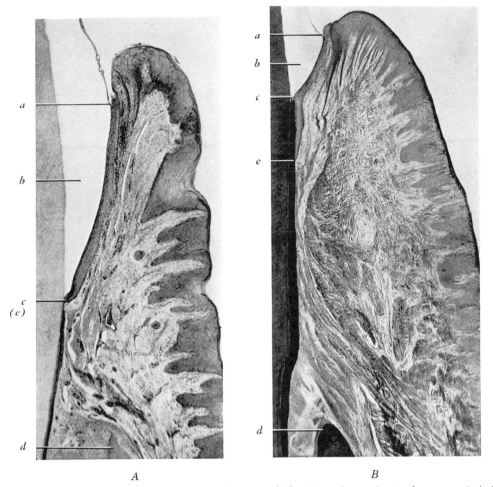

A   B

Figure 120. *A,* Epithelial attachment on the enamel (first stage in passive tooth exposure). Apical end of attachment is at cementoenamel junction. *B,* Epithelial attachment on enamel and cementum (second stage in passive tooth exposure). Apical end of attachment has proliferated along cementum. *a,* Bottom of gingival sulcus; *b,* enamel; *c,* cementoenamel junction; *d,* alveolar crest; *e,* apical end of epithelial attachment. (From Orban, B.: *Periodontics,* 1958, The C. V. Mosby Company.)

All protective curvatures are most functional when the teeth are in proper alignment. It should be quite plain that when teeth are malposed their curvatures are displaced and ineffective.

The curvatures are rather uniform at the cervical third of all of the maxillary teeth and on the buccal portion of mandibular posterior teeth (Figs. 122, 123 and 124).

The normal curvature from the cementoenamel junction to the crest of contour is approximately 0.5 mm. in extent. When the long axis of the tooth is placed vertically, it is found that this curvature is fairly constant and may be recognized as average or normal for the maxillary teeth, labially or buccally and lingually, and for the mandibular posterior teeth on the buccal surfaces. The curvature lingually of mandibular posterior teeth extends about a millimeter beyond the cervical line. In this instance, however, the extreme curvature does not contribute to the stasis of

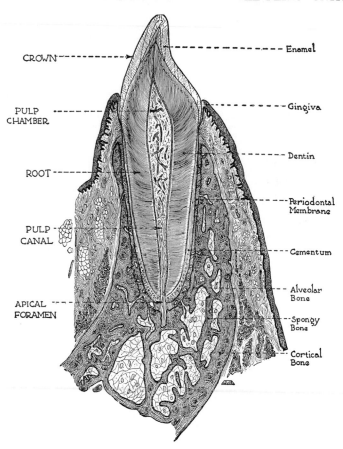

CROWN

PULP
CHAMBER

ROOT

PULP
CANAL

APICAL
FORAMEN

Enamel

Gingiva

Dentin

Periodontal
Membrane

Cementum

Alveolar
Bone

Spongy
Bone

Cortical
Bone

Figure 121. Diagrammatic representation of the dental tissues. (From Noyes, Schour and Noyes, *Dental Histology and Embryology,* Lea & Febiger.)

food material at the cervix because of the activity of the tongue in keeping the lingual surfaces of these teeth clean.

Figure 122 demonstrates the fact that the maxillary central incisor and canine have curvatures labially and lingually which are almost identical. *Because the canines have a more massive development of the cingulum, clinical observation only gives an impression of greater curvature. This is an optical illusion which is dispelled when the outline of the canine is properly compared with other teeth on a graph.*

The maxillary premolar and molar show the same limited curvatures. The crest of curvature lingually on all posterior teeth is at or near the middle third of the crowns.

When curvatures are found that are greater in extent than 0.5 mm., rarely is the curvature as much as 1 mm., except lingually on mandibular posterior teeth and occasionally lingually on maxillary posterior teeth. In these instances, the crest of contour will be found at the middle third of the crowns instead of at the cervical third (Figs. 123 and 124).

The eye is easily confused at times when viewing certain aspects of the teeth because of the abrupt sweep of curvatures as they travel from the cervical line

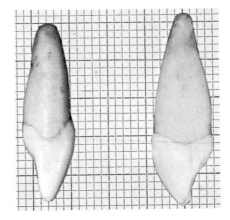

Figure 122. The maxillary central incisor exhibits a curvature of approximately 0.5 mm. labially and somewhat less lingually at the cervical third of the crown. Many specimens will show equal curvature on the two sides.

The maxillary canine exhibits approximately the same curvature. Note the limitation of the curvature at the cingulum area above the cervical line.

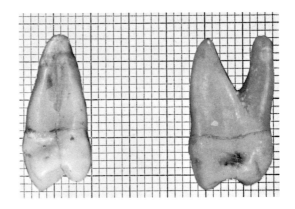

Figure 123. The maxillary first premolar has a curvature of approximately 0.5 mm. buccally and lingually. The crest of curvature buccally is located at the cervical third of the crown and lingually at the middle third.

The maxillary first molar has curvatures of the same degree at similar points on both sides.

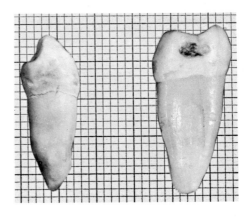

Figure 124. Mandibular first premolar and first molar. Both teeth have a curvature of approximately 0.5 mm. buccally at the cervical third of the crown and a curvature of approximately 1 mm. lingually, with the crest of curvature at the middle third.

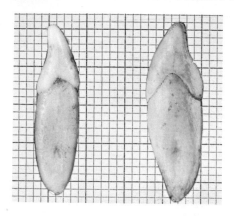

Figure 125. Mandibular central incisor and canine. The central incisor curvature labially and lingually is less than 0.5 mm. in extent, and the crest of curvature is near the cervical line. The canine also exhibits less than 0.5 mm. curvatures, although the crest of curvature is higher up on the crown; within the confines of the cervical third, however.

toward occlusal and incisal surfaces, *i.e.*, the buccal surfaces of mandibular posterior teeth, the lingual surfaces of posterior maxillary teeth, or the labial surfaces of canines. When the actual photographs are placed on a background of squares, with the long axis of each tooth held vertically, one readily sees that the extent of curvature from the cervical line to the crest of curvature facially or lingually is slight. Quite often, in restorative procedures, it is greatly overestimated and reproduced.

Figure 125 shows a mandibular central incisor and canine from the mesial aspect. Here the curvature at the cervical third is less than that of the other teeth in the mouth, occasionally appearing so slight that it is hardly distinguishable. The canine often has very little more curvature immediately above the cervical line than the mandibular central of lateral incisor.

Summary of Protective Contours of Tooth Crowns, Facially and Lingually

All tooth crowns will exhibit some curvature above the cervical line. This curvature is sometimes called the *cervical ridge.* Although the extent of curvature will vary in different individuals, apparently it is not normal for the curvatures on permanent teeth to extend out over 1 mm. beyond the cervical line, and usually the curvature will be less.

The curvatures on the labial, buccal and lingual surfaces of all maxillary teeth and on the buccal surfaces of mandibular posterior teeth will be rather uniform in any one mouth; the average curvature is about 0.5 mm.

Mandibular posterior teeth will have a lingual curvature of approximately 1 mm., with the crest of curvature at the middle third of the crown instead of at the cervical third. It is not uncommon for maxillary posterior teeth to have similar curvatures on the lingual aspect. (Compare the lingual curvatures in Figs. 123 and 124.)

Mandibular anterior teeth will have less curvature on the crown above the cervical line than any of the other teeth. Usually it is less than 0.5 mm., and occasionally it is so slight that it is hardly distinguishable. The canines may show a little more curvature than central and lateral incisors.

5. CURVATURES OF THE CERVICAL LINES ON MESIAL AND DISTAL SURFACES [CEMENTOENAMEL JUNCTION] INDICATING THE CURVATURE AND HEIGHT OF ATTACHMENT (NORMALLY) OF THE INTERPROXIMAL TISSUE

The dentist is interested from a clinical point of view in keeping the investment tissues about the teeth in a normal healthy state. Carelessness in operative procedure can cause abrupt breaks in the epithelial attachment resulting in chronic irritation and ultimate breakdown of the tissues.

The height of normal gingival tissue between the teeth, that is, mesially and distally on approximating teeth, is directly dependent upon the heights of the epithelial attachment. Normal attachment follows the curvature of the cementoenamel junction if the teeth are in normal alignment and contact. This does not mean that the cementoenamel junction and the epithelial attachment are at the same level, but it does mean that they tend to follow the same curvature even though the epithelial attachment may be higher on the crown on its enamel surface (Fig. 129). A comparison of the curvatures of the cementoenamel junction mesially and distally on the teeth is therefore in order. Measurement and comparisons are shown in Figures 130, 131 and 132.

The extent of curvature seems to depend upon the height of the contact area above the crown cervix and also upon the diameter of the crown labiolingually or buccolingually. The crowns of anterior teeth, which are narrower and longer from these aspects, show the greatest curvature (Fig. 131). In using the words "height" and "above," the supposition is made that in either the maxillary or the mandibular arch the occlusal surfaces of the teeth are above the cervices. Any point approaching the incisal edge or occlusal surface of a crown is considered above the cervix, and the height is increased as it approaches occlusal levels.

Periodontal attachment which follows the cervical curvatures seems to be about as high on mandibular anterior teeth as on their counterparts in the maxillary arch. Although the crowns of the mandibular anterior teeth average 1 mm. less in labiolingual diameter (the lateral incisors excepted), the contact areas are higher accordingly, being near the incisal edges on centrals and laterals. Consequently, measurements will usually show less than 1 mm. variation in cervical curvatures between maxillary and mandibular anterior teeth.

Posterior teeth will show little variation in either arch. Figure 130 is a diagrammatic drawing of the outlines of the teeth on one side of the arch when viewed from the labial and buccal aspects. These outlines have been placed so that a direct comparison can be made with the graphs below them. The graphs demonstrate the relative height of individual attachments in the average normal case. They are based on cases having upper central incisors with crowns 10.5 to 11 mm. in length. Unless the teeth were very large or very small, the graphs would not vary from those illustrated by more than 0.5 mm.

The curvature of the cementoenamel junction will usually be about 1 mm. *less* on the *distal* side of the tooth than on the mesial. If the maxillary central incisor has a 3.5 mm. curvature mesially, the distal curvature may be 2.5 mm., etc.

In order to secure scientific data regarding comparative curvatures, it was

(Text continued on page 123.)

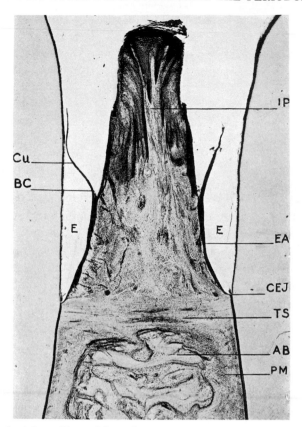

Figure 126. Interdental papilla and bone between two lower premolars of a child aged fourteen years. This photomicrograph shows the topographic relation between interdental papilla, epithelial attachment to the enamel of both bicuspids, transseptal fibers, interdental bone, and periodontal membrane. *IP,* interdental papilla; *EE,* space formerly occupied by the enamel; *EA,* epithelial attachment to the enamel; *Cu,* enamel cuticle; *BC,* bottom of gingival crevice; *CEJ,* cementoenamel junction; *TS,* transseptal fibers; *AB,* alveolar bone; *PM,* periodontal membrane. Magnification × 24. (Kronfeld, *Dental Histology and Comparative Dental Anatomy,* Lea & Febiger.)

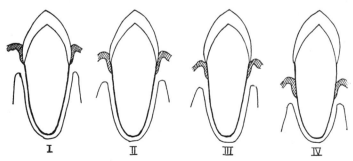

Figure 127. Four different stages of the relations existing between the tooth and the surrounding tissues, especially the epithelial attachment. I, Bottom of the gingival crevice on the enamel; deepest point of the epithelial attachment at the cementoenamel junction (see Fig. 120, A). II, Bottom of the crevice still on the enamel, but deepest point of attachment already on the cementum. III, Bottom of the crevice exactly at the cementoenamel junction and the epithelial attachment on the cementum. IV, Bottom of the crevice on the cementum with the deepest point of the epithelial attachment shifted farther apically (Fig. 128). (Mueller and Orban, J. Am. Dent. A.)

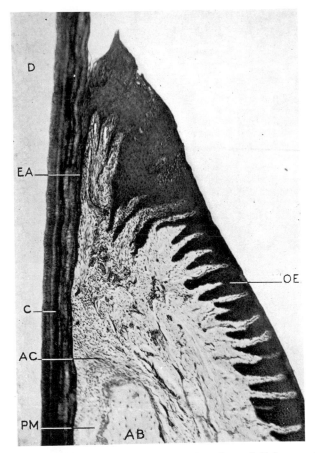

Figure 128. Epithelial attachment and gingival crevice of an adult human tooth. Lingual side of a lower bicuspid; age, fifty-two years. The bottom of the gingival crevice is located on the root surface. *D,* Dentin; *C,* cementum; *EA,* epithelial attachment to the cementum; *OE,* oral epithelium; *AC,* alveolar crest fibers; *PM,* periodontal membrane; *AB,* alveolar bone. Magnification × 55. (Kronfeld, *Dental Histology and Comparative Dental Anatomy,* Lea & Febiger.)

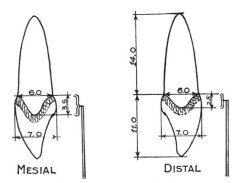

Figure 129. Curvatures of the cervical line (cementoenamel junction) mesially and distally on the maxillary central incisor, demonstrating the points of measurement in determining the relation between the curvatures of the cervical line mesially and distally. Other points of measurement of the crown and root, when the student observes the mesial and distal aspects, are outlined. The shaded area in the form of a band on the enamel follows the cervical curvature and represents the epithelial attachment of gingival tissue to the enamel of the crown. Compare with Figure 121.

121

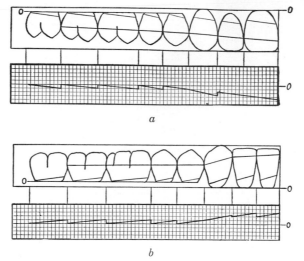

Figure 130. Schematic drawings of the crowns of maxillary and mandibular teeth with associated graphs of the usual extent of curvatures of the cervical line mesially and distally. *a,* Maxillary teeth. *b,* Mandibular teeth. Compare the graph of cervical curvatures with a line drawn through the center of contact areas. Note that the graph tends to run somewhat parallel to this line.

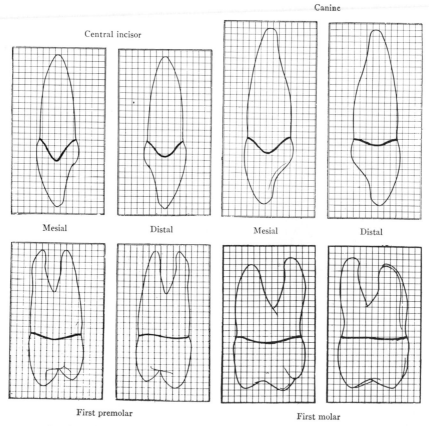

Figure 131. Graphs of typical forms of maxillary teeth accenting the outlines of cervical lines mesially and distally.

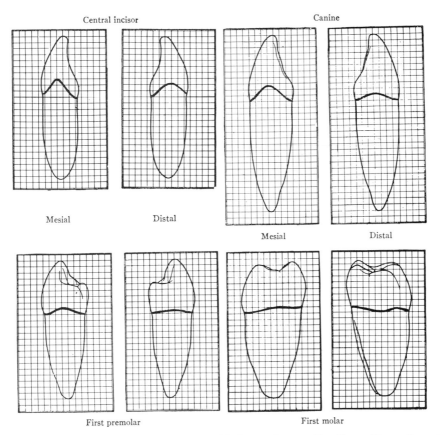

Figure 132. Graphs of typical forms of mandibular teeth accenting the outlines of cervical lines mesially and distally.

necessary to examine many tooth speciments. It was found that, usually, a graph of the curvatures from the median line distally could be staggered as in Figure 130. It will be noticed that, in the posterior teeth, the variation in curvature is slight and the amount of curvature is minor, the variance ranging from 1 mm. toward the occlusal surface to a slight curvature in the opposite direction. (Note the distal aspect of the mandibular first molar, Fig. 132.)

Figures 131 and 132 are graphs of maxillary and mandibular teeth demonstrating typical cervical lines mesially and distally.

THE PERMANENT TEETH

THE ANATOMY of the permanent teeth
will be described in detail in Chapters VI through XII.

Chapter VI

THE PERMANENT
MAXILLARY INCISORS

THE MAXILLARY incisors are *four* in number. The maxillary *central* or *first* incisors are centered in the maxilla, one on either side of the median line, with the mesial surface of each in contact with the mesial surface of the other. The maxillary and mandibular central incisors are the only neighboring teeth in the dental arches with mesial surfaces in contact. The right and left maxillary *lateral* or *second* incisors are distal to the central incisors.

The maxillary central incisor is larger than the lateral incisor. These teeth supplement each other in function, and they are similar anatomically. The incisors are shearing or cutting teeth. Their major function is to punch and cut food material during the process of mastication. These teeth have incisal *ridges* or *edges* rather than cusps such as are found on the canines and posterior teeth.

It might be well at this point to differentiate between the two terms, "incisal *ridge*" and "incisal *edge*." The incisal ridge is that portion of the crown which makes up the actual incisal portion. When an incisor is newly erupted, the incisal portion is rounded and merges with the mesio- and distoincisal angles and the labial and lingual surfaces. This ridge portion of the crown is called the *incisal ridge*. The term "edge" implies an angle formed by the merging of two flat surfaces. Therefore an incisal edge does not exist on an incisor until occlusal wear has created a flattened surface linguoincisally, which surface forms an angle with the labial surface. The *incisal edge* is formed by the junction of the linguoincisal surface, sometimes called the "incisal surface," and the labial surface. (Fig. 133.)

Preceding the description of each tooth in this and subsequent chapters, the chronology of *calcification* and *eruption* for the tooth will be given as in the table

125

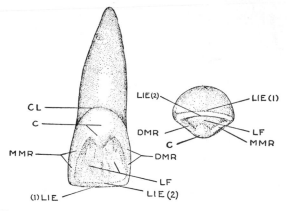

Figure 133. Maxillary right central incisor—lingual aspect and incisal aspect. *CL,* cervical line; *C,* cingulum; *MMR,* mesial marginal ridge; *LIE* (1), labioincisal edge, and *LIE* (2), linguoincisal edge (these (1) and (2), border the *incisal ridge*); *LF,* lingual fossa; *DMR,* distal marginal ridge.

below. A table of measurements as suggested by the author for carving technique will follow. Average measurements of each tooth as found in the table should be memorized. Knowing the proportions of the individual tooth helps one learn the proportions of one tooth to another.

Outline drawings of the five aspects of the teeth, and following that tooth carving, are explained more fully in a laboratory manual.*

MAXILLARY CENTRAL INCISOR

Maxillary Central Incisor

First evidence of calcification . . .   3 to 4 months
Enamel completed . . . .   4 to 5 years
Eruption . . . .   7 to 8 years
Root completed . . . . 10 years

Measurement Table

	Cervico-incisal Length of Crown	Length of Root	Mesio-distal Diameter of Crown	Mesio-distal Diameter of Crown at Cervix	Labio- or Bucco-lingual Diameter of Crown	Labio- or Bucco-lingual Diameter at Cervix	Curvature of Cervical Line—Mesial	Curvature of Cervical Line—Distal
Dimensions suggested for carving technic	10.5*	13.0	8.5	7.0	7.0	6.0	3.5	2.5

* Millimeters.

An Atlas of Tooth Form, W. B. Saunders Company.

The maxillary central incisor is the widest mesiodistally of any of the anterior teeth. The labial face is less convex than the maxillary lateral incisor or canine, which gives the central incisor a squared or rectangular appearance. From this aspect the crown nearly always looks symmetrical and regularly formed, having a nearly straight incisal edge, a cervical line with even curvature toward the root, a mesial side with straight outline, the distal side more curved. The mesial incisal angle is relatively sharp, the distal incisal angle rounded.

Although the *labial* surface of the crown is usually convex, especially toward the cervical third, some central incisors will be flat at the middle and incisal portions. The enamel surface is relatively smooth. When the tooth is newly erupted, or if little wear is evident, mamelons will be seen on the incisal ridge. The middle one is the smallest. The developmental lines on the labial surface which divide the surface into three parts are most noticeable at the middle portion if they can be distinguished at all.

Lingually, the surface form of the maxillary central incisor is more irregular. The largest part of the middle and incisal portions of the lingual area is concave. The concavity is bordered by mesial and distal marginal ridges, the lingual portion of the incisal ridge, and the convexity rootwise of the cingulum. The lingual topography gives a scooplike form to the crown.

The maxillary central incisor usually develops normally. One anomaly which sometimes occurs is a short root. Another variation is an unusually long crown. (Fig. 144, specimens 4, 6, 7, 8.)

The maxillary central incisors are the most prominent teeth in the mouth. There are *two* basic forms: The first is relatively wide at the cervix when viewed from the labial aspect, in comparison with the mesiodistal width at the contact areas (Fig. 141, specimens 1 and 2); the second form is relatively narrow at the cervix, where the root joins the crown, in comparison with the mesiodistal width at the contact areas (Fig. 141, specimens 5 and 7).

In the description of the central incisor an attempt will be made to strike an average between the extremes of the two forms.

Detailed Description of the Maxillary Central Incisor
from All Aspects

Labial Aspect (Figs. 134 and 141)

The crown of the average central incisor will be 10 to 11 mm. long from the highest point on the cervical line to the lowest point on the incisal edge. The mesiodistal measurement will be 8 to 9 mm. wide at the contact areas. The mesiodistal measurement, where the root joins the crown, will be 1.5 to 2 mm. less. The crests of curvature mesially and distally on the crown represent the areas at which the central incisor contacts its neighbors. Any change in the position of this crest of contour influences the point of contact.

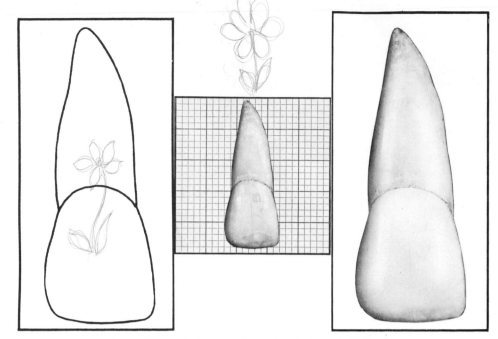

Figure 134. Maxillary right central incisor—labial aspect.

The mesial outline of the crown is only slightly convex, with the crest of curvature (representing the contact area) approaching the mesioincisal angle. (See "Proximal Contact Areas," Chapter V.)

The distal outline of the crown is more convex than the mesial outline, the crest of curvature being higher toward the cervical line. The distoincisal angle is not so sharp as the mesioincisal angle, the extent of curvature depending upon the typal form of the tooth.

The incisal outline is usually regular and straight in a mesiodistal direction after the tooth has been in function long enough to obliterate the mamelons. The incisal outline tends to curve downward toward the center of the crown outline, making the crown length greater at the center than at the two mesial angles.

The cervical outline of the crown follows a semicircular direction with the curvature rootwise, from the point at which the root outline joins the crown mesially to the point at which the root outline joins the crown distally.

The root of the central incisor from the labial aspect is cone-shaped, in most instances with a blunt apex, the outline mesially and distally being regular. The root is usually 2 or 3 mm. longer than the crown, although it varies considerably. (See illustrations of typical central incisors and those of variations from the labial aspect, Figs. 141 and 144.)

A line drawn through the center of the root and crown of the maxillary central incisor tends to parallel the mesial outline of the crown and root.

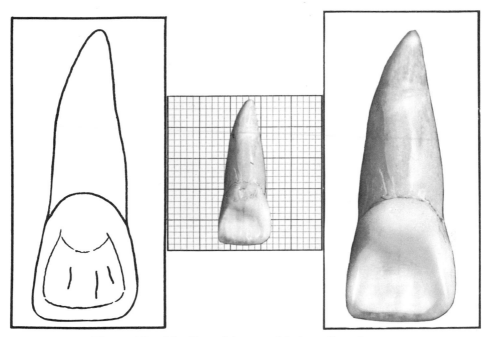

Figure 135. Maxillary right central incisor – lingual aspect.

Lingual Aspect (Fig. 135)

The lingual outline of the maxillary central incisor is the reverse of that found on the labial aspect. The lingual aspect of the crown is different, however, when one is comparing the surface of the lingual aspect with that of the labial aspect. From the labial aspect the surface of the crown is smooth generally. The lingual aspect has convexities and a concavity. The outline of the cervical line is similar, but immediately below the cervical line a smooth convexity is to be found; this is called the *cingulum.*

Mesially and distally confluent with the cingulum are the *marginal ridges.* Between the marginal ridges, below the cingulum, a shallow concavity is present which is called the *lingual fossa.* Outlining the lingual fossa, the linguoincisal edge is raised somewhat, being on a level with the marginal ridges mesially and distally, completing the lingual portion of the incisal ridge of the central incisor.

From the foregoing description one notes that the lingual fossa is bordered mesially by the mesial marginal ridge, incisally by the lingual portion of the incisal ridge, distally by the distal marginal ridge and cervically by the cingulum. Usually there are developmental grooves extending from the cingulum into the lingual fossa.

The crown and root taper lingually, making the crown calibration at the two labial line angles greater than the calibration at the two lingual line angles.

The lingual portion of the root is narrower than the labial portion. A cross sec-

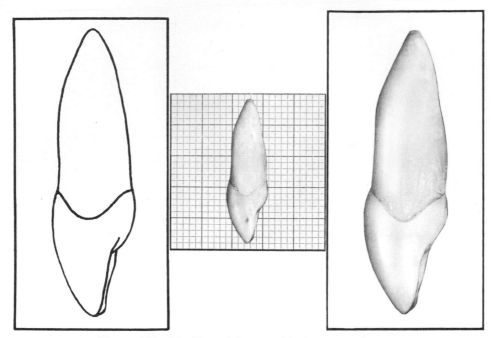

Figure 136.   Maxillary right central incisor — mesial aspect.

tion of the root at the cervix shows the root to be generally triangular with rounded angles: one side is toward the labial, and mesial and distal sides point toward the lingual. The mesial side of the triangle is longer than the distal side (Fig. 321, specimens C, 3, 4, 5, 6).

Mesial Aspect (Figs. 136 and 142)

The mesial aspect of this tooth illustrates the fundamental form of an incisor: The crown is wedge-shaped, or triangular, with the base of the triangle at the cervix and the apex at the incisal ridge.

Usually a line drawn through the crown and the root from the mesial aspect through the center of the tooth at the cervical line will tend to bisect the apex of the root and also the incisal ridge of the crown. The incisal ridge of the crown is on a line with the center of the root. This alignment is characteristic of maxillary central and lateral incisors. A straight line drawn through the center of the crown and root from the mesial or distal aspects will rarely if ever pass through the lingual surface. Maxillary incisors are occasionally seen with the incisal ridges lingual to the line (Fig. 144, specimen 1).

Labially and lingually, immediately coronal to the cervical line are the crests of curvature of these surfaces. These crests of contour give the crown its greatest labiolingual measurement.

Normally, the curvature labially or lingually is a mere 0.5 mm. in extent (Fig. 136).

The labial outline of the crown from the crest of curvature to the incisal edge is very slightly convex. The lingual outline is convex at the point where it joins the crest of curvature at the cingulum; it then becomes concave at the mesial marginal ridge, and it becomes slightly convex again at the linguoincisal ridge and the incisal edge.

The cervical line which outlines the cementoenamel junction mesially on the maxillary central incisor curves incisally to a noticeable degree. The cervical curvature is greater on the mesial surface of this tooth than on any surface of any other tooth in the mouth. This curvature varies in extent, depending upon the length of the crown and the measurement of the crown labiolingually. On an average central incisor of 10.5 to 11 mm. in crown length, the curvature will be 3 to 4 mm. (See "Curvatures of the Cervical Lines," Chapter V.)

The root of this tooth from the mesial aspect is cone-shaped, with the labial outline a straighter line than the lingual. The apex of the root is bluntly rounded.

Distal Aspect (Fig. 137)

There is little difference between the distal and mesial outlines of this tooth. When looking at the central incisor from the distal aspect, one may note that the crown gives the impression of being somewhat thicker toward the incisal third. Because of the slope of the labial surface distolingually, more of that surface is seen from the distal aspect; this creates the illusion of greater thickness.

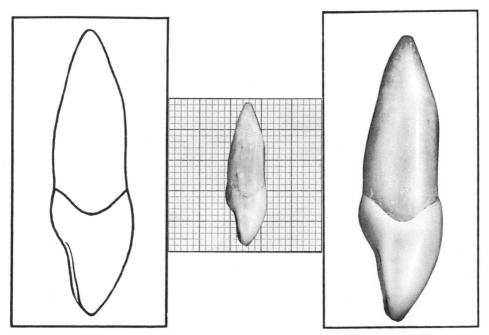

Figure 137.   Maxillary right central incisor—distal aspect.

The curvature of the cervical line outlining the cementoenamel junction is less on the distal than on the mesial. This is characteristic of most of the teeth.

Incisal Aspect (Figs. 138 and 143)

The specimen of this tooth is posed so that the incisal edge is centered over the root. A view of the crown from this aspect superposes it over the root entirely, so that the latter is not visible.

The labial face of the crown, from this aspect, is relatively broad and flat in comparison with the lingual surface, especially toward the incisal third. Nevertheless, the cervical portion of the crown is convex, although the arc described is broad.

The incisal ridge may be seen clearly, and a differentiation between the incisal edge and the remainder of the incisal ridge, with its slope toward the lingual, is easily distinguished.

The outline of the lingual portion tapers lingually toward the cingulum. The cingulum of the crown makes up the cervical portion of the lingual surface.

The mesiolabial and distolabial line angles are prominent from the incisal aspect. The relative positions of these line angles should be compared with the mesiolingual and distolingual line angles—which are represented by the borders of the mesial and distal marginal ridges. The mesiodistal size of the crown at the labial line angles is greater than the same dimension at the lingual line angles.

The crown of this tooth shows more bulk from the incisal aspect than one would expect from viewing it from the mesial or distal aspect. There are relatively broad

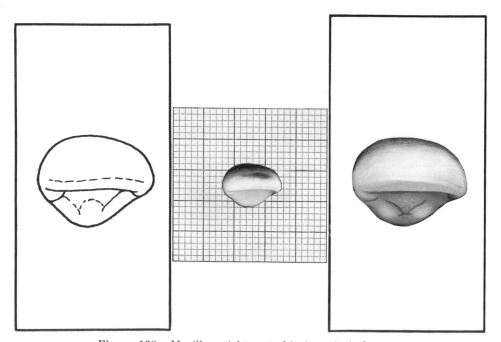

Figure 138. Maxillary right central incisor—incisal aspect.

surfaces at the site of contact areas mesially and distally. Comparison should also be made between the dimensions of the crown labiolingually and mesiodistally.

Bilaterally, the outline of the incisal aspect is rather uniform. The lingual portion shows some variation, however, in that a line drawn from the mesioincisal angle to the center of the cingulum lingually will be a longer line than one drawn from the same point on the cingulum to the distoincisal angle. In a general way the crown conforms to a triangular outline which was reflected by the outline of the root cross section at the cervix mentioned formerly.

MAXILLARY LATERAL INCISOR

Maxillary Lateral Incisor

First evidence of calcification ... 1 year
Enamel completed .... 4 to 5 years
Eruption .... 8 to 9 years
Root completed .... 11 years

Measurement Table

	Cervico-incisal Length of Crown	Length of Root	Mesio-distal Diam-eter of Crown	Mesio-distal Diam-eter of Crown at Cervix	Labio- or Bucco-lingual Diameter of Crown	Labio- or Bucco-lingual Diameter at Cervix	Curvature of Cervical Line— Mesial	Curvature of Cervical Line— Distal
Dimensions suggested for carving technic	9.0*	13.0	6.5	5.0	6.0	5.0	3.0	2.0

* Millimeters.

The maxillary lateral incisor supplements the central incisor in function, and they resemble each other in form. The lateral incisor is smaller in all dimensions except root length. Since it resembles the maxillary central incisor in form, direct comparisons will be made with the central incisor in its description.

This tooth differs from the central incisor in this—its development may vary considerably. Maxillary lateral incisors vary in form more than any other tooth in the mouth except the third molar. If the variation is too great, it is considered a developmental anomaly. A not uncommon situation is to find maxillary lateral incisors with a nondescript, pointed form; such teeth are called "peg-shaped" laterals (Fig. 153, specimens 7 and 8). In some individuals the lateral incisors are missing entirely; in these cases the maxillary central incisor is often in contact distally with the canine.

One type of malformed maxillary lateral incisor will have a large pointed tubercle as part of the cingulum; some will have deep developmental grooves which extend down on the root lingually with a deep fold in the cingulum; some will show twisted roots, distorted crowns, etc. (Fig. 153).

(Text continued on page 138.)

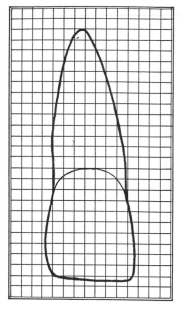

LABIAL

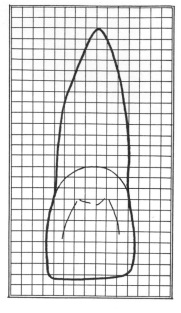

LINGUAL

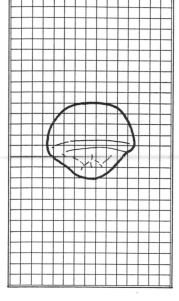

INCISAL

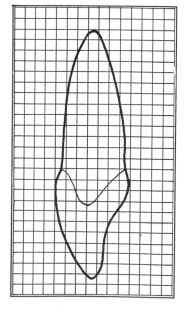

MESIAL

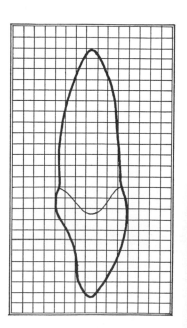

DISTAL

Figure 139. Maxillary right central incisor. Graph outlines of five aspects. In incisal view, labial aspect is at top of drawing.

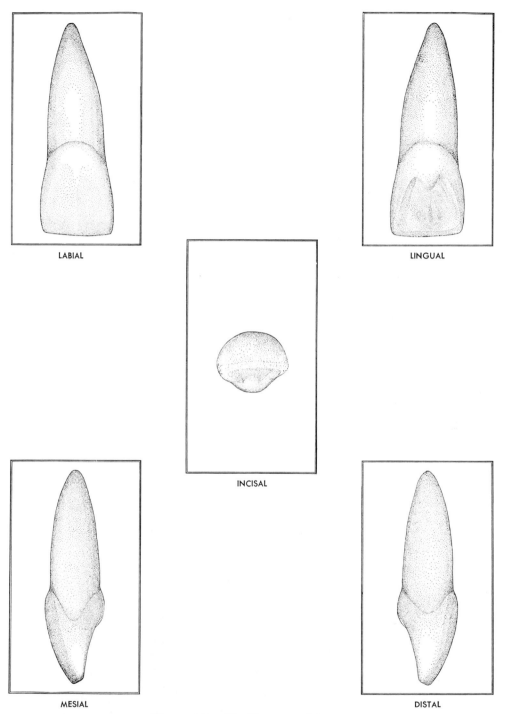

LABIAL

LINGUAL

INCISAL

MESIAL

DISTAL

Figure 140.   Maxillary central incisor.

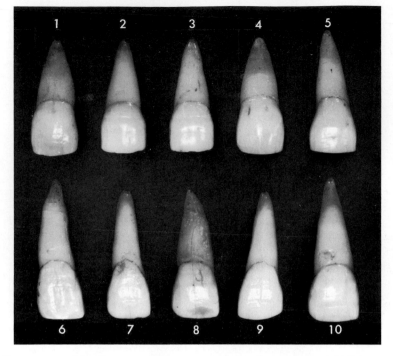

Figure 141.   Maxillary central incisor — ten typical specimens — labial aspect.

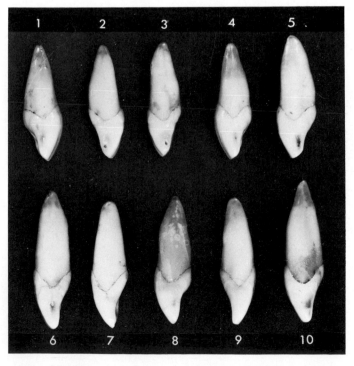

Figure 142.   Maxillary central incisor — ten typical specimens — mesial aspect.

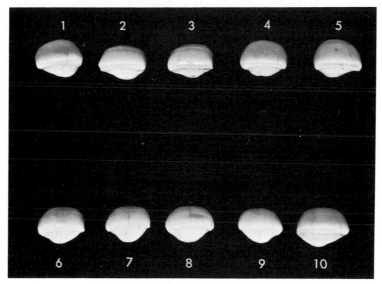

Figure 143. Maxillary central incisor—ten typical specimens—incisal aspect.

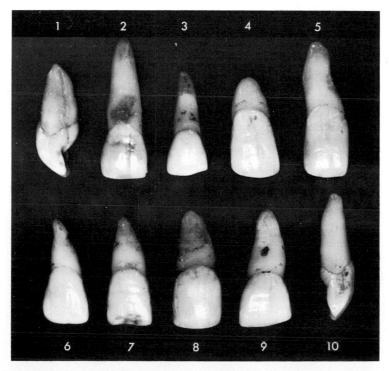

Figure 144. Maxillary central incisor—ten specimens showing uncommon variations. 1, Extreme lingual inclination of incisal portion of crown. Note developmental groove traversing root part of crown. 2, Root extremely long. 3, Specimen small in all dimensions. 4, Crown extremely long—root very short. 5, Specimen malformed—crown unusually long—cervix very wide. 6, Root short and tapering. 7, Same as specimen 6. 8, Crown nearly as wide at the cervix as at contact areas—crown long—root short. 9, Root with unusual curvature. 10, Crown and root narrow labiolingually.

Detailed Description of the Maxillary Lateral Incisor
from All Aspects

Labial Aspect (Figs. 145 and 151)

Although the labial aspect of the maxillary lateral incisor may appear to favor that of the central incisor, usually it has more curvature, with a rounded incisal ridge and rounded incisal angles mesially and distally. Although the crown is smaller in all dimensions, its proportions usually correspond to those of the central incisor.

The mesial outline of the crown from the labial aspect resembles that of the central incisor, with a more rounded mesioincisal angle. The crest of contour mesially is usually at the point of junction of the middle and incisal thirds; occasionally, in the so-called square forms, the mesioincisal angle is almost as sharp as that found on most maxillary central incisors (Fig. 151, specimens 4 and 5). However, a more rounded mesioincisal angle is more frequently seen.

The distal outline of the crown from the labial aspect differs somewhat from that of the central incisor. The distal outline is always more rounded, and the crest of contour is more cervical, usually in the center of the middle third. Some forms describe a semicircular outline distally from the cervix to the center of the incisal ridge (Fig. 151, specimens 3 and 7).

The labial surface of the crown is more convex than that of the central incisor except in some square and flat-faced forms.

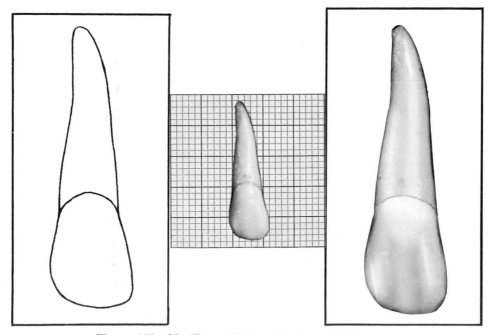

Figure 145. Maxillary right lateral incisor—labial aspect.

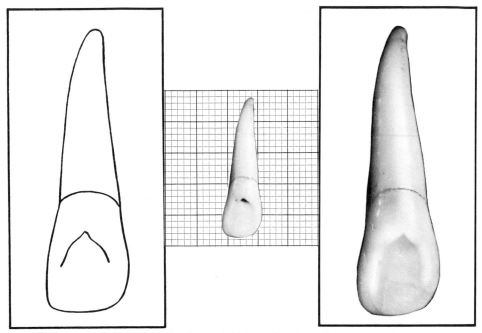

Figure 146. Maxillary right lateral incisor – lingual aspect.

This tooth is relatively narrow mesiodistally, usually about 2 mm. narrower than the central incisor. The crown on the average will measure from 2 to 3 mm. shorter cervicoincisally than that of the central incisor, although the root is as long if not somewhat longer than that of the central incisor.

As a rule its root length is greater in proportion to its crown length than that of the central incisor. The root is often about one and one-half times the length of the crown.

The root tapers evenly from the cervical line to a point approximately two-thirds of its length apically. In most cases it curves sharply from this location in a distal direction and ends in a pointed apex. Although the curvature distally is typical, some roots are straight (Fig. 151, specimens 4, 7 and 9), and some may be found curving mesially.

Lingual Aspect (Fig. 146)

Mesial and distal marginal ridges are marked, and the cingulum is usually prominent, with a tendency toward deep developmental grooves within the lingual fossa, where it joins the cingulum. The linguoincisal ridge is well developed, and the lingual fossa is more concave and circumscribed that that found on the central incisor.

The tooth tapers toward the lingual, resembling a central incisor in this respect. It is not uncommon to find a deep developmental groove at the side of the cingulum, usually on the distal side, which may extend up on the root for part or all of its length. Faults in the enamel of the crown are often found in the deep portions of these developmental grooves (Fig. 153, specimens 3 and 4).

Mesial Aspect (Figs. 147 and 152)

The mesial aspect of the maxillary lateral incisor is similar to that of a small central incisor except that the root appears longer. The crown is shorter; the root is relatively longer, and the labiolingual measurement of the crown and root is a millimeter or so less than the maxillary central incisor of the same mouth.

The curvature of the cervical line is marked in the direction of the incisal ridge, although because of the small size of the crown the actual extent of curvature is less than that found on the central incisor. The heavy development of the incisal ridge accordingly makes the incisal portion appear somewhat thicker than that of the central incisor.

The root appears as a tapered cone from this aspect, with a bluntly rounded, apical end. This varies in individuals, sometimes being quite blunt, while at other times it is pointed. In a good many cases the labial outline of the root from this aspect is straight. As in the central incisor, a line drawn through the center of the root tends to bisect the incisal ridge of the crown.

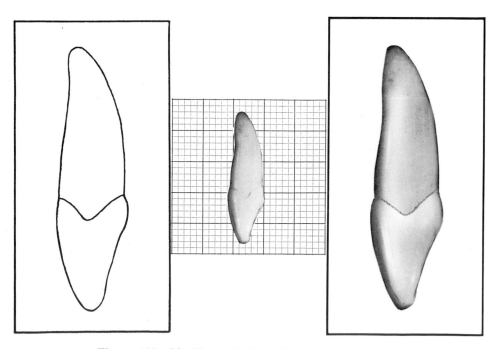

Figure 147.   Maxillary right lateral incisor—mesial aspect.

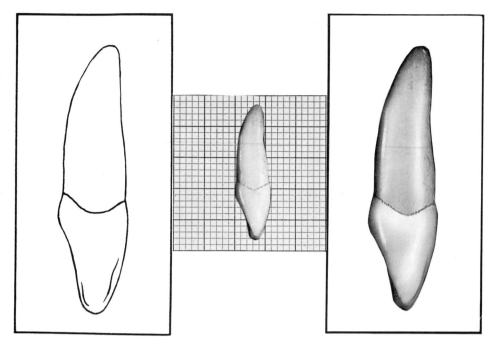

Figure 148.   Maxillary right lateral incisor—distal aspect.

Distal Aspect (Fig. 148)

Because of the placement of the crown on the root, the width of the crown distally appears thicker than it does on the mesial aspect from marginal ridge to labial face. The curvature of the cervical line is usually a millimeter or so less in depth than on the mesial side. It is not uncommon to find a developmental groove distally on this crown extending on the root for part or all of its length.

Incisal Aspect (Figs. 149 and 150)

The incisal aspect of this tooth sometimes resembles that of the central incisor, or it may resemble that of a small canine. If the tooth conforms in development to its central incisor neighbor in other respects, it will, from the incisal aspect, resemble a central incisor except in size (Fig. 150, specimens 5 and 9). The cingulum, however, may be large, as may also the incisal ridge; the labiolingual dimension may be greater than usual in comparison with the mesiodistal dimension. If these variations are present, the tooth has a marked resemblance to a canine (Fig. 150, specimen 3).

All maxillary lateral incisors exhibit more convexity labially and lingually from the incisal aspect than maxillary central incisors.

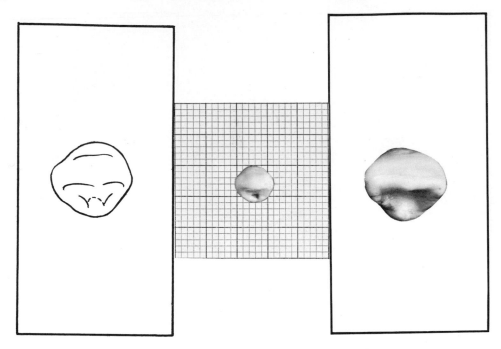

Figure 149.   Maxillary right lateral incisor – incisal aspect.

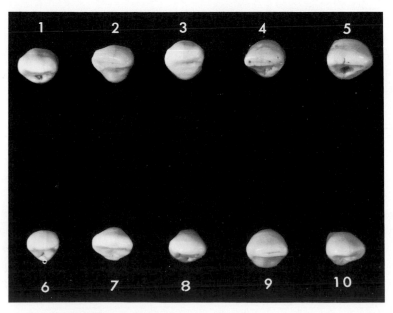

Figure 150.   Maxillary lateral incisor – ten typical specimens – incisal aspect.

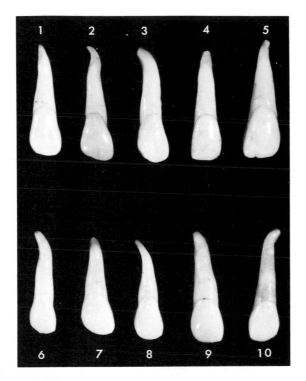

Figure 151. Maxillary lateral incisor—ten typical specimens—labial aspect.

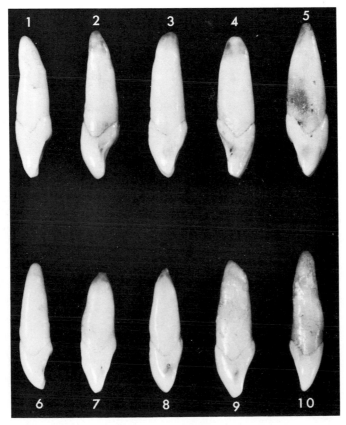

Figure 152. Maxillary lateral incisor—ten typical specimens—mesial aspect.

143

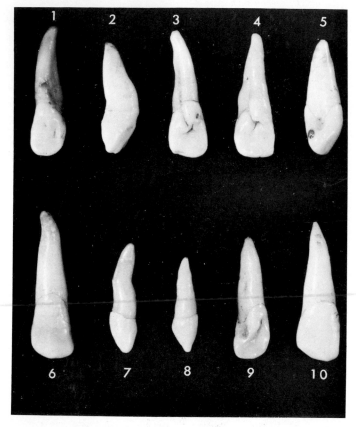

Figure 153. Maxillary lateral incisor—ten specimens showing uncommon variations. 1, Odd twist to crown and root. 2, Malformed generally. 3, Deep developmental groove distally; note pit in lingual fossa. 4, Same as specimen 3 with pit and groove connected. 5, Deep concavity above contact area of the crown. 6, Abnormally large but well formed. 7, Single-cusp development and malformed root—so-called "peg lateral incisor." 8, Same as specimen 7 except root is straight. 9, Same as specimen 5, with deep lingual pit in addition. 10, Resemblance to a small maxillary central incisor more marked than the average.

Chapter VII

THE PERMANENT
MANDIBULAR INCISORS

THE MANDIBULAR incisors are *four* in number. The mandibular *central* or *first* incisors are centered in the mandible, one on either side of the median line, with the mesial surface of each one in contact with the mesial surface of the other. The right and left mandibular *lateral* or *second* incisors are distal to the central incisors. They are in contact with the central incisors mesially and with the canines distally.

The mandibular incisors have smaller mesiodistal dimensions than any of the other teeth. The central incisor is somewhat smaller than the lateral incisor, which is the reverse of the situation in the maxilla.

These teeth are similar in form and have smooth crown surfaces which show few traces of developmental lines. Mamelons on the incisal ridges are worn off soon after eruption, if the occlusion is normal, leaving the incisal ridges smooth and straight (compare specimens 7 and 8, Fig. 162). The contact areas are near the incisal ridges mesially and distally, and lines drawn through the contact areas are near the same level on both central and lateral incisors. The mandibular incisors show uniform development, with few instances of malformations or anomalies.

The anatomic form of these teeth differs entirely from that of the maxillary incisors. The inclination of the crowns differs from the mesial and distal aspects; the labial faces are inclined lingually so that the incisal ridges are lingual to a line bisecting the root. After normal wear has taken place, obliterating the mamelons, the incisal surfaces thus created show a labial inclination when the occlusion has been normal. It will be remembered that the incisal surfaces of maxillary incisors have a lingual inclination. With this arrangement the incisal planes of the mandibular and maxillary incisors are parallel with each other, fitting together during incising action.

145

MANDIBULAR CENTRAL INCISOR

Normally, the mandibular central incisor is the smallest tooth in the dental arch. The crown has little more than half the mesiodistal diameter of the maxillary central incisor; however, the labiolingual diameter is only about 1 mm. less. The lines of greatest stress are brought to bear on the mandibular incisors in a labiolingual direction.

Mandibular Central Incisor

First evidence of calcification . . . 3 to 4 months
Enamel completed . . . . 4 to 5 years
Eruption . . . . 6 to 7 years
Root completed . . . . 9 years

Measurement Table

	Cervico-incisal Length of Crown	Length of Root	Mesiodistal Diameter of Crown	Mesiodistal Diameter of Crown at Cervix	Labio- or Buccolingual Diameter of Crown	Labio- or Buccolingual Diameter of Crown at Cervix	Curvature of Cervical Line— Mesial	Curvature of Cervical Line— Distal
Dimensions suggested for carving technic	9.0*	12.5	5.0	3.5	6.0	5.3	3.0	2.0

* Millimeters.

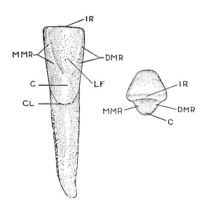

Figure 154. Mandibular right central incisor —lingual aspect and incisal aspect. *IR,* incisal ridge; *DMR,* distal marginal ridge; *LF,* lingual fossa; *CL,* cervical line; *C,* cingulum; *MMR,* mesial marginal ridge.

The single root is very narrow mesiodistally and corresponds to the narrowness of the crown, although the root and crown are wide labiolingually. The length of the root is as great, if not greater, than that of the maxillary central incisor.

Detailed Description of the Mandibular Central Incisor
from All Aspects

Labial Aspect (Figs. 155 and 162)

The labial aspect of the mandibular central incisor is regular, tapering evenly from the sharp mesial and distal incisal angles to the apical portion of the root. The incisal ridge of the crown is straight and is at approximately a right angle to the long axis of the tooth. Usually the mesial and distal outlines of the crown make a straight drop downward from the incisal angles to the contact areas, which are incisal to the junction of incisal and middle thirds of the crown. The mesial and distal sides of the crown taper evenly from the contact areas to the narrow cervix, which is a short arc.

The mesial and distal root outlines are straight with the mesial and distal outlines of the crown down to the apical portion. The apical third of the root terminates in a small pointed taper, in most cases curving distally. Sometimes the roots are straight (Fig. 162, specimens 2 and 10).

The labial face of the mandibular central incisor crown is ordinarily smooth, with a flattened surface at the incisal third; the middle third is more convex, narrowing down to the convexity of the root at the cervical portion.

Except in newly erupted teeth, central incisors show few traces of developmental lines.

The labial surface of the root of the mandibular central incisor is regular and convex.

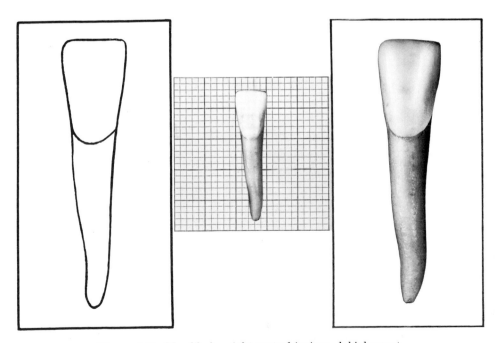

Figure 155. Mandibular right central incisor—labial aspect.

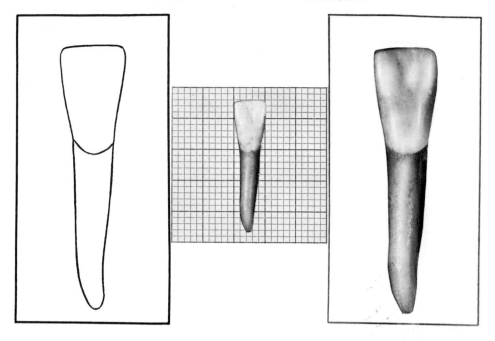

Figure 156. Mandibular right central incisor—lingual aspect.

Lingual Aspect (Fig. 156)

The *lingual* surface of the crown is smooth, with a very slight concavity at the incisal third between the inconspicuous marginal ridges. In some instances the marginal ridges are more prominent near the incisal edges (Fig. 164, specimens 3 and 9). In these cases the concavity between the marginal ridges is more distinct.

The lingual surface becomes flat and then convex as progression is made from the incisal third to the cervical third.

No developmental lines mark the cingulum development on this tooth at the cervical third. No other tooth in the mouth, except the mandibular lateral incisor, shows so few developmental lines and grooves. The outlines and surfaces of the mandibular incisors are regular and symmetrical.

Mesial Aspect (Figs. 157, 160, 161 and 163)

The curvature labially and lingually above the cervical line is less than that found on maxillary incisors.

The outline of the labial face of the crown is straight above the cervical curvature, sloping rapidly from the crest of curvature to the incisal ridge. The lingual outline of the crown is a straight line inclined labially for a short distance above the smooth convexity of the cingulum; the straight outline joins a concave line at the middle third of the crown, which extends upward to join the rounded outline of a narrow incisal ridge. The incisal ridge is rounded or worn flat, and its center is lingual to the center of the root.

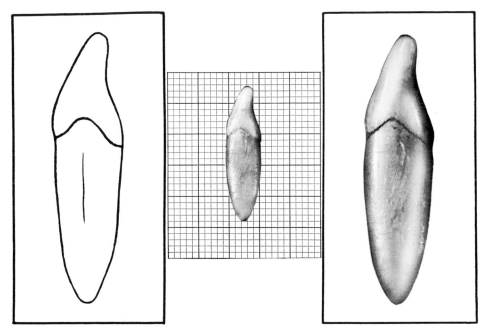

Figure 157. Mandibular right central incisor — mesial aspect.

The curvature of the cervical line on the mesial surface is marked, curving incisally approximately one-third the length of the crown.

The root outlines from the mesial aspect are straight with the crown outline from the cervical line, keeping the root diameter uniform through the cervical third and part of the middle third; the outline of the root begins to taper in the middle third area, tapering rapidly in the apical third to either a bluntly rounded or a pointed root end.

The mesial surface of the crown is convex and smooth at the incisal third and becomes broader and flatter at the middle third cervical to the contact area; it then becomes quite flat, with a tendency toward concavity immediately below the middle third of the crown and above the cervical line (Fig. 163, specimens 5, 8 and 10).

The mesial surface of the root is flat just below the cervical line. Most of these roots have a broad developmental depression for most of the root length. The depressions usually are deeper at the junction of the middle and apical thirds (Fig. 163, specimens 7 and 9).

Distal Aspect (Fig. 158)

The cervical line representing the cementoenamel junction curves incisally about 1 mm. less than on the mesial.

The distal surface of the crown and root of the mandibular central incisor is similar to that of the mesial surface. The developmental depression on the distal surface of the root may be more marked, with a deeper and more well-defined developmental groove at its center.

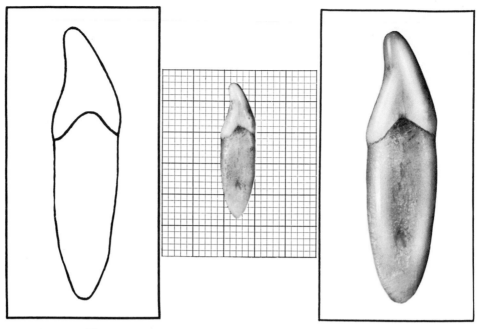

Figure 158.   Mandibular right central incisor—distal aspect.

Incisal Aspect (Figs. 159 and 164)

This aspect illustrates the bilateral symmetry of the mandibular central incisor. The mesial half of the crown is almost identical with the distal half.

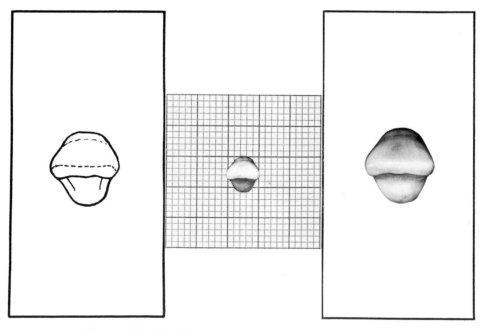

Figure 159.   Mandibular right central incisor—incisal aspect.

The incisal edge is almost at right angles to a line bisecting the crown labiolingually. This feature is characteristic of the tooth and serves as a mark of identification in differentiation between mandibular central and lateral incisors (see "Mandibular Lateral Incisor"). Note the comparison between the diameter of these crowns labiolingually and their diameters mesiodistally. The labiolingual diameter is always *greater*.

The labial surface of the crown is wider mesiodistally than the lingual surface. The crown is usually wider labially than lingually at the cervical third, which latter area is represented by a smooth cingulum.

The labial surface of the crown at the incisal third, although rather broad and flat in comparison with the cervical third, has a tendency toward *convexity*, whereas the lingual surface of the crown at the incisal third has an inclination toward *concavity*.

When this tooth is posed from the incisal aspect so that the line of vision is on a line with the long axis of the tooth, more of the labial surface may be seen than of the lingual surface.

MANDIBULAR LATERAL INCISOR

The mandibular lateral incisor is the second mandibular tooth from the median line, right or left (Figs. 166 to 174). It resembles the mandibular central incisor so closely that a detailed description of each aspect of the lateral incisor is unnecessary. Direct comparison will be made with the mandibular central incisor, and the variations will be mentioned.

Mandibular Lateral Incisor

First evidence of calcification ... 3 to 4 months
Enamel completed .... 4 to 5 years
Eruption .... 7 to 8 years
Root completed .... 10 years

Measurement Table

	Cervico-incisal Length of Crown	Length of Root	Mesio-distal Diameter of Crown	Mesio-distal Diameter of Crown at Cervix	Labio- or Bucco-lingual Diameter of Crown	Labio- or Bucco-lingual Diameter of Crown at Cervix	Curvature of Cervical Line—Mesial	Curvature of Cervical Line—Distal
Dimensions suggested for carving technic	9.5*	14.0	5.5	4.0	6.5	5.8	3.0	2.0

* Millimeters.

(Text continued on page 154.)

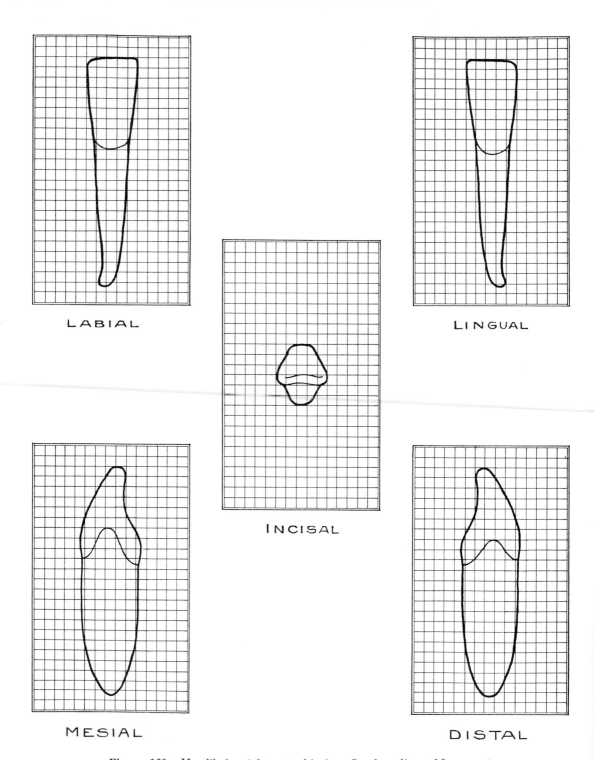

LABIAL

LINGUAL

INCISAL

MESIAL

DISTAL

Figure 160.   Mandibular right central incisor. Graph outlines of five aspects.

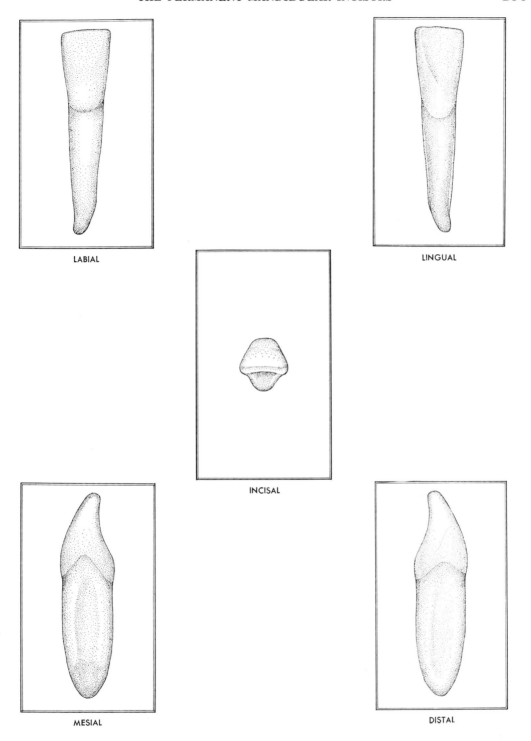

Figure 161. Mandibular right central incisor.

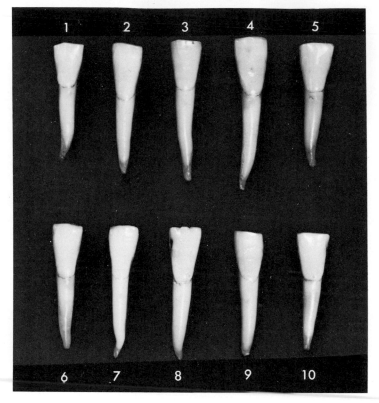

Figure 162. Mandibular central incisor—ten typical specimens—labial aspect.

The mandibular lateral incisor is somewhat larger than the mandibular central incisor (compare measurements) but, generally speaking, its outline closely resembles the central.

The labial and lingual aspects show the added fraction of approximately 1 mm. of crown diameter mesiodistally added to the distal half. This, however, is not invariable (see Fig. 172, specimens 3 and 6).

The mesial side of the crown is often longer than the distal side, causing the incisal ridge, which is straight, to slope downward in a distal direction (Fig. 172, specimen 1). The distal contact area is more toward the cervical than the mesial contact area to contact properly the mesial contact area of the mandibular canine.

Except as to size, there is no marked difference between the mesial and distal surfaces of central and lateral incisors. Even the cuvatures of the cervical lines mesially and distally are similar in extent. There is a tendency toward a deeper concavity immediately above the cervical line on the distal surface of the mandibular lateral incisor.

Although the crown of the mandibular lateral incisor is somewhat longer than that of the central incisor (usually a fraction of a millimeter), the root may be considerably longer. The tooth is, therefore, in most instances, a little larger in all dimensions. The root form is similar to that of the central incisor, including the developmental depressions mesially and distally.

The *incisal aspect* of the mandibular lateral incisor provides a feature which can usually serve to identify this tooth. The incisal edge is not at approximate right angles to a line bisecting the crown and root labiolingually, as was found when studying the central incisor: The edge follows the curvature of the mandibular dental arch, giving the crown of the mandibular lateral incisor the appearance of being twisted slightly on its root base. It is interesting to note that the labiolingual root axes of mandibular central and lateral incisors remain almost parallel in the alveolar process, even though the incisal ridges are not directly in line (see mandibular alveoli, Chapter XIV, Fig. 359).

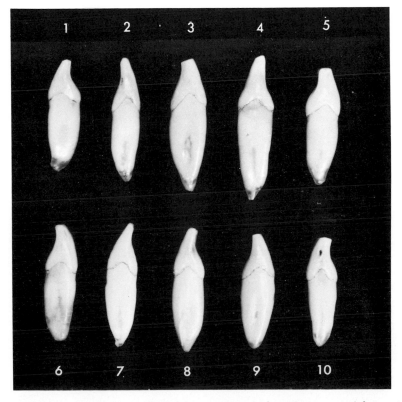

Figure 163. Mandibular central incisor—ten typical specimens—mesial aspect.

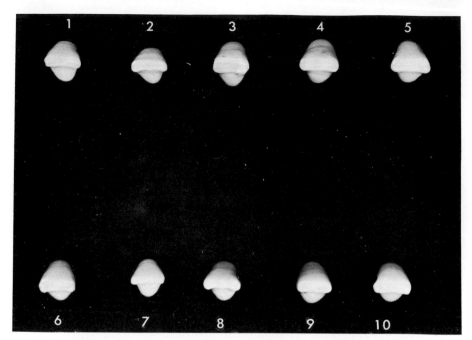

Figure 164. Mandibular central incisor — ten typical specimens — incisal aspect.

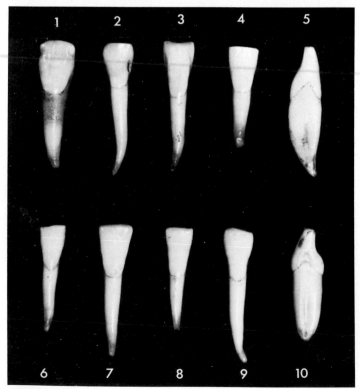

Figure 165. Mandibular central incisor — ten specimens showing uncommon variations. 1, Crown and root very broad mesiodistally, malformed enamel at incisal third of crown. 2, Crown wide at incisal third, with short crown. Root length extreme. 3, Unusual contours at middle third of crown, cervix narrow. 4, Well-formed crown, short root. 5, No curvature labially at cervical third, extreme labial curvature at root end. 6, Specimen well formed but undersized. 7, Contact areas pointed at incisal edge. Crown and root very long. 8, Crown long and narrow, root short. 9, Crown measurement at cervical third same as root, crown and root of extreme length. 10, Crown and root very wide labiolingually, greater curvature than average above cervical line at the cervical third of the crown.

156

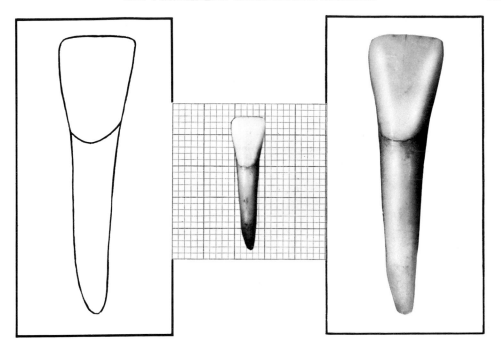

Figure 166. Mandibular right lateral incisor — labial aspect.

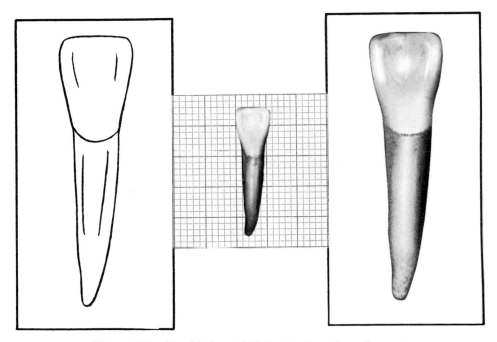

Figure 167. Mandibular right lateral incisor — lingual aspect.

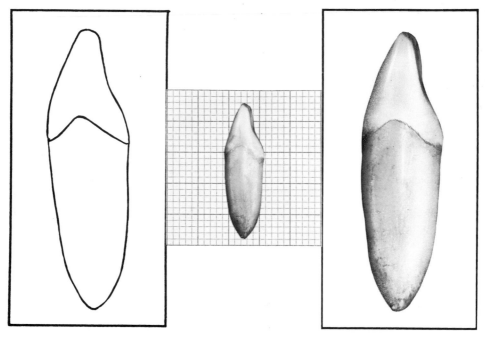

Figure 168. Mandibular right lateral incisor — mesial aspect.

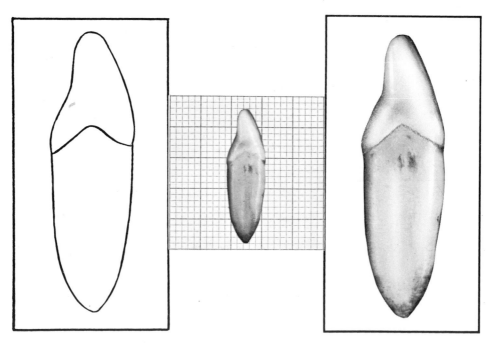

Figure 169. Mandibular right lateral incisor — distal aspect.

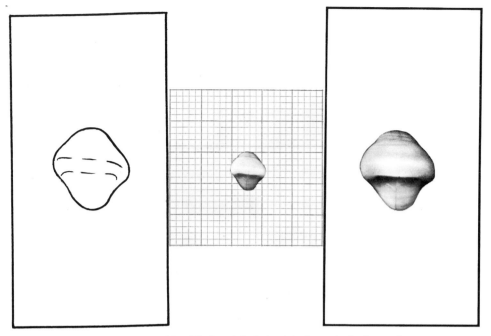

Figure 170. Mandibular right lateral incisor—incisal aspect.

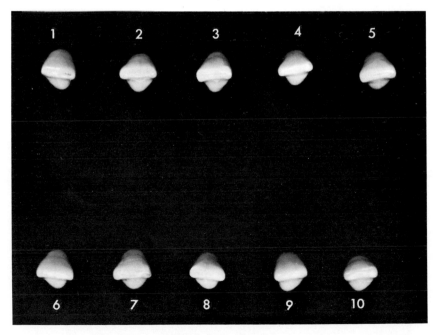

Figure 171. Mandibular lateral incisor—ten typical specimens—incisal aspect.

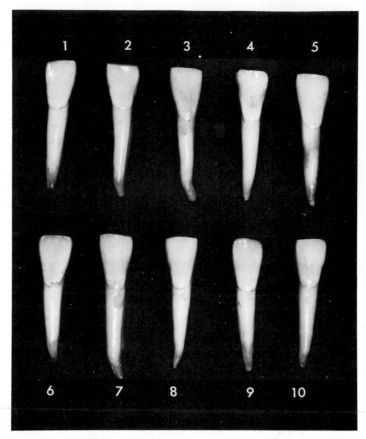

Figure 172. Mandibular lateral incisor — ten typical specimens — labial aspect.

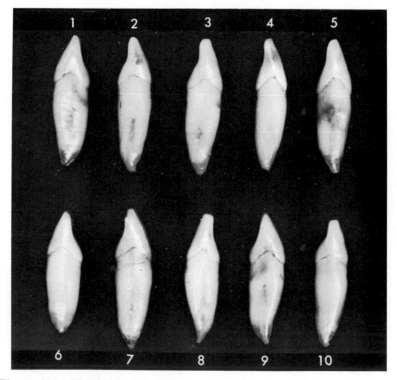

Figure 173. Mandibular lateral incisor — ten typical specimens — mesial aspect.

160

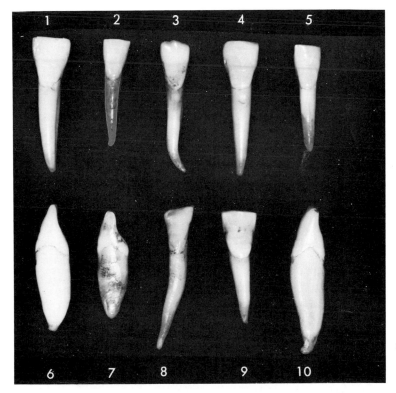

Figure 174. Mandibular lateral incisor — ten specimens showing uncommon variations. 1, Tooth very large, cervix constricted in comparison with crown width. 2, Specimen well formed, smaller than average. 3, Root extra long, extreme curvature at apical third, mesial and middle mamelons intact on incisal ridge. 4, Extreme mesiodistal measurement for crown length, contact areas very broad cervicoincisally. 5, Specimen undersized. 6, Incisal ridge thin, little or no curvature at cervical third of crown. 7, Incisal edge labial to center of root, root rounded, cingulum with more curvature above root than average. 8, Malformed crown and root, root with extreme length. 9, Crown very wide, root short. 10, Very slight curvature at cervical third of crown, entire tooth oversize, malformation at root end.

Chapter VIII

THE PERMANENT CANINES,
MAXILLARY AND MANDIBULAR

THE MAXILLARY and mandibular canines bear a close resemblance to each other, and their functions are closely related. The four canines are placed at the "corners" of the mouth, each one the third tooth from the median line, right and left, in the maxilla and mandible. They are the longest teeth in the mouth; the crowns are usually as long as those of the maxillary central incisors, and the single roots are longer than those of any of the other teeth. The middle labial lobes have been highly developed incisally into strong well-formed cusps. Crowns and roots are markedly convex on most surfaces.

The shape of the crowns, with their single pointed cusps, their locations in the mouth, and the extra anchorage furnished by the long, strongly developed roots, makes these canines resemble those of the Carnivora. This resemblance to the prehensile teeth of Carnivora gives rise to the term *canine*.

Because of the labiolingual thickness of crown and root and the anchorage in the alveolar process of the jaws, these teeth are perhaps the most stable in the mouth. The crown portions of the canines are shaped in a manner which promotes cleanliness. This self-cleansing quality, along with the efficient anchorage in the jaws, tends to preserve these teeth throughout life. When teeth are lost, the canines are usually the last ones to go. They are very valuable teeth, either when considered as units of the natural dental arches, or as possible assistants in stabilizing replacements of lost teeth in prosthetic procedures.

Both maxillary and mandibular canines have another quality which must not be overlooked: The positions and forms of these teeth and their anchorage in the bone, along with the bone ridge over the labial portions of the roots, called the *canine eminence*, have a cosmetic value. They help to form a foundation that insures normal

162

facial expression at the "corners" of the mouth. Loss of all of these teeth makes it extremely difficult, if not impossible, to make replacements that will restore the natural appearance of the face for any length of time. It would therefore be difficult to place a value on the canines, their importance being made manifest by their efficiency in function, their stability, and their help in maintaining natural facial expression.

In *function*, the canines assist the incisors and the premolars, since they are located between those groups. The canine crowns have some characteristics of functional form which will bear a resemblance to incisor form, and some which resemble the premolar form.

MAXILLARY CANINE

Maxillary Canine

First evidence of calcification . . .   4 to 5 months
Enamel completed . . . .   6 to 7 years
Eruption . . . . 11 to 12 years
Root completed . . . . 13 to 15 years

Measurement Table

	Cervico-incisal Length of Crown	Length of Root	Mesio-distal Diam-eter of Crown	Mesio-distal Diam-eter of Crown at Cervix	Labio- or Bucco-lingual Diameter of Crown	Labio- or Bucco-lingual Diameter at Cervix	Curvature of Cervical Line— Mesial	Curvature of Cervical Line— Distal
Dimensions suggested for carving technic	10.0*	17.0	7.5	5.5	8.0	7.0	2.5	1.5

* Millimeters.

The outline of the labial or lingual aspect of the maxillary canine is a series of curves or arcs except for the angle made by the tip of the cusp. This cusp has a mesial incisal ridge and a distoincisal ridge.

The mesial half of the crown makes contact with the lateral incisor, and the distal half contacts the first premolar. Therefore the contact areas of the maxillary canine are at different levels cervicoincisally.

From a labial view, the mesial half of the crown resembles a portion of an incisor, whereas the distal half resembles a portion of a premolar. This tooth seems to be a compromise in the change from anterior to posterior teeth in the dental arch.

It is apparent that the construction of this tooth has reinforcement, labiolingually, to offset directional lines of the force brought against it when in use. The incisal portion is thicker labiolingually than that of either the maxillary central or the lateral incisor.

The labiolingual measurement of the crown is about 1 mm. greater than that of the maxillary central incisor. The mesiodistal measurement is approximately 1 mm. less.

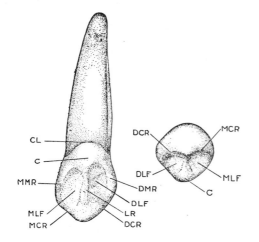

Figure 175. Maxillary right canine—lingual aspect—incisal aspect. *CL*, cervical line; *C*, cingulum; *MMR*, mesial marginal ridge; *MLF*, mesiolingual fossa; *MCR*, mesial cusp ridge; *DCR*, distal cusp ridge; *LR*, lingual ridge; *DLF*, distolingual fossa; *DMR*, distal marginal ridge.

The cingulum shows greater development than that of the central incisor.

The root of the maxillary canine is usually the longest of any root with the possible exception of that of the mandibular canine, which may be as long at times. The root is thick labiolingually, with developmental depressions mesially and distally which help to furnish the secure anchorage this tooth has in the maxilla.

Detailed Description of the Maxillary Canine from All Aspects

Labial Aspect (Figs. 176 and 183)

The crown and root are narrower mesiodistally than those of the maxillary central incisor. The difference is about 1 mm. in most mouths. The cervical line labially is convex, with the convexity toward the root portion.

Mesially, the outline of the crown may be convex from the cervix to the center of the mesial contact area; or the crown may exhibit a slight concavity above the contact area from the labial aspect. The center of the contact area mesially is approximately at the junction of middle and incisal thirds of the crown.

Distally, the outline of the crown is usually concave between the cervical line and the distal contact area. The distal contact area is usually at the center of the middle third of the crown. The two levels of contact areas mesially and distally should be noted.

Unless the crown has been worn unevenly, the cusp tip is on a line with the center of the root. The cusp has a mesial slope and a distal slope, the mesial slope being the shorter of the two. Both slopes show a tendency toward concavity before wear has taken place (Fig. 183, specimens 5 and 6). These depressions are developmental in character.

The labial surface of the crown is smooth, with no developmental lines of note except shallow depressions mesially and distally, dividing the three labial lobes. The middle labial lobe shows much greater development than the other lobes. This produces a ridge on the labial surface of the crown. A line drawn over the crest of this ridge, from the cervical line to the tip of the cusp, is a curved one inclined mesially at its center. All areas mesial to the crest of this ridge exhibit convexity except for

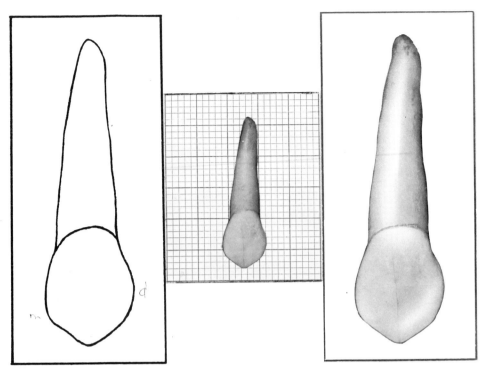

Figure 176.   Maxillary left canine—labial aspect.

insignificant developmental lines in the enamel. Distally to the labial ridge there is a tendency toward concavity at the cervical third of the crown, although convexity is noted elsewhere in all areas approaching the labial ridge.

The root of the maxillary canine appears slender from the labial aspect when compared with the bulk of the crown; it is conical in form with a pointed apex. It is not uncommon for this root to have a sharp curve in the vicinity of the apical third. This curvature may be in a mesial or distal direction—in most instances the latter (Fig. 183, compare specimens 1 and 6). The labial surface of the root is smooth and convex at all points.

Lingual Aspect (Fig. 177)

The crown and root are narrower lingually than labially.

The cervical line from this aspect differs somewhat from the curvature found labially. The cervical line shows a more even curvature. The line may be straight for a short interval at this point.

The cingulum is large, and in some instances is pointed like a small cusp. In the latter types, definite ridges are found on the lingual surface of the crown below the cingulum and between strongly developed marginal ridges. Although depressions are to be found between these ridge forms, there are seldom any deep developmental grooves.

Very often a well-developed lingual ridge is seen which is confluent with the

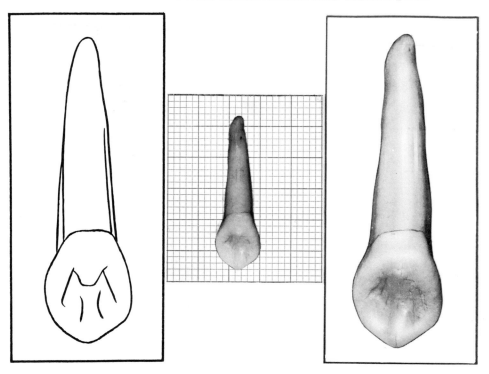

Figure 177. Maxillary left canine—lingual aspect.

cusp tip; this extends to a point near the cingulum. There may be shallow concavities between this ridge and the marginal ridges. When these concavities are present, they are called mesial and distal lingual fossae.

Sometimes the lingual surface of the canine crown is so smooth that fossae or minor ridges are difficult to distinguish. There is a tendency toward concavities, however, where the fossae are usually found and heavy marginal ridges with a well formed cingulum are to be expected. The smooth cingulum, marginal ridges and the lingual portion of the incisal ridges are confluent usually, with little evidence of developmental grooves.

The lingual portion of the root of the maxillary canine is narrower than the labial portion. Because of this formation, much of the mesial and distal surfaces of the root is visible from the lingual aspect. Developmental depressions mesially and distally may be seen on most of these roots, extending most of the root length. The lingual ridge of the root is narrow but it is smooth and convex at all points from the cervical line to the apical end.

Mesial Aspect (Figs. 178 and 184)

The mesial aspect of the maxillary canine presents the outline of the functional form of an anterior tooth. It shows greater bulk generally, however, and greater labiolingual measurement than any of the other anterior teeth.

The outline of the crown is wedge-shaped, the greatest measurement being at the cervical third and the wedge point being represented by the tip of the cusp.

The curvature of the crown below the cervical line labially and lingually corresponds in extent to the curvature of maxillary central and lateral incisors. Nevertheless, the crest of that curvature is found at a level more incisal, since the middle labial and the lingual lobes are more highly developed (Fig. 184, specimens 5 and 10). Many canines show a flattened area labially at the cervical third of the crown, which appears as a straight outline from the mesial aspect. It is questionable just how much wear has to do with this effect (Fig. 184, specimens 1 and 2).

Below the cervical third of the crown, the labial face may be represented by a line only slightly convex from the crest of curvature at the cervical third to the tip of the cusp. The line usually becomes straighter as it approaches the cusp.

The entire labial outline from the mesial aspect exhibits more convexity from the cervical line to the cusp tip than the maxillary central incisor does from cervix to incisal edge.

The lingual outline of the crown from the mesial aspect may be represented by a convex line describing the cingulum, which convexity straightens out as the middle third is reached, becoming convex again in the incisal third (Fig. 184, specimen 10).

The cervical line which outlines the base of the crown from this aspect curves toward the cusp, on the average, approximately 2.5 mm.

The outline of the root from this aspect is conical, with a tapered or pointed apex.

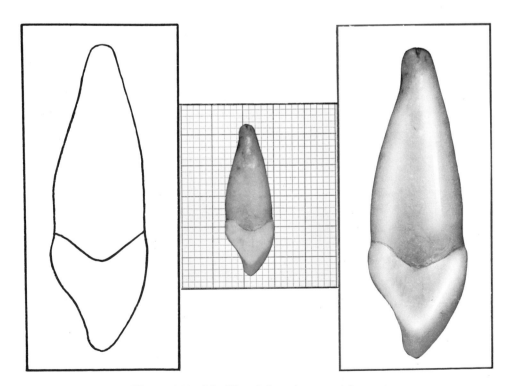

Figure 178. Maxillary left canine—mesial aspect.

The root may curve labially toward the apical third. The labial outline of the root may be almost perpendicular, with most of the taper appearing on the lingual side (Fig. 184, specimens 4 and 9).

The position of the tip of the cusp in relation to the long axis of the root is different from that of maxillary central and lateral incisors. Although the specimen illustrations in Figures 178 and 179 do not illustrate this difference, the specimens shown in Figure 184 show it conclusively. A line bisecting the cusp is labial to a line bisecting the root. Lines bisecting the roots of central and lateral incisors also bisect the incisal ridges.

The mesial surface of the canine crown presents convexities at all points except for a small circumscribed area above the contact area, where the surface is concave or flat between that area and the cervical line.

The mesial surface of the root appears broad, with a shallow developmental depression for part of the root length. Developmental depressions on the roots help to anchor the teeth in the alveoli and help to prevent rotation and displacement.

Distal Aspect (Fig. 179)

The distal aspect of the maxillary canine shows somewhat the same form as the mesial aspect, with the following variations: The cervical line exhibits less curvature toward the cusp ridge; the distal marginal ridge is heavier and more irregular in outline; the surface displays more concavity, usually, above the contact area, and the developmental depression on the distal side of the root is more pronounced.

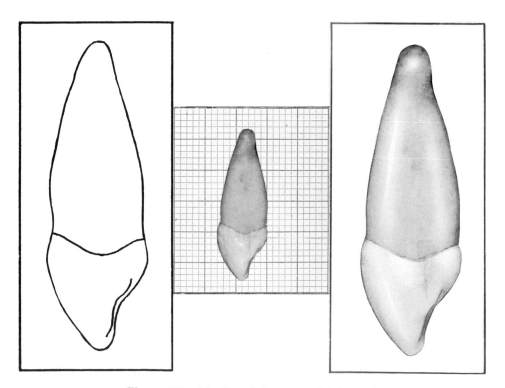

Figure 179.   Maxillary left canine – distal aspect.

Incisal Aspect (Figs. 180, 181, 182, 185)

The incisal aspect of the maxillary canine emphasizes the proportions of this tooth mesiodistally and labiolingually. In general, the labiolingual dimension is greater than the mesiodistal. Occasionally the two measurements are about equal (Fig. 185, specimen 8). Other instances appear with the crown larger than usual in a labiolingual direction (Fig. 185, specimen 10).

From the incisal aspect, if the tooth is correctly posed so that the long axis of the root is directly in the line of vision, the tip of the cusp is labial to the center of the crown labiolingually and mesial to the center mesiodistally.

If the tooth were to be sectioned labiolingually, beginning at the center of the cusp of the crown, the two sections would show the root rather evenly bisected, with the mesial portion carrying a narrower portion of the crown mesiodistally than that carried by the distal section of the tooth. (Note the proportions demonstrated by the fracture line in the enamel of specimen 9, Fig. 185.) Nevertheless, the mesial section shows a crown portion with greater labiolingual bulk. The crown of this tooth gives the impression of having all of the distal portion extended to make contact with the first premolar.

The ridge of the middle labial lobe is very noticeable labially from the incisal aspect. It attains its greatest convexity at the cervical third of the crown, becoming broader and flatter at the middle and incisal thirds.

The cingulum development makes up the cervical third of the crown lingually. The outline of the cingulum may be described by a shorter arc than the one labially

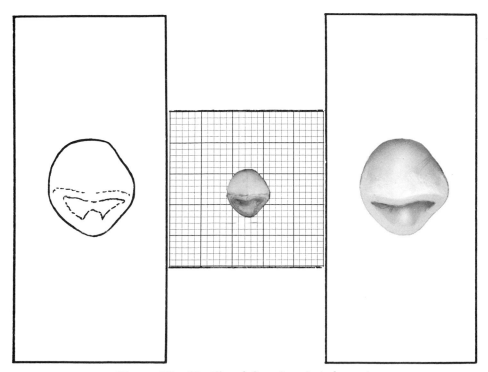

Figure 180.   Maxillary left canine—incisal aspect.

(Text continued on page 172.)

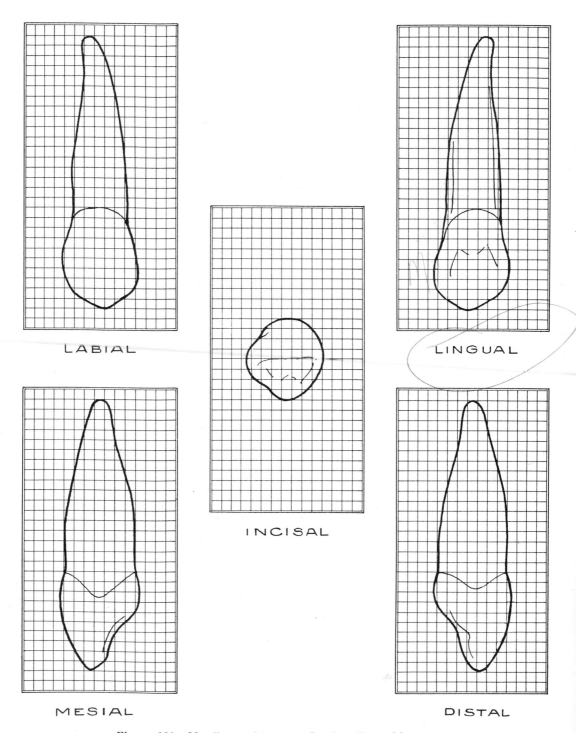

LABIAL

INCISAL

LINGUAL

MESIAL

DISTAL

Figure 181.   Maxillary right canine. Graph outlines of five aspects.

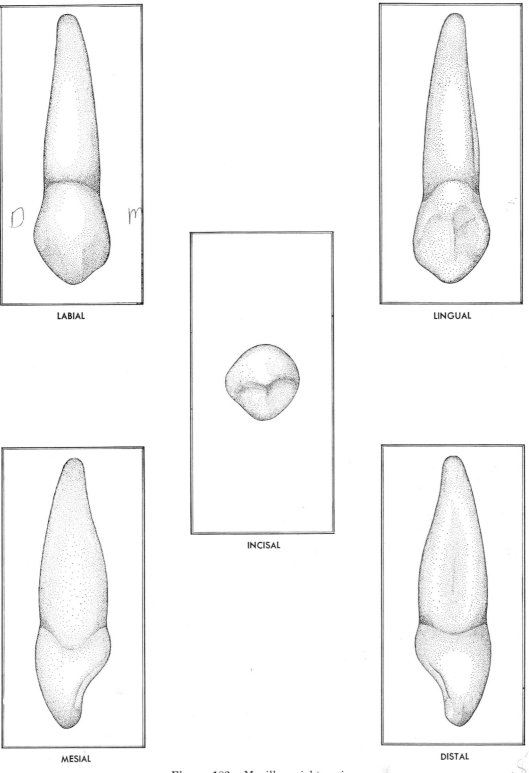

Figure 182. Maxillary right canine.

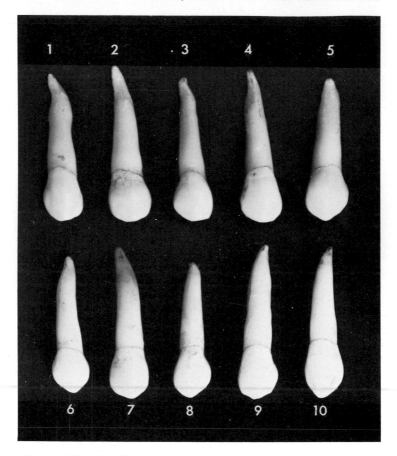

Figure 183.   Maxillary canine—ten typical specimens—labial aspect.

from this aspect. This comparison coincides with the relative mesiodistal dimensions of the root lingually and labially.

A line bisecting the cusp and cusp ridges drawn in a mesiodistal direction is almost straight and bisects the short arcs representative of the mesial and distal contact areas. This fact emphasizes the close relation between maxillary canines and some lateral incisors, since they resemble each other in this characteristic (compare specimen 7, Fig. 185, with specimen 1, Fig. 150, Chapter VI). As was mentioned in Chapter VI, there are two types of maxillary lateral incisors: Some resemble canines from the incisal aspect and some resemble central incisors. The latter are supposed to be in the majority. Naturally the lateral incisors that resemble canines are those which are relatively wide labiolingually, and those that resemble central incisors are those which are narrow in that direction.

The incisal aspect of most canines, maxillary or mandibular, may be outlined in many cases by a series of arcs. Specimen 6, Figure 185, for example, could be drawn almost perfectly with the aid of a "French curve," a drawing instrument used by draftsmen to draw arcs of varying degrees.

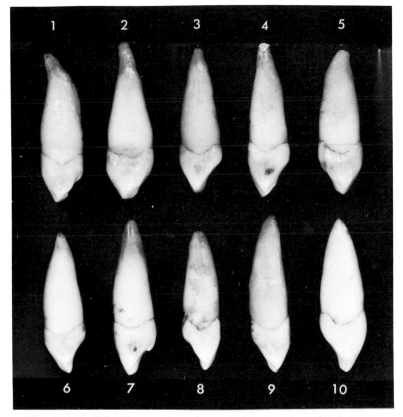

Figure 184.   Maxillary canine—ten typical specimens—mesial aspect.

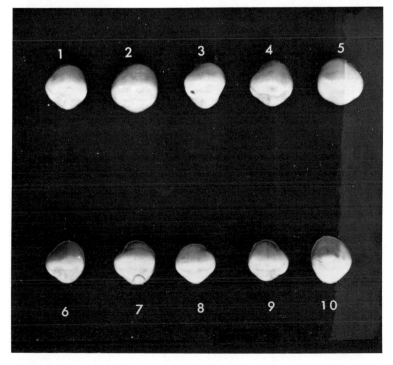

Figure 185.   Maxillary canine—ten typical specimens—incisal aspect.

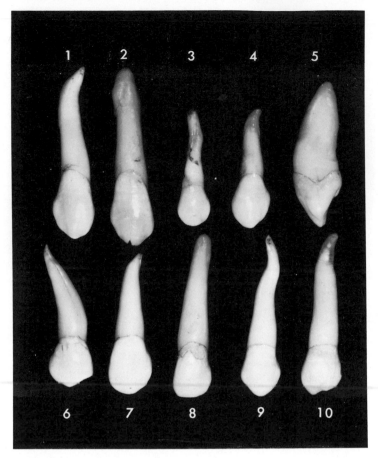

Figure 186. Specimens of maxillary canine—variations. 1, Crown extremely long, with extreme mesial curvature at apical third of the root. 2, Entire tooth unusually long. Note hypercementosis at root end. 3, Very short crown, root small and malformed. 4, Mesiodistal dimension of crown at contact area extreme, calibration at cervix narrow in comparison; root short for crown of this size. 5, Extreme labiolingual calibration, root with unusual curvature. 6, Tooth malformed generally. 7, Large crown, short root. 8, Root overdeveloped and very blunt at apex. 9, Odd curvature to root, extra length. 10, Crown poorly formed, root extra long.

MANDIBULAR CANINE

Because maxillary and mandibular canines bear a close resemblance to each other, direct comparisons will be made with the maxillary canine in describing the mandibular canine.

MANDIBULAR CANINE

First evidence of calcification	4 to 5 years
Enamel completed	6 to 7 years
Eruption	9 to 10 years
Root completed	12 to 14 years

Measurement Table

	Cervico-incisal Length of Crown	Length of Root	Mesiodistal Diameter of Crown	Mesiodistal Diameter of Crown at Cervix	Labio- or Bucco-lingual Diameter of Crown	Labio- or Bucco-lingual Diameter of Crown at Cervix	Curvature of Cervical Line— Mesial	Curvature of Cervical Line— Distal
Dimensions suggested for carving technic	11.0*	16.0	7.0	5.5	7.5	7.0	2.5	1.0

* Millimeters.

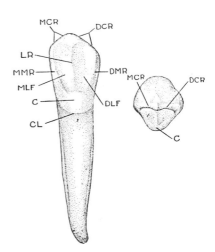

Figure 187. Mandibular right canine—lingual aspect—incisal aspect. *DCR,* Distal cusp ridge; *DMR,* distal marginal ridge; *DLF,* distolingual fossa; *CL,* cervical line; *C,* cingulum; *MLF,* mesiolingual fossa; *MMR,* mesial marginal ridge; *LR,* lingual ridge; *MCR,* mesial cusp ridge.

The mandibular canine crown is narrower mesiodistally than that of the maxillary canine, although it is just as long in most instances and in many instances is longer by 0.5 to 1 mm. The root may be as long as the maxillary canine, but usually it is somewhat shorter. The labiolingual diameter of crown and root is usually a fraction of a millimeter less.

The lingual surface of the crown is smoother, with less cingulum development and less bulk to the marginal ridges. The lingual portion of this crown resembles the form of the lingual surfaces of mandibular lateral incisors.

The cusp of the mandibular canine is not so well developed as that of the maxillary canine, and the cusp ridges are thinner labiolingually. Usually the cusp tip is on a line with the center of the root, from the mesial or distal aspect, but sometimes it lies lingual to the line.

A variation in the form of the mandibular canine is *bifurcated* roots. This variation is not rare (Fig. 198, specimens 1, 2, 5 and 6).

Detailed Description of Mandibular Canine from All Aspects

Labial Aspect (Figs. 188 and 195)

The mesiodistal dimensions of the mandibular canine are less than those of the maxillary canine. The difference is usually about 1 mm. The mandibular canine is

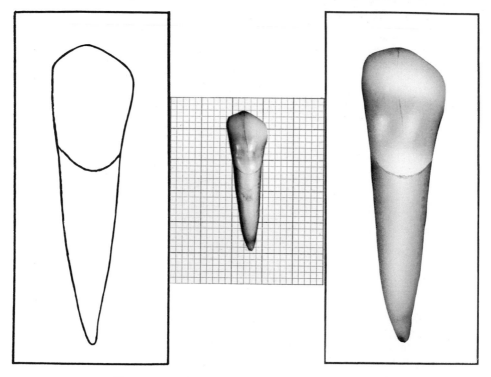

Figure 188.   Mandibular left canine—labial aspect.

broader mesiodistally than either of the mandibular incisors; for example, about 1 mm. wider than the mandibular lateral incisor.

The essential differences between mandibular and maxillary canines viewed from the labial aspect may be described as follows:

The crowns of the mandibular canines *appear* longer. Sometimes they are longer, but the effect of greater length is emphasized by the narrowness of the crown mesiodistally and the height of the contact areas above the cervix.

The mesial outline of the crown of the mandibular canine is nearly straight with the mesial outline of the root, the mesial contact area being near the mesioincisal angle.

When the cusp ridges have not been affected by wear, the cusp angle is on a line with the center of the root, as on the maxillary canine. The mesial cusp ridge is the shorter.

The distal contact area of the mandibular canine is more toward the incisal than that of the maxillary canine.

The cervical line labially has a semicircular curvature apically.

Many mandibular canines give the impression from this aspect of being bent distally on the root base. The maxillary canine crowns are more likely to be in line with the root.

The mandibular canine root is shorter by 1 or 2 mm. on the average than that of the maxillary canine, and its apical end is more sharply pointed. When curvature of root ends is present, it is often in a mesial direction. (Fig. 195, specimens 1, 2, 3, 4.)

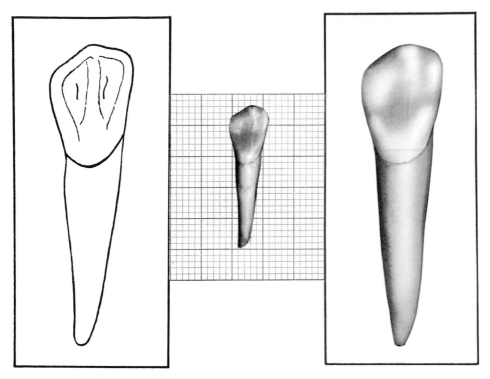

Figure 189.   Mandibular left canine — lingual aspect.

Lingual Aspect (Fig. 189)

In comparing the lingual aspect of the mandibular canine with the maxillary canine the following differences are noted:

The lingual surface of the crown of the mandibular canine is flatter, simulating the lingual surfaces of mandibular incisors. The cingulum is smooth and poorly developed. The marginal ridges are less distinct. This is true also of the lingual ridge except toward the cusp tip, where it is raised. Generally speaking, the lingual surface of the crown is smooth and regular.

The lingual portion of the root is narrower relatively than that of the maxillary canine. It narrows down to little more than half the width of the labial portion.

Mesial Aspect (Figs. 190 and 196)

The characteristic differences between the two teeth in question from the mesial aspect are as follows:

The mandibular canine has less curvature labially on the crown, with very little curvature directly above the cervical line. The curvature at the cervical portion is, as a rule, less than 0.5 mm.

The lingual outline of the crown is curved in the same manner as that of the maxillary canine, but it differs in degree. The cingulum is not so pronounced, and the incisal portion of the crown is thinner labiolingually, which allows the cusp to appear

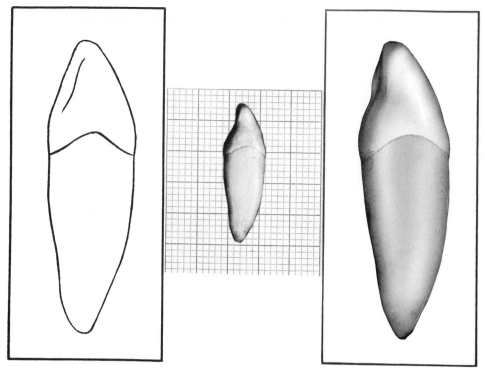

Figure 190.   Mandibular left canine—mesial aspect.

more pointed and the cusp ridge more slender. The tip of the cusp is more nearly centered over the root, with a lingual placement in some cases comparable to the placement of incisal ridges on mandibular incisors.

The cervical line curves more toward the incisal portion than does the cervical line on the maxillary canine.

The roots of the two teeth are quite similar from the mesial aspect, with the possible exception of a more pointed root tip. The developmental depression mesially on the root of the mandibular canine is more pronounced and sometimes quite deep.

Distal Aspect (Fig. 191)

There is little difference from the distal aspect between mandibular and maxillary canines except those features mentioned under *mesial aspect,* which are common to both.

Incisal Aspect (Figs. 192 and 197)

The outlines of the crowns of mandibular and maxillary canines from the incisal aspect are often similar. The main differences are these:

The mesiodistal dimension of the mandibular canine is less than the labiolingual dimension. In this, there is a similarity, but the outlines of the mesial surface is less curved. The cusp tip and mesial cusp ridge are more likely to be inclined in a lingual direction, in the mandibular canine with the distal cusp ridge and the contact area extension distinctly so. It will be remembered that the cusp ridges of the maxillary canine with the contact area extensions were more nearly in a straight line mesiodistally from the incisal aspect.

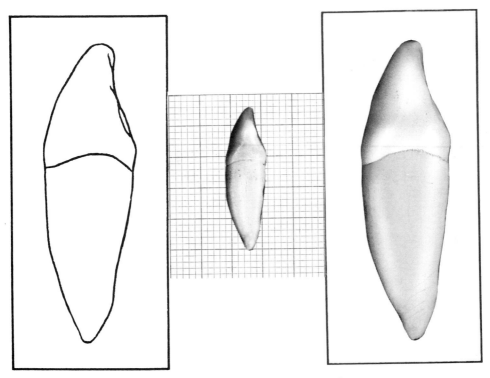

Figure 191. Mandibular left canine — distal aspect.

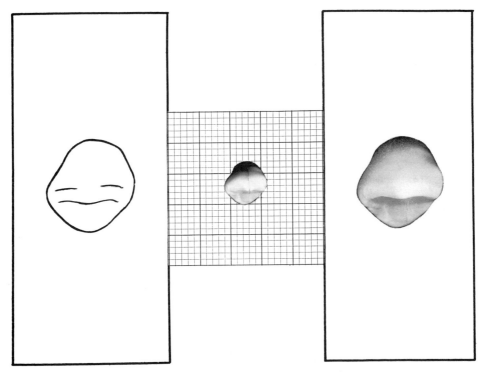

Figure 192. Mandibular left canine — incisal aspect.

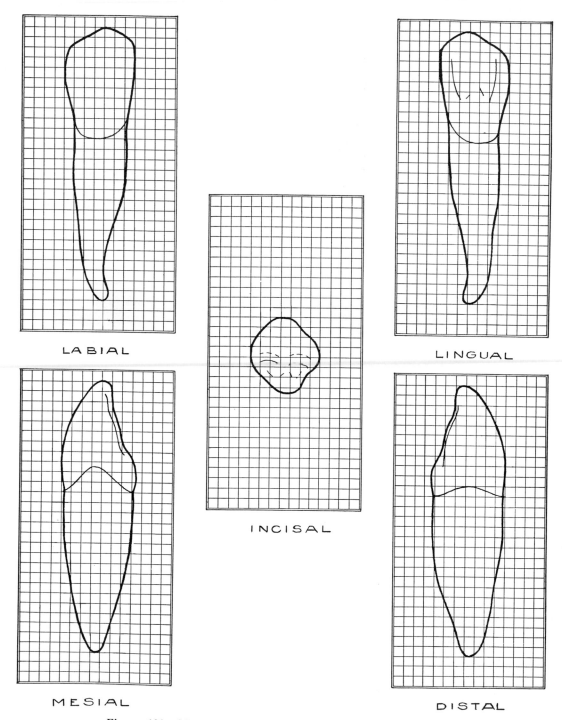

Figure 193.   Mandibular right canine. Graph outlines of five aspects.

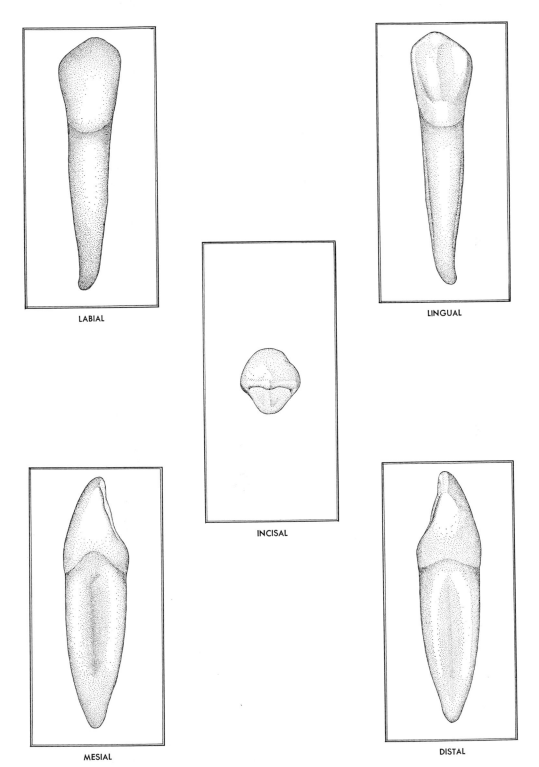

LABIAL

LINGUAL

INCISAL

MESIAL

DISTAL

Figure 194: Maxillary right canine.

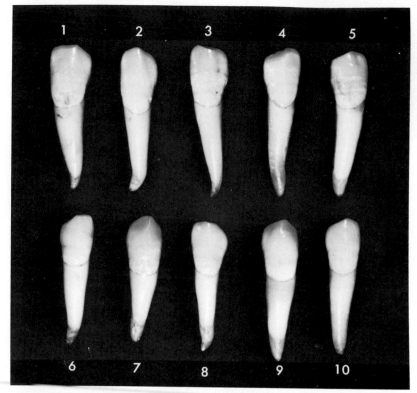

Figure 195.   Mandibular canine—ten typical specimens—labial aspect.

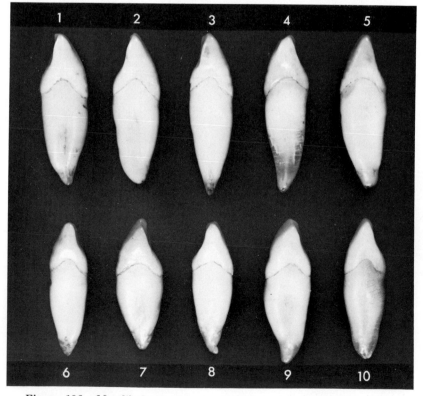

Figure 196.   Mandibular canine—ten typical specimens—mesial aspect.

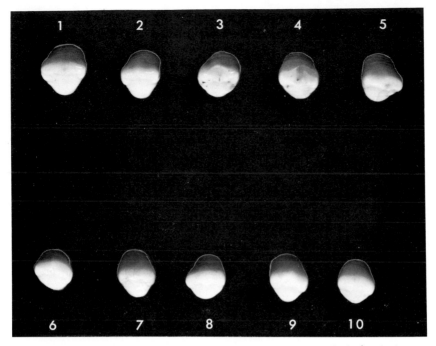

Figure 197. Mandibular canine — ten typical specimens — incisal aspect.

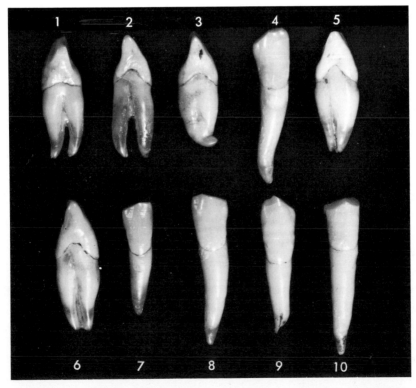

Figure 198. Specimens of mandibular canine — variations. 1, Well-formed crown; two roots, one lingual and one labial. 2, Same as specimen 1, with longer roots. 3, Well-formed crown portion, poorly formed root. 4, Root longer than average, with extreme curvature. 5, Deep developmental groove dividing the root. 6, Same as specimen 5. 7, Crown resembling mandibular lateral incisor, root short. 8, Root extra long, with odd mesial curvature starting at cervical third. 9, Crown extra long and irregular in outline. Root short and poorly formed at apex. 10, Crown with straight mesial and distal sides, wide at cervix, with a root of extreme length.

183

Chapter IX

THE PERMANENT
MAXILLARY PREMOLARS

THE MAXILLARY premolars are four in number: two in the right maxilla and two in the left maxilla. They are posterior to the canines and immediately anterior to the molars.

The premolars are so named because they are anterior to the molars in the permanent dentition. In zoology, the premolars are those teeth which succeed the deciduous molars regardless of the number to be succeeded. The term *bicuspid,* which is widely used when one describes human teeth, presupposes two cusps, a supposition which makes the term misleading, since mandibular premolars in the human subject may show a variation in the number of cusps from one to three. Among Carnivora, in the study of comparative dental anatomy, premolar forms differ so greatly that a more descriptive single term than premolar is out of the question. Since the term *premolar* is the one most widely used by all sciences interested in dental anatomy, human and comparative, it is the one which will be given preference here.

The maxillary premolars are developed from the same number of lobes as anterior teeth, which is four. The primary difference in development is the well-formed lingual cusp, developed from the lingual lobe, which is represented by the cingulum development on incisors and canines. The middle buccal lobe on the premolars, corresponding to the middle labial lobe of the canines, remains highly developed, the maxillary premolars resembling the canines when viewed from the buccal aspect. The buccal cusp of the maxillary first premolar, especially, is long and sharp, assisting the canine as a prehensile or tearing tooth. The mandibular first premolar assists the mandibular canine in the same manner.

The *second* premolars, both maxillary and mandibular, have cusps less sharp than the others, and their cusps intercusp with opposing teeth when the jaws are brought together; this makes them more efficient as grinding teeth and they function much like the molars.

The maxillary premolar crowns are shorter than those of the maxillary canines, and the roots are shorter also. The root lengths resemble those of the molars. The crowns are a little longer than those of the molars.

Because of the cusp development buccally and lingually, the marginal ridges are in a more horizontal plane and are considered part of the occlusal surface of the crown rather than of the lingual surface, as in the case of incisors and canines.

When premolars have two roots, one is placed buccally and one lingually.

MAXILLARY FIRST PREMOLAR

Maxillary First Premolar

First evidence of calcification .... 1½ to   1¾ years
Enamel completed ....   5 to 6   years
Eruption .... 10 to 11   years
Root completed .... 12 to 13   years

Measurement Table

	Cervico-occlusal Length of Crown	Length of Root	Mesio-distal Diam-eter of Crown	Mesio-distal Diam-eter of Crown at Cervix	Labio- or Bucco-lingual Diameter of Crown	Labio- or Bucco-lingual Diameter at Cervix	Curvature of Cervical Line— Mesial	Curvature of Cervical Line— Distal
Dimensions suggested for carving technic	8.5*	14.0	7.0	5.0	9.0	8.0	1.0	0.0

* Millimeters.

The maxillary first premolar has two cusps, a buccal and a lingual, each being sharply defined. The buccal cusp is usually about 1 mm. longer than the lingual cusp. The crown is angular and the buccal line angles prominent.

The crown is shorter than the canine by 1.5 to 2 mm. on the average. Although this tooth resembles the canine from the buccal aspect, it differs in that the contact areas mesially and distally are at about the same level. The root is shorter. If the buccal cusp form has not been changed by wear, the mesial slope of the cusp is longer than the distal slope. The opposite arrangement is true of the maxillary canine. Generally the first premolar is not so wide in a mesiodistal direction as the canine.

Most maxillary first premolars have two roots (Fig. 208) and two pulp canals. When only one root is present, two pulp canals are usually found anyway.

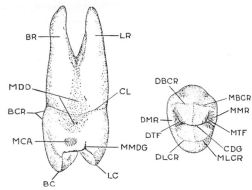

Figure 199. Maxillary right first premolar—mesial aspect and occlusal aspect. *LR*, lingual root; *CL*, cervical line; *MMDG*, mesial marginal developmental groove; *LC*, lingual cusp; *BC*, buccal cusp; *MCA*, mesial contact area; *BCR*, buccal cervical ridge; *MDD*, mesial developmental depression; *BR*, buccal root; *MBCR*, mesiobuccal cusp ridge; *MMR*, mesial marginal ridge; *MTF*, mesial triangular fossa (shaded area); *CDG*, central developmental groove; *MLCR*, mesiolingual cusp ridge; *DLCR*, distolingual cusp ridge; *DTF*, distal triangular fossa; *DMR*, distal marginal ridge; *DBCR*, distobuccal cusp ridge.

The maxillary first premolar has some characteristics common to all posterior teeth. Briefly, these characteristics as differentiated from those of anterior teeth are as follows:

1. Greater relative faciolingual measurement as compared with the mesiodistal measurement.

2. Broader contact areas.

3. Contact areas more nearly at the same level.

4. Less curvature of the cervical line from all aspects.

5. Shorter crown, cervico-occlusally in posterior teeth when compared with anterior teeth.

Detailed Description of the Maxillary First Premolar from All Aspects

Buccal Aspect (Figs. 200, 205, 206 and 207)

From this aspect the crown is roughly trapezoidal (Chapter IV, Fig. 102, *c*). The crown exhibits little curvature at the cervical line. The crest of curvature of the cervical line buccally is near the center of the root buccally.

The mesial outline of the crown is slightly concave from the cervical line to the mesial contact area. The contact area is represented by a relatively broad curvature, the crest of which lies immediately occlusal to the halfway point from the cervical line to the tip of the buccal cusp.

The mesial slope of the buccal cusp is rather straight and longer than the distal slope, which is shorter and more curved. This arrangement places the tip of the buccal cusp distal to a line bisecting the buccal surface of the crown. The mesial slope of the buccal cusp is sometimes notched; in other instances a concave outline is noted at this point (Fig. 207, specimens 7, 9 and 10).

The distal outline of the crown below the cervical line is straighter than that of the mesial, although it may be somewhat concave also. The distal contact area is represented by a broader curvature than is found mesially, and the crest of curvature of the contact area tends to be a little more occlusal when the tooth is posed with its long axis vertical. Even so, the contact areas are more nearly level with each other than those found on anterior teeth.

The width of the crown of the maxillary first premolar mesiodistally is about 2 mm. less at the cervix than at its width at the points of its greatest mesiodistal measurement.

The buccal cusp is long, coming to a pointed tip and resembling the canine in this respect.

The buccal surface of the crown is convex, showing strong development of the middle buccal lobe. The continuous ridge from cusp tip to cervical margin on the buccal surface of the crown is called the *buccal ridge*.

Mesial and distal to the buccal ridge, at or occlusal to the middle third, developmental depressions are usually seen which serve as demarcations between the middle buccal lobe and the mesio- and distobuccal lobes. Although the latter lobes show less development, they are nevertheless prominent and serve to emphasize strong mesiobuccal and distobuccal line angles on the crown (Chapter IV, Fig. 98, *e*).

The roots are 3 or 4 mm. shorter than those of the maxillary canine, although the outline of the buccal portion of the root form bears a close resemblance.

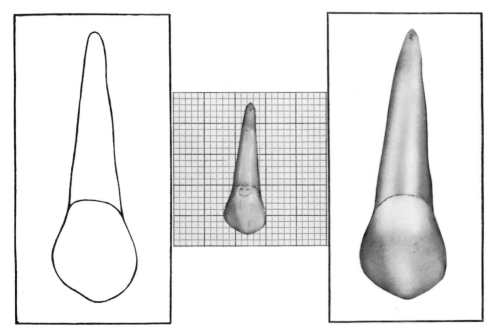

Figure 200. Maxillary left first premolar—buccal aspect.

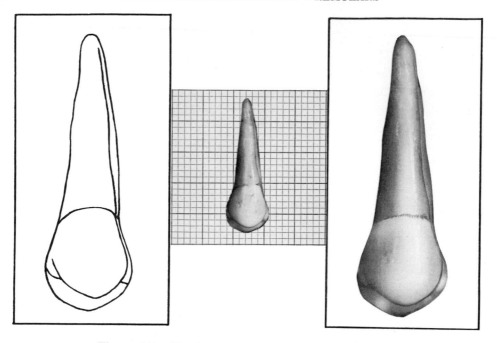

Figure 201. Maxillary left first premolar — lingual aspect.

Lingual Aspect (Figs. 201, 205 and 206)

From the lingual aspect, the gross outline of the maxillary first premolar is the reverse of the gross outline of the buccal aspect.

The crown tapers toward the lingual, since the lingual cusp is narrower mesiodistally than the buccal cusp. The lingual cusp is smooth and spheroidal from the cervical portion to the area near the cusp tip. The cusp tip is pointed, with mesial and distal slopes meeting at an angle of about 90 degrees.

Naturally the spheroidal form of the lingual portion of the crown is convex at all points. Sometimes the crest of the smooth lingual portion which terminates at the point of the lingual cusp is called the *lingual ridge*.

The mesial and distal outlines of the lingual portion of the crown are convex, these outlines being continuous with the mesial and distal slopes of the lingual cusp, straightening out as they join the mesial and distal sides of the lingual root at the cervical line.

The cervical line lingually is regular, with slight curvature toward the root and the crest of curvature centered on the root. Since the lingual portion of the crown is narrower than the buccal portion, it is possible to see part of the mesial and distal surfaces of crown and root from the lingual aspect, according to the posing of the tooth and the line of vision.

Since the lingual cusp is not so long as the buccal cusp, the tips of both cusps, with their mesial and distal slopes, may be seen from the lingual aspect.

The lingual portion of the root, or the lingual portion of the lingual root if two roots are present, is smooth and convex at all points. The apex of the lingual root of a two-root specimen tends to be more blunt than the buccal root apex.

Mesial Aspect (Figs. 202, 205, 206 and 208)

The mesial aspect of the crown of the maxillary first premolar is also roughly trapezoidal. However, the longest of the uneven sides is toward the cervical portion and the shortest toward the occlusal portion (Chapter IV, Fig. 102,e).

Another characteristic which is representative of all posterior maxillary teeth is that the tips of the cusps are well within the confines of the root trunk (for a definition of root trunk, see Figures 246, 251 and also the Glossary). That is, the measurement from the tip of the buccal cusp to the tip of the lingual cusp is less than the buccolingual measurement of the root at the cervix.

Most maxillary first premolars have two roots, one buccal and one lingual; these are clearly outlined from the mesial aspect.

The cervical line may be regular in outline (Fig. 208, specimen 1) or irregular (Fig. 208, specimen 4). In either case the curvature occlusally is less (about 1 mm. on the average) than the cervical curvature on the mesial of any of the anterior teeth. The extent of the curvature of the cervical line mesially on these teeth is constant within a fraction of a millimeter and is similar to the average curvature to the mesial of all posterior teeth.

The buccal outline of the crown from the mesial aspect curves outward below the cervical line; the crest of curvature is often located approximately at the junction of cervical and middle thirds. Or the crest of curvature may be located within the cervical third (Fig. 208, specimens 1 and 10). From the crest of curvature the buccal outline continues as a line of less convexity to the tip of the buccal cusp, which is directly below the center of the buccal root (when two roots are present).

The lingual outline of the crown may be described as a smoothly curved line starting at the cervical line and ending at the tip of the lingual cusp. The crest of this curvature is most often near the center of the middle third. Some specimens show a more abrupt curvature at the cervical third (Fig. 208, specimens 2 and 9).

The tip of the lingual cusp is on a line, in most cases, with the lingual border of the lingual root. The lingual cusp is always shorter than the buccal cusp, the average difference being about 1 mm. This difference, however, may be greater (Fig. 208, specimens 1, 4 and 10). From this aspect it is noted that the cusps of the maxillary first premolar are long and sharp, with the mesial marginal ridge at about the level of the junction of the middle and occlusal thirds.

A distinguishing feature of this tooth is found on the mesial surface of the crown. Immediately cervical to the mesial contact area, centered on the mesial surface, is a marked depression, which continues up to and includes the cervical line (Fig. 199). This *mesial developmental depression* is bordered buccally and lingually by the mesiobuccal and mesiolingual line angles. The concavity continues upward beyond the cervical line, joining a deep developmental depression between the roots which ends at the root bifurcation. On single-root specimens, the concavity on the crown and root is plainly seen also, although it may not be so deeply marked. Maxillary second premolars do not have this feature.

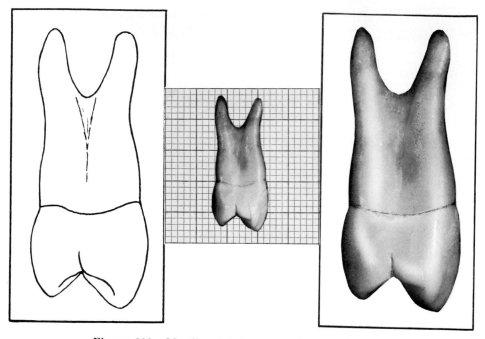

Figure 202.   Maxillary left first premolar—mesial aspect.

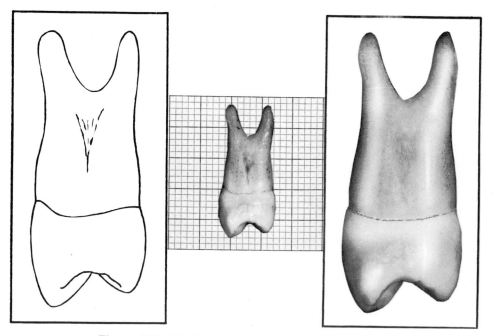

Figure 203.   Maxillary left first premolar—distal aspect.

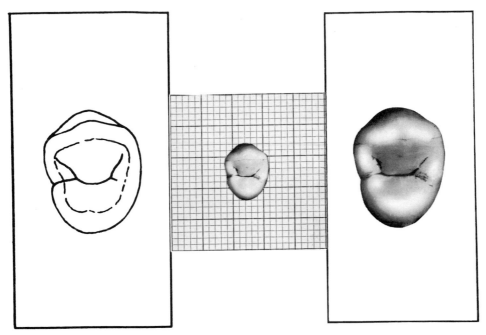

Figure 204. Maxillary left first premolar—occlusal aspect.

Another distinguishing feature of the maxillary first premolar is a well-defined developmental groove in the enamel of the mesial marginal ridge. This groove is in alignment with the developmental depression on the mesial surface of the root but is not usually connected with it. This marginal groove is continuous with the central groove of the occlusal surface of the crown, crossing the marginal ridge immediately lingual to the mesial contact area and terminating a short distance cervical to the mesial marginal ridge on the mesial surface (Fig. 208, specimen 10).

The buccal outline of the buccal root, above the cervical line, is straight, with a tendency toward a lingual inclination. On those buccal roots which have a buccal inclination above the root bifurcation, the outline may be relatively straight up to the apical portion of the buccal root, or it may curve buccally at the middle third. Buccal roots may take a buccal or lingual inclination, apical to middle thirds.

The lingual outline of the lingual root is rather straight above the cervical line. It may not exhibit much curvature between the cervix and the apex. Many cases, however, show considerable curvature to lingual roots apical to the middle thirds. It may take a buccal or lingual inclination (Fig. 208, specimens 1, 2 and 9).

The root trunk is long on this tooth, making up about half of the root length. The bifurcation on those teeth with two roots begins at a more occlusal point mesially than distally. Generally speaking, when bifurcated, the root is bifurcated for half its total length.

Except for the deep developmental groove and depression at or below the bifurcation, the mesial surface of the root portion of this tooth is smoothly convex buccally and lingually. Even when one root only is present, the developmental depression is very noticeable for most of the root length. The latter instances show roots with

(Text continued on page 195.)

INDIVIDUAL TOOTH FORM

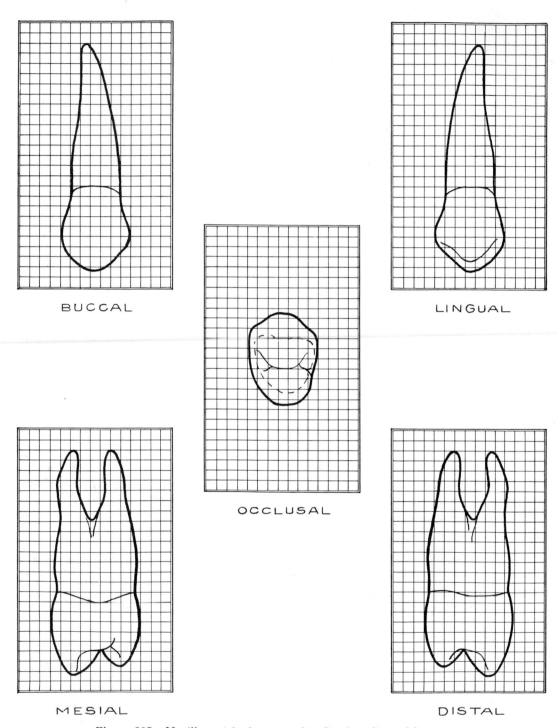

BUCCAL

LINGUAL

OCCLUSAL

MESIAL

DISTAL

Figure 205.   Maxillary right first premolar. Graph outlines of five aspects.

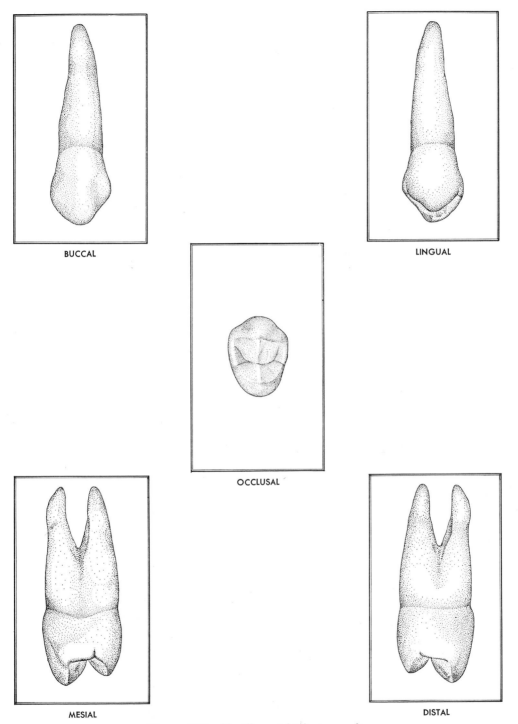

BUCCAL

LINGUAL

OCCLUSAL

MESIAL

DISTAL

Figure 206. Maxillary right first premolar.

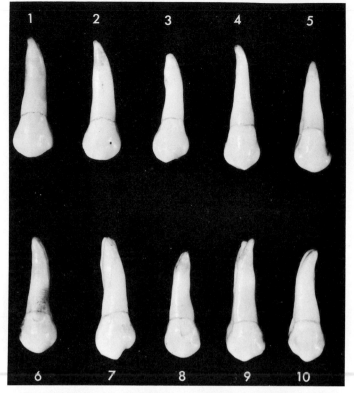

Figure 207.   Maxillary first premolars — ten typical specimens — buccal aspect.

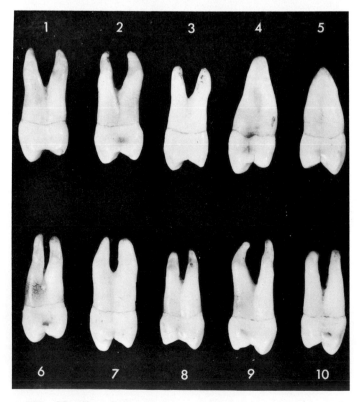

Figure 208.   Maxillary first premolars — ten typical specimens — mesial aspect.

buccal and lingual outlines ending in a blunt apex above the center of the crown (Fig. 208, specimens 4 and 5).

Distal Aspect

From the distal aspect the anatomy of crown and root of the maxillary first premolar differs from that of the mesial aspect as follows.

The crown surface is convex at all points except for a small flattened area just cervical to the contact area and buccal to the center of the distal surface.

The curvature of the cervical line is less on the distal than on the mesial surface, often showing a line straight across from buccal to lingual.

There is no evidence of a deep developmental groove crossing the distal marginal ridge of the crown. If a developmental groove should be noticeable, it is shallow and insignificant.

The root trunk is flattened on the distal surface above the cervical line with no outstanding developmental signs.

The bifurcation of the roots is abrupt near the apical third, with no developmental groove leading to it such as one finds mesially.

Occlusal Aspect (Figs. 204, 205, 206, 209, 211 and 212)

The occlusal aspect of the maxillary first premolar resembles roughly a six-sided or hexagonal figure (Fig. 211). The six sides are made up of the mesiobuccal

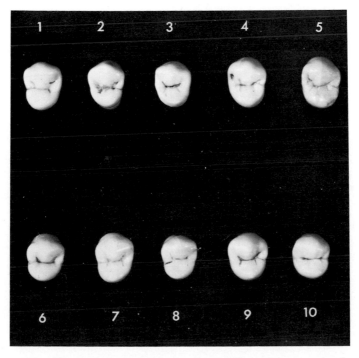

Figure 209. Maxillary first premolars—ten typical specimens—occlusal aspect.

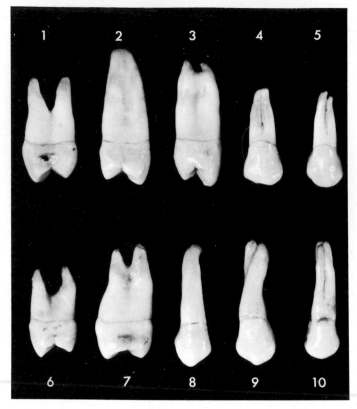

Figure 210. Maxillary first premolars—ten specimens showing uncommon variations. 1, Constricted occlusal surface, short roots. 2, Single root of extreme length. 3, Constricted occlusal surface, mesial developmental groove indistinct on mesial surface of root. 4, Short root form, with two buccal roots fused. 5, Short root form, with two buccal roots showing bifurcation. 6, Short roots, with considerable separation. 7, Buccolingual calibration greater than usual. 8, Root extremely long, distal contact area high. 9, Twisted buccal root. 10, Three roots fused; uncommonly long also.

(which is mesial to the buccal ridge), mesial, mesiolingual (which is mesial to the lingual ridge), distolingual, distal and distobuccal. This hexagonal figure is not, however, equilateral. The two buccal sides are nearly equal, the mesial side is shorter than the distal side and the mesiolingual side is shorter than the distolingual side (Fig. 211).

The relation and position of various anatomic points are to be considered from the occlusal aspect. A drawing of the outline of this occlusal aspect, when placed within a rectangle the dimensions of which represent the mesiodistal and buccolingual width of the crown, demonstrates the relative positions of the mesial and distal contact areas and also those of the buccal and lingual ridges (Fig. 212). (See also Fig. 204.)

The crest of the distal contact area is somewhat buccal to that of the mesial contact area, and the crest of the buccal ridge is somewhat distal to that of the

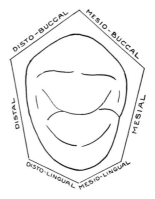

Figure 211. Maxillary first premolar—hexagonal figure—occlusal aspect.

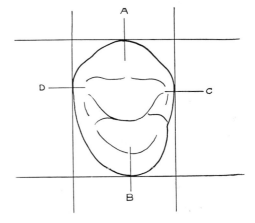

Figure 212. Maxillary first premolar—occlusal aspect. *A*, crest of buccal ridge. *B*, crest of lingual ridge. *C*, crest of mesial contact area. *D*, crest of distal contact area.

lingual ridge. The crests of curvature represent the highest points on the buccal and lingual ridges and the mesial and distal contact areas.

Close observation of the crown from this aspect reveals the following characteristics (Fig. 212).

1. The distance from the buccal crest (*A*) to the mesial crest (*C*) is slightly longer than the distance from the buccal crest to the distal crest (*D*).

2. The distance from the mesial crest to the lingual crest is much shorter than the distance from the distal crest to the lingual crest.

3. The crown is wider on the buccal than on the lingual.

4. The buccolingual dimension of the crown is much greater than the mesiodistal dimension.

The occlusal surface of the maxillary first premolar is circumscribed by the cusp ridges and marginal ridges. The mesiobuccal and distobuccal cusp ridges are in line with each other, and their alignment is in a distobuccal direction. In other words, even though they are in the same alignment, the distobuccal cusp ridge is buccal to the mesiobuccal cusp ridge (Fig. 213).

The angle formed by the convergence of the mesiobuccal cusp ridge and the

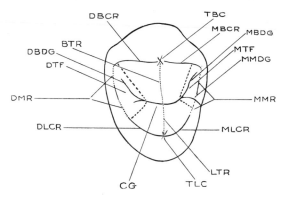

Figure 213. Maxillary first premolar—occlusal aspect. *TBC,* tip of buccal cusp; *MBCR,* mesiobuccal cusp ridge; *MBDG,* mesiobuccal developmental groove; *MTF,* mesial triangular fossa; *MMDG,* mesial marginal developmental groove; *MMR,* mesial marginal ridge; *MLCR,* mesiolingual cusp ridge; *LTR,* lingual triangular ridge; *TLC,* tip of lingual cusp; *CG,* central groove; *DLCR,* distolingual cusp ridge; *DMR,* distal marginal ridge; *DTF,* distal triangular fossa; *DBDG,* distobuccal developmental groove; *BTR,* buccal triangular ridge; *DBCR,* distobuccal cusp ridge. (Compare with Fig. 199.)

mesial marginal ridge approaches a right angle. The angle formed by the convergence of the distobuccal cusp ridge and the distal marginal ridge is acute. The mesiolingual and distolingual cusp ridges are confluent with the mesial and distal marginal ridges; these cusp ridges are curved, following a semicircular outline from the marginal ridges to their convergence at the tip of the lingual cusp.

When looking at the occlusal aspect of the maxillary first premolar, posing the tooth so that the line of vision is in line with the long axis, one sees more of the buccal surface of the crown than of the lingual surface. It should be remembered that when one looks at the tooth from the mesial aspect, the tip of the buccal cusp is nearer the center of the root trunk than is the lingual cusp.

The occlusal surface of this tooth has no supplemental grooves in most cases, a fact which makes the surface relatively smooth. A well-defined central developmental groove divides the surface evenly buccolingually. This groove is called the *central developmental groove.* It is located at the bottom of the central sulcus of the occlusal surface, extending from a point just mesial to the distal marginal ridge to the mesial marginal ridge, where it joins the *mesial marginal developmental groove;* this latter crosses the mesial marginal ridge and ends on the mesial surface of the crown (see "Mesial Aspect").

Two collateral developmental grooves join the central groove just inside the mesial and distal marginal ridges. These grooves are called the *mesiobuccal developmental groove* and the *distobuccal developmental groove.* The junctions of the grooves are deeply pointed and are named the *mesial* and *distal developmental pits.*

Just distal to the mesial marginal ridge, the triangular depression which harbors the mesiobuccal developmental groove is called the *mesial triangular fossa.* The depression in the occlusal surface, just mesial to the distal marginal ridge, is called the *distal triangular fossa.*

Although no supplemental grooves are present in most instances, smooth developmental depressions may be visible radiating from the central groove and giving the occlusal surface an uneven appearance.

The *buccal triangular ridge* of the buccal cusp is prominent, arising near the center of the central groove and converging with the tip of the buccal cusp. The *lingual triangular ridge* is less prominent; it also arises near the center of the central groove and converges with the tip of the lingual cusp.

The lingual cusp is pointed more sharply than the buccal cusp.

MAXILLARY SECOND PREMOLAR

Maxillary Second Premolar

First evidence of calcification .... 2 to 2¼ years
Enamel completed .... 6 to 7 years
Eruption .... 10 to 12 years
Root completed .... 12 to 14 years

Measurement Table

	Cervico-occlusal Length of Crown	Length of Root	Mesio-distal Diam-eter of Crown	Mesio-distal Diam-eter of Crown at Cervix	Labio- or Bucco-lingual Diameter of Crown	Labio- or Bucco-lingual Diameter at Cervix	Curvature of Cervical Line—Mesial	Curvature of Cervical Line—Distal
Dimensions suggested for carving technic	8.5*	14.0	7.0	5.0	9.0	8.0	1.0	0.0

* Millimeters.

The maxillary second premolar supplements the maxillary first premolar in function (Figs. 214 to 222). The two teeth resemble each other so closely that detailed description of each aspect of the second premolar will be unnecessary. Direct comparison will be made between it and the first premolar, variations being mentioned.

Compare, therefore, the accompanying illustrations of the two teeth and observe the following variations:

The maxillary second premolar is less angular, giving a more rounded effect to the crown from all aspects. It has a single root.

Considerable variations in the relative sizes of the two teeth may be seen, since the second premolar does not appear true to form as often as does the first premolar. The maxillary second premolar may have a crown which is noticeably smaller cervico-occlusally and also mesiodistally. On the other hand, it may be larger in those dimensions. Usually the root length of the second premolar is as great, if not a millimeter or so greater, than that of the first premolar. The two teeth have about the same dimensions *on the average*, except for the tendency toward greater length to the second premolar root.

From the buccal aspect it may be noticed that the buccal cusp of the second premolar is not so long as that of the first premolar, and it appears less pointed. Also, the mesial slope of the buccal cusp ridge is usually shorter than the distal slope. The opposite is true of the first premolar.

In a good many instances the crown and root are thicker at the cervix. This is not, however, the rule (Fig. 219, specimens 5, 6, 7 and 9). The buccal ridge of the crown may not be so prominent.

From the lingual aspect little variation may be seen except that the lingual cusp is longer, making the crown longer on the lingual side.

The mesial aspect shows the difference in cusp length between the two teeth. The cusps of the second premolar are shorter, with the buccal and lingual cusps more nearly the same length. There may be greater distance between cusp tips—a condition which lengthens the occlusal surface buccolingually.

There is no deep developmental depression on the mesial surface of the crown as on the first premolar; the crown surface is convex instead. A shallow developmental groove appears on the single tapered root.

There is no deep developmental groove crossing the mesial marginal ridge, and except for the variation in root form there is no outstanding variation to be noted when one views the distal aspect.

From the *occlusal* aspect, some differences are to be noted: The outline of the crown is more rounded or oval, rather than angular. There are, of course, exceptions. The central developmental groove is shorter and more irregular, and there is a tendency toward multiple supplementary grooves radiating from the central groove. These supplementary grooves terminate in shallow depressions in the enamel which may extend out to the cusp ridges.

This arrangement makes for an irregular occlusal surface and gives the surface a very wrinkled appearance.

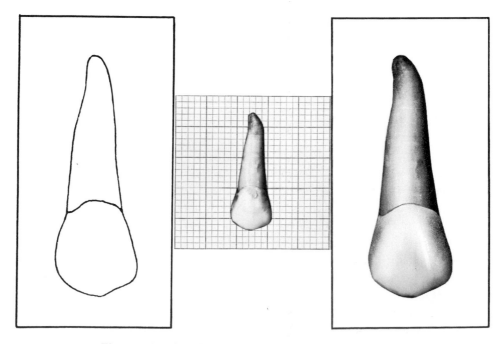

Figure 214.   Maxillary left second premolar—buccal aspect.

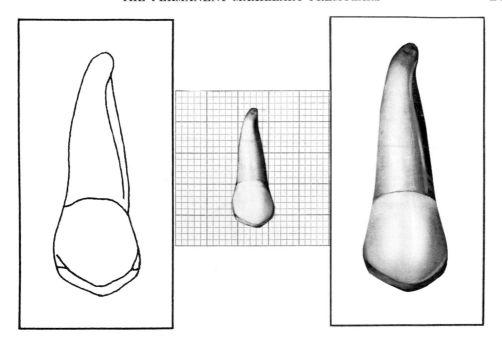

Figure 215. Maxillary left second premolar — lingual aspect.

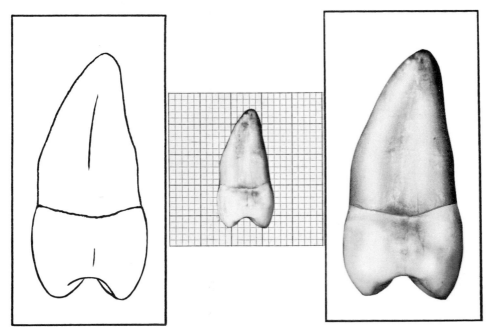

Figure 216. Maxillary left second premolar — mesial aspect.

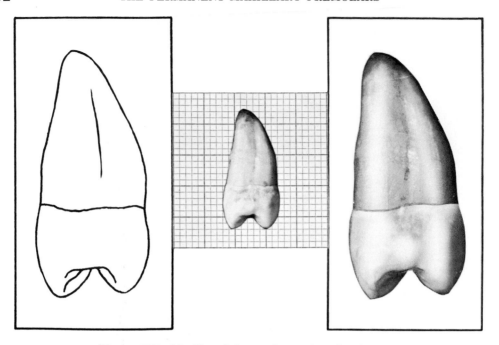

Figure 217. Maxillary left second premolar—distal aspect.

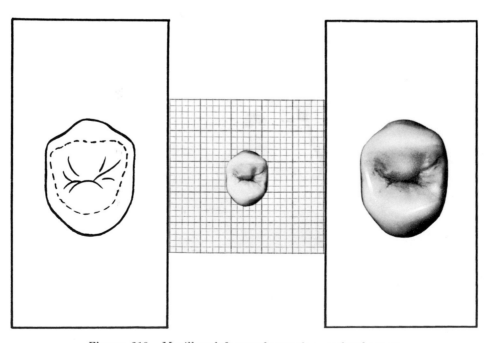

Figure 218. Maxillary left second premolar—occlusal aspect.

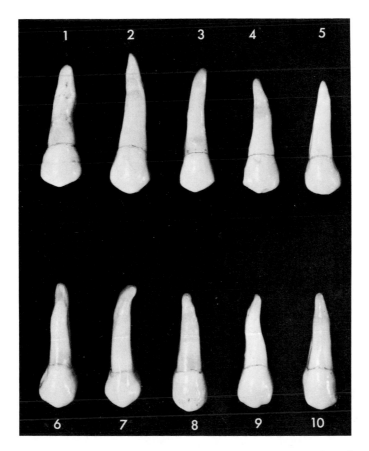

Figure 219.   Maxillary second premolars—ten typical specimens—buccal aspect.

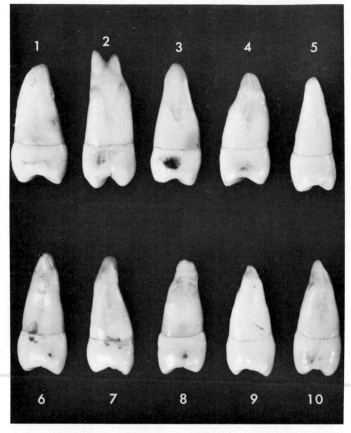

Figure 220.   Maxillary second premolars—ten typical specimens—mesial aspect.

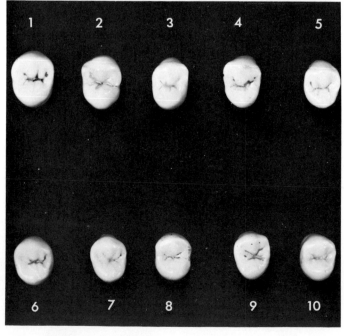

Figure 221.   Maxillary second premolars—ten typical specimens—occlusal aspect.

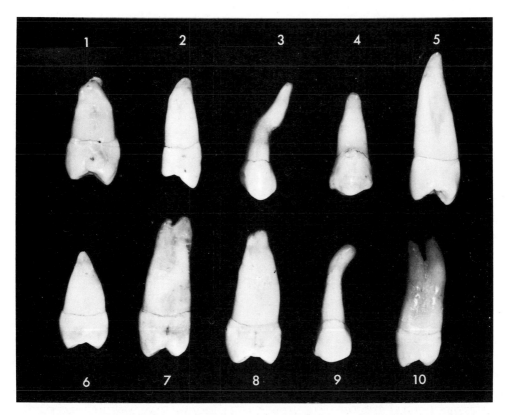

Figure 222. Maxillary second premolars—ten specimens showing uncommon variations. 1, Root dwarfed and malformed. 2, Broad occlusal surface, lingual outline of crown straight. 3, Malformed root. 4, Crown very broad mesiodistally, root dwarfed. 5, Root extremely long. 6, Root dwarfed and very pointed at apex. 7, Root extremely long, bifurcation at root end. 8, Crown wider than usual buccolingually, curvature at cervical third extreme. 9, Root malformed, thick at apical third. 10, Root unusually long, bifurcated at apical third.

Chapter X

THE PERMANENT
MANDIBULAR PREMOLARS

mand. 2nd p. molars
developed 5 lobes

THE MANDIBULAR premolars are four in number: Two are situated in the right side of the mandible and two in the left side. They are immediately posterior to the mandibular canines and anterior to the molars.

The mandibular first premolars are developed from four *lobes* as were the maxillary premolars. The mandibular second premolars are, in most instances, developed from five lobes, three buccal and two lingual lobes.

The first premolar has a large buccal *cusp,* which is long and well formed, with a small nonfunctioning lingual cusp that in some specimens is no larger than the cingulum found on some maxillary canines (Fig. 232, specimens 3 and 8; Fig. 234, specimens 4 and 7). The second premolar has three well-formed cusps in most cases, one large buccal cusp and two smaller lingual cusps. The form of both mandibular premolars fails to conform to the implications of the term "bicuspid," which term implies two functioning cusps.

The mandibular first premolar has many of the characteristics of a small canine, since its sharp buccal cusp is the only part of it occluding with maxillary teeth. It functions with the mandibular canine. The mandibular second premolar has more of the characteristics of a small molar, because its lingual cusps are well developed, a fact which places both marginal ridges high and which produces a more efficient occlusion with antagonists in the opposite jaw. It functions by being supplementary to the mandibular first molar.

The first premolar is always the smaller of the two *mandibular* premolars, whereas the opposite is true, in many cases, of the *maxillary* premolars.

MANDIBULAR FIRST PREMOLAR

The mandibular first premolar is the fourth tooth from the median line and the first posterior tooth in the mandible. This tooth is situated between the canine and second premolar and has some characteristics similar to each of them.

The characteristics which resemble those of the *mandibular canine* are as follows:

1. The buccal cusp is long and sharp and is the only occluding cusp.

2. The buccolingual measurement is similar to that of the canine.

3. The occlusal surface slopes sharply lingually in a cervical direction.

4. The mesiobuccal cusp ridge is shorter than the distobuccal cusp ridge.

5. The outline form of the occlusal aspect resembles the outline form of the incisal aspect of the canine.

Mandibular First Premolar

First evidence of calcification .... 1¾ to 2 years
Enamel completed 5   to 6 years
Eruption 10   to 12 years
Root completed 12   to 13 years

Measurement Table

	Cervico-occlusal Length of Crown	Length of Root	Mesio-distal Diameter of Crown	Mesio-distal Diameter of Crown at Cervix	Labio- or Bucco-lingual Diameter of Crown	Labio- or Bucco-lingual Diameter of Crown at Cervix	Curvature of Cervical Line—Mesial	Curvature of Cervical Line—Distal
Dimensions suggested for carving technic	8.5*	14.0	7.0	5.0	7.5	6.5	1.0	0.0

* Millimeters.

The characteristics which resemble those of the *second mandibular premolar* are as follows:

1. Except for the longer cusp, the outline of crown and root from the buccal aspect resembles the second premolar.

2. The contact areas, mesially and distally, are near the same level.

3. The curvatures of the cervical line mesially and distally are similar.

4. It has more than one cusp.

Although the root of the mandibular first premolar is shorter than that of the mandibular second premolar, it is closer to the length of the second premolar root than it is to that of the mandibular canine.

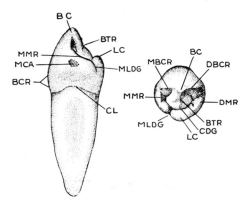

Figure 223. Mandibular right first premolar—mesial aspect and occlusal aspect. *BC*, buccal cusp; *BTR*, buccal triangular ridge; *LC*, lingual cusp; *MLDG*, mesiolingual developmental groove; *CL*, cervical line; *BCR*, buccal cervical ridge; *MCA*, mesial contact area; *MMR*, mesial marginal ridge; *BC*, buccal cusp; *DBCR*, distobuccal cusp ridge; *DMR*, distal marginal ridge; *BTR*, buccal triangular ridge; *CDG*, central developmental groove; *LC*, lingual cusp; *MLDG*, mesiolingual developmental groove; *MMR*, mesial marginal ridge; *MBCR*, mesiobuccal cusp ridge.

Detailed Description of the Mandibular First Premolar from All Aspects

Buccal Aspect (Figs. 224, 229, 230 and 231)

From the buccal aspect, the form of the mandibular first premolar crown is nearly symmetrical bilaterally. The middle buccal lobe is well developed, resulting in a large, pointed buccal cusp. The mesial cusp ridge is shorter than the distal cusp ridge. The contact areas are broad from this aspect; they are almost at the same level mesially and distally, this level being a little more than half the distance from cervical line to cusp tip. The measurement mesiodistally at the cervical line is small when it is compared with the measurement at the contact areas.

From the buccal aspect, the crown is roughly trapezoidal (Chapter IV, Fig. 102, *c*). The cervical margin is represented by the shortest of the uneven sides.

The crown exhibits little curvature at the cervical line buccally, a fact caused by the slight curvature of the cervical line on the mesial and distal surfaces of the tooth. The crest of curvature of the cervical line buccally approaches the center of the root buccally.

The mesial outline of the crown is straight or slightly concave above the cervical line to a point where it joins the curvature of the mesial contact area. The center of the contact area mesially is occlusal to the cervical line, a distance equal to a little more than half the crown length. The outline of the mesial slope of the buccal cusp usually shows some concavity unless wear has obliterated the original form.

The tip of the buccal cusp is pointed and is, in most cases, located a little mesial to the center of the crown buccally (Fig. 231, specimens 3, 7, 8 and 9). The mandibular canine has the same characteristic to a greater degree.

The distal outline of the crown is slightly concave above the cervical line to a point where it is confluent with the curvature describing the distal contact area. This curvature is broader than that describing the curvature of the mesial contact area. The distal slope of the buccal cusp usually exhibits some concavity.

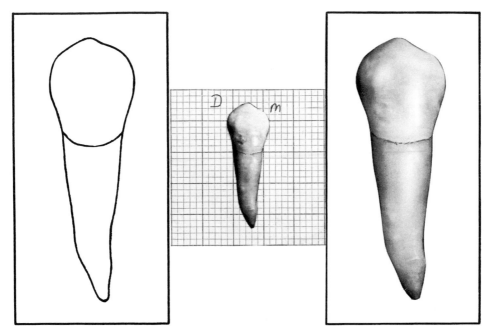

Figure 224. Mandibular right first premolar — buccal aspect.*

The cervix of the mandibular first premolar crown is narrow mesiodistally when compared with the crown width at the contact areas.

The root of this tooth is 3 or 4 mm. shorter than that of the mandibular canine, although the outline of the buccal portion of the root bears a close resemblance to the canine.

The buccal surface of the crown is more convex than in the maxillary premolars, especially at the cervical and middle thirds.

The development of the middle buccal lobe is outstanding, and it has a pointed buccal cusp. Developmental depressions are often seen between the three lobes (Fig. 231, specimens 2, 3, 8 and 10).

The continuous ridge from the cervical margin to the cusp tip is called the *buccal ridge.*

In general, the enamel of the buccal surface of the crown is smooth and shows no developmental grooves and few developmental lines. If the latter are present, they are seen as very fine horizontal cross lines at the cervical portion.

Lingual Aspect (Figs. 225, 229 and 230)

The crown of the mandibular first premolar tapers toward the lingual, since the lingual measurement mesiodistally is less than that buccally. The lingual cusp is always small. The major portion of the crown is made up of the middle buccal lobe (Fig. 233). This makes it resemble the canine.

The crown and the root taper markedly toward the lingual, so that most of the mesial and distal surfaces of both may be seen from the lingual aspect.

The occlusal surface slopes greatly toward the lingual in a cervical direction

*The specimen in this photograph shows a mesial inclination of the root. Mandibular premolars and canines have this tendency although most of the roots of these teeth will curve, if at all, in a distal direction.

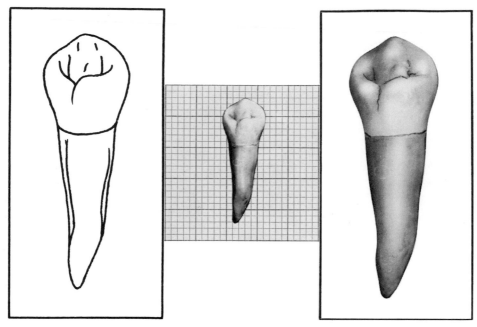

Figure 225. Mandibular right first premolar – lingual aspect.

down to the short lingual cusp. Most of the occlusal surface of this tooth can therefore be seen from this aspect.

The cervical portion of the crown lingually is narrow and convex, with concavities in evidence between the cervical line and the contact areas on the lingual portion of mesial and distal surfaces. The contact areas and marginal ridges are pronounced and extend out above the narrow cervical portion of the crown.

Although the lingual cusp is short and poorly developed (resembling a strongly developed cingulum at times), it usually shows a pointed tip. This cusp tip is in alignment with the buccal triangular ridge of the occlusal surface, which is in plain view. The mesial and distal occlusal fossae are on each side of the triangular ridge. (See Fig. 223.)

A characteristic of the lingual surface of the mandibular first premolar is the *mesiolingual developmental groove.* This groove acts as a line of demarcation between the mesiobuccal lobe and the lingual lobe and extends into the mesial fossa of the occlusal surface.

The root of this tooth is much narrower on the lingual side, and there is a narrow ridge, smooth and convex, the full length of the root. This formation allows most of the mesial and distal surfaces of the root to be seen. Often developmental depressions in the root may be seen with developmental grooves mesially. The root of this tooth tapers from the cervix to a pointed apex.

Mesial Aspect (Figs. 226, 229, 230 and 232)

From the mesial aspect, the mandibular first premolar shows an outline which is fundamental and characteristic of all mandibular posterior teeth when viewed from the mesial or distal aspect. The crown outline is roughly rhomboidal (Chapter IV, Fig. 102, *e*), and the tip of the buccal cusp is nearly centered over the root. The convexity of the lingual outline of the lingual lobe is lingual to the lingual outline of the root. The lingual surface of the crown presents an overhang above the root trunk in a lingual direction. The tip of the lingual cusp will be on a line approximately with the lingual border of the root. This differs from the condition found in maxillary posterior teeth, where both buccal and lingual cusp tips are well within the confines of the root trunks.

The mandibular first premolar, when viewed from the mesial aspect, often shows the buccal cusp centered over the root (Fig. 226). In other instances the buccal cusp tip is a little buccal to the center, corresponding to the typical placement of buccal cusps on all mandibular posterior teeth.

The buccal outline of the crown from this aspect is prominently curved from the cervical line to the tip of the buccal cusp; the crest of curvature is near the middle third of the crown. This accented convexity and the location of the crest of contour are characteristic of all mandibular posterior teeth on the buccal surfaces.

The lingual outline of the crown, representative of the lingual outline of the lingual cusp, is a curved outline of less convexity than that of the buccal surface. The crest of curvature lingually approaches the middle third of the crown, the curvature ending at the tip of the lingual cusp which is in line with the lingual border of the root.

The distance from the cervical line lingually to the tip of the lingual cusp is about two-thirds of that from the cervical line buccally to the tip of the buccal cusp.

The mesiobuccal lobe development is prominent from this aspect; it creates by its form the mesial contact area and the mesial marginal ridge, which in turn has a

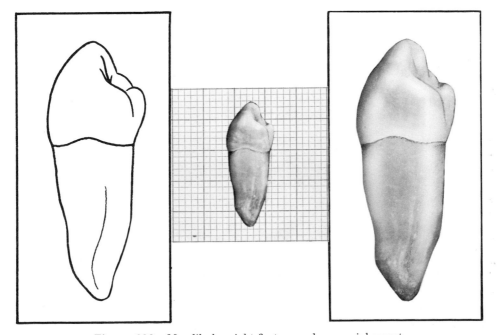

Figure 226. Mandibular right first premolar — mesial aspect.

sharp inclination lingually in a cervical direction. The lingual border of the mesial marginal ridge merges with the developmental depression mesiolingually; this harbors the mesiolingual developmental groove.

Some of the occlusal surface of the crown mesially may be seen with the mesial portion of the buccal triangular ridge. The slope of this ridge parallels the mesial marginal ridge, although the crest of the triangular ridge is above it. The sulcus formed by the convergence of buccal and lingual triangular ridges is directly above the mesiolingual groove from this aspect.

The cervical line on the mesial surface is rather regular, curving occlusally. The crest of the curvature is centered buccolingually, the average curvature being about 1 mm. in extent. It may, however, be a fraction of a millimeter, or the line may be straight across buccolingually.

The surface of the crown mesially is smooth except for the mesiolingual groove. The surface is plainly convex at the mesial contact area, which is centered on a line with the tip of the buccal cusp. Immediately below the convexity of the contact area, the surface is sharply concave between that area and the cervical line. The distance between the contact area and the cervical line is very short.

The root outline from the mesial aspect is a tapered form from the cervix, ending in a relatively pointed apex in line with the tip of the buccal cusp. The lingual outline may be straight, the buccal outline more curved.

The mesial surface of the root is smooth and flat from the buccal margin to the center. From this point, it too converges sharply toward the root center lingually, often displaying a deep developmental groove in this area. Shallow grooves are nearly always in evidence, and occasionally a deep developmental groove will end in a bifurcation at the apical third (Fig. 234, specimens 5 and 7).

Distal Aspect (Figs. 227, 229 and 230)

The distal aspect of the mandibular first premolar differs from the mesial aspect in some respects. The distal marginal ridge is higher above the cervix, and it does not have the extreme lingual slope of the mesial marginal ridge, being more nearly at right angles to the axis of crown and root. The marginal ridge is confluent with the lingual cusp ridge; it has no developmental groove on the mesial marginal ridge. The major portion of the distal surface of the crown is smoothly convex, the spheroidal form having an unbroken curved surface. Below this curvature and just above the cervical line, a concavity is to be noted which is linear in form and which extends buccolingually. The distal contact area is broader than the mesial, although it is centered in the same relation to the crown outlines. The center of the distal contact area is at a point midway between buccal and lingual crests of curvature and midway between the cervical line and the tip of the buccal cusp.

The curvature of the cervical line distally may be the same as that found mesially, although less curvature distally is the general rule when one is describing all posterior teeth.

The surface of the root distally exhibits more convexity than was found mesially. A shallow developmental depression is centered on the root, but rarely does it contain a deep developmental groove.

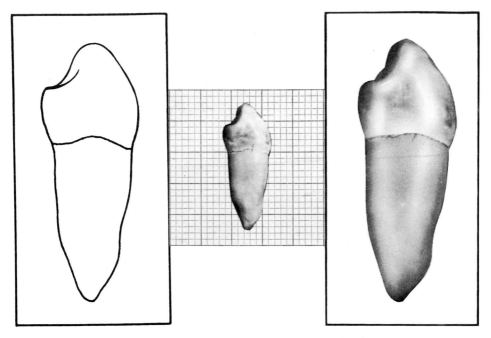

Figure 227. Mandibular right first premolar — distal aspect.

The distal surface slopes from the buccal margin toward the center of the root lingually, but the slope is more gradual than that found mesially.

Occlusal Aspect (Figs. 228, 229, 230 and 233)

The occlusal aspects of many specimens show considerable variation in the gross outlines of this tooth. Both mandibular premolars exhibit more variations in form occlusally than the maxillary premolars.

The usual outline form of the mandibular first premolar from the occlusal aspect is roughly diamond-shaped and similar to the incisal aspect of mandibular canines (Fig. 233, specimens 1, 3, 4, 7, 8, 9 and 10). Some of these teeth have a circular form similar to that of some mandibular second premolars (specimen 2); others conform to the gross outlines of the more common second premolars (specimens 5 and 6).

The characteristics common to all mandibular first premolars, regardless of type, when viewed from the occlusal aspect are these:

1. The middle buccal lobe makes up the major bulk of the tooth.

2. The buccal ridge is prominent.

3. The mesiobuccal and distobuccal line angles are prominent even though rounded.

4. The curvatures representing the contact areas, immediately lingual to the buccal line angles, are relatively broad, the distal area being the broader of the two.

5. The crown converges sharply to the center of the lingual surface, starting from points approximating the mesial and distal contact areas. This formation makes that part of the crown represented by buccal cusp ridges, marginal ridges and lingual

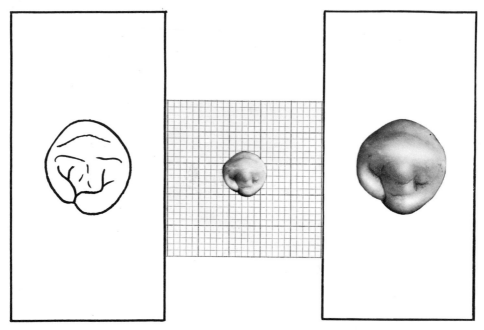

Figure 228. Mandibular right first premolar—occlusal aspect.

lobe triangular in form, with the base of the triangle at the buccal cusp ridges and the point of the triangle at the lingual cusp.

6. The marginal ridges are well developed.

7. The lingual cusp is small.

8. The occlusal surface shows a heavy buccal triangular ridge and a small lingual triangular ridge.

9. The occlusal surface harbors two depressions which are called the *mesial* and *distal fossae* because of their irregularity of form, although they correspond in location to the mesial and distal triangular fossae of other posterior teeth.

The most common type of mandibular first premolars shows a mesiolingual developmental depression and groove. These constrict the mesial surface of the crown and create a smaller mesial contact area which is in contact with the mandibular canine. The distal portion of the crown is described by a larger arc which creates a broader contact area in contact with the second mandibular premolar, which has a broader proximal surface than the canine.

The mesial fossa is more linear in form, being more sulcate and containing the *mesial developmental groove*, which extends buccolingually. This groove is confluent with its extension, which becomes the *mesiolingual developmental groove* as it passes over to the mesiolingual surface. The distal fossa is more circular in most cases and is circumscribed by the distobuccal cusp ridge, the distal marginal ridge, the buccal triangular ridge and the distolingual cusp ridge.

The distal fossa may contain a distal developmental groove which is crescent-shaped (Fig. 233, specimen 2). It may harbor a distal developmental pit with accessory supplemental grooves radiating from it (specimen 10), or it may contain a linear groove running mesiodistally with an arrangement resembling the typical triangular fossa (specimens 4, 5 and 6).

Because of the position of this crown over the root, most of the buccal surface may be seen from the occlusal aspect, whereas very little of the lingual surface is in view.

MANDIBULAR SECOND PREMOLAR

Mandibular Second Premolar

First evidence of calcification .... 2¼ to 2½ years
Enamel completed .... 6 to 7 years
Eruption .... 11 to 12 years
Root completed .... 13 to 14 years

Measurement Table

	Cervico-occlusal Length of Crown	Length of Root	Mesio-distal Diam-eter of Crown	Mesio-distal Diam-eter of Crown at Cervix	Labio- or Bucco-lingual Diameter of Crown	Labio- or Bucco-lingual Diameter of Crown at Cervix	Curvature of Cervical Line—Mesial	Curvature of Cervical Line—Distal
Dimensions suggested for carving technic	8.0*	14.5	7.0	5.0	8.0	7.0	1.0	0.0

* Millimeters.

The mandibular second premolar resembles the mandibular first premolar from the buccal aspect only. Although the buccal cusp is not so pronounced, the mesiodistal measurement of the crown and its general outline are similar. The tooth is larger and has better development in other respects. There are two common forms which this tooth assumes: The first form, which probably occurs most often, is the *three-cusp* type, which appears more angular from the occlusal aspect (Fig. 239). The second form is the *two-cusp* type, which appears more rounded from the occlusal aspect. (Fig. 242, specimens 1, 2, 7 and 10.)

The two types differ mainly in the occlusal design. The outlines and general appearance from all other aspects are similar.

The single root of the second premolar is larger and longer than that of the first premolar. The root is seldom if ever bifurcated, although some specimens show a deep developmental groove buccally (Fig. 240, specimens 3 and 8). Often a flattened area appears in this location.

(Text continued on page 220.)

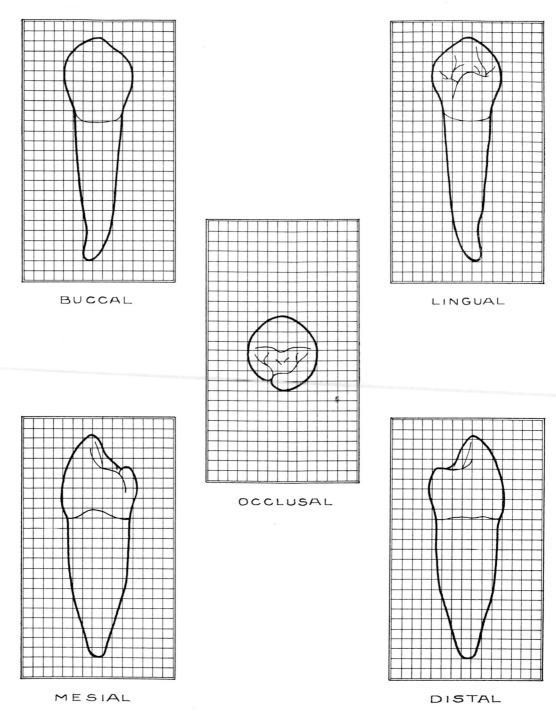

Figure 229.   Mandibular right first premolar. Graph outlines of five aspects.

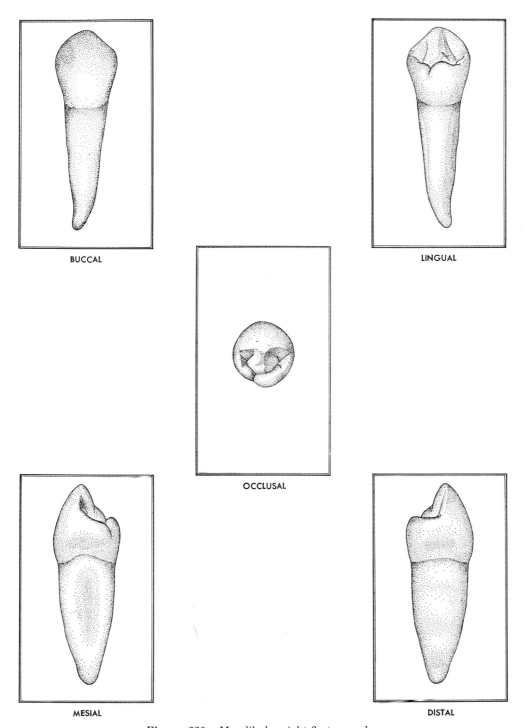

BUCCAL

LINGUAL

OCCLUSAL

MESIAL

DISTAL

Figure 230. Mandibular right first premolar.

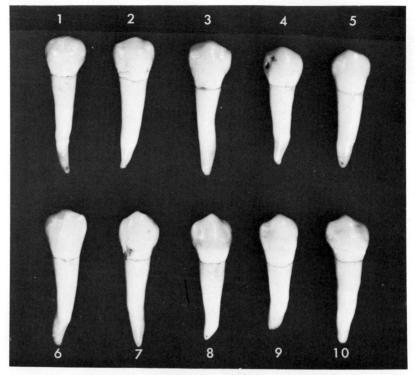

Figure 231.   Mandibular first premolar—ten typical specimens—buccal aspect.

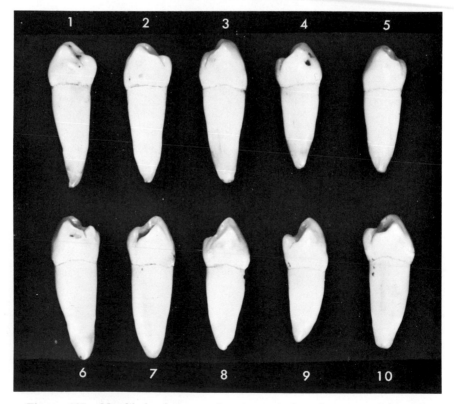

Figure 232.   Mandibular first premolar—ten typical specimens—mesial aspect.

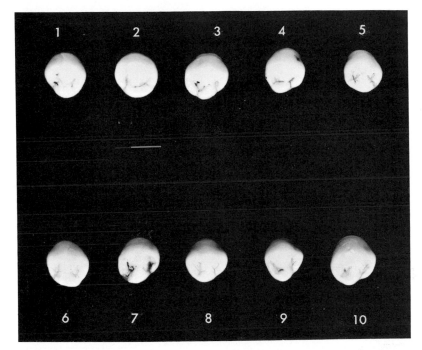

Figure 233. Mandibular first premolar – ten typical specimens – occlusal aspect.

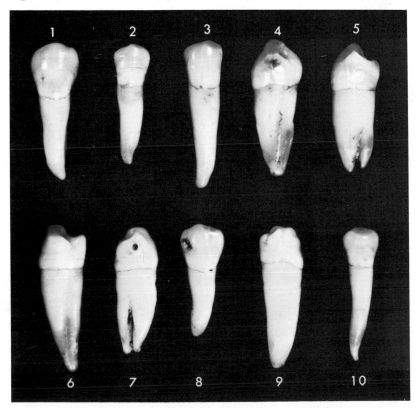

Figure 234. Mandibular first premolar – ten specimens showing uncommon variations. 1, Crown oversize. 2, Crown and root diminutive. 3, Mesial and distal sides of crown straight, cervix wide mesio-distally, root extra long. 4, Unusual formation of lingual portion of crown, root with deep developmental groove mesially. 5, Bifurcated root. 6, Lingual cusp long, little lingual curvature, root of extra length. 7, No lingual cusp, root bifurcated. 8, Dwarfed root. 9, Crown poorly formed, root unusually long. 10, Very long curved root for crown so small.

219

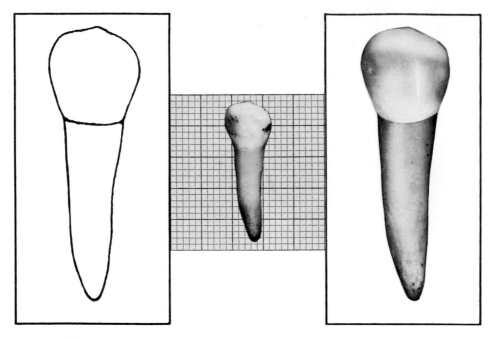

Figure 235. Mandibular left second premolar (bicuspid) — buccal aspect.

Detailed Description of the Mandibular Second Premolar from All Aspects

In describing the separate aspects of this tooth, direct comparisons are made with the mandibular first premolar except for the occlusal aspect.

Buccal Aspect (Figs. 235 and 240)

From the buccal aspect the mandibular second premolar presents a shorter buccal cusp than the first premolar, with mesiobuccal and distobuccal cusp ridges presenting angulation of less degree. The contact areas, both mesial and distal, are broad. The contact areas appear to be higher because of the short buccal cusp.

The root is broader mesiodistally than that of the first premolar, the extra breadth appearing for most of its length, and the root ends in an apex which is more blunt. In other respects the two teeth are quite similar from this aspect.

Lingual Aspect (Fig. 236)

From the lingual aspect, the second premolar crown shows considerable variation from the crown portion of the first premolar. The variations are as follows:

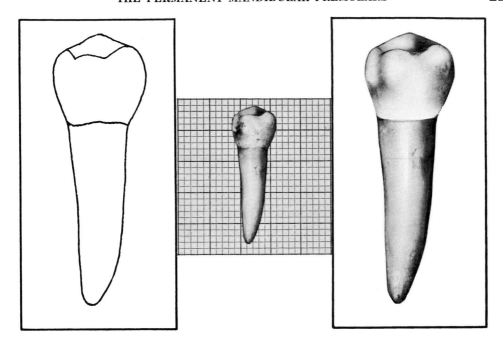

Figure 236. Mandibular left second premolar—lingual aspect.

1. The lingual lobes are developed to a greater degree, making the cusp or cusps (depending on the type) longer.

2. Less of the occlusal surface may be seen from this aspect. Nevertheless, since the lingual cusps are not as long as the buccal cusp, part of the buccal portion of the occlusal surface may be seen.

3. In the three-cusp type, the lingual development brings about the greatest variation between the two teeth. There are a mesiolingual and a distolingual cusp, the former being the larger and the longer one in most cases. There is a groove between them extending a very short distance on the lingual surface and usually centered over the root (Fig. 242, specimen 8).

In the two-cusp type, the single lingual cusp development attains equal height with the three-cusp type. The two-cusp type has no groove, but it shows a developmental depression distolingually where the lingual cusp ridge joins the distal marginal ridge (Fig. 242, specimen 3).

The lingual surface of the crown of all mandibular second premolars is smooth and spheroidal, having a bulbous form above the constricted cervical portion.

The root is wide lingually, although not quite so wide as the buccal portion. There is less difference in dimension than was found on the first premolar, a fact which creates much less convergence toward the lingual.

Since in most instances the lingual portion of the crown converges little from the buccal portion, less of the mesial and distal sides of this tooth may be seen from this aspect than are seen from the lingual aspect of the first premolar.

The lingual portion of the root is smoothly convex for most of its length.

Mesial Aspect (Figs. 237 and 241)

The second premolar differs from the first premolar from the mesial aspect as follows:

1. The crown and root are wider buccolingually than in the first premolar.

2. The buccal cusp is not so nearly centered over the root trunk, and it is shorter.

3. The lingual lobe development is greater.

4. The marginal ridge is at right angles to the long axis of the tooth.

5. Less of the occlusal surface may be seen.

6. There is no mesiolingual developmental groove on the crown portion.

7. The root is longer and in most cases slightly convex on the mesial surface. (This convexity is not, however, always present. See Fig. 241, specimens 6, 7 and 8.)

8. The apex of the root is usually more blunt.

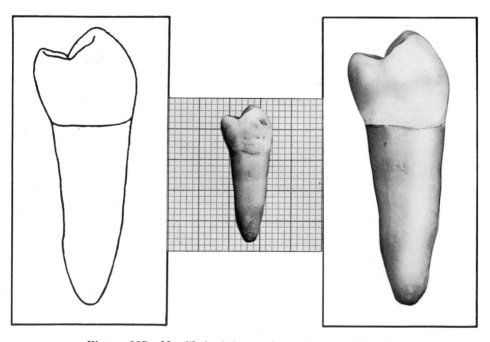

Figure 237.   Mandibular left second premolar — mesial aspect.

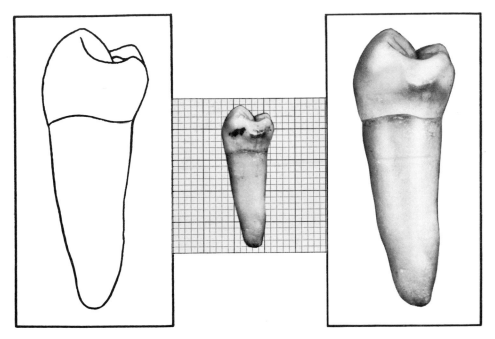

Figure 238. Mandibular left second premolar—distal aspect.

Distal Aspect (Fig. 238)

This aspect of the mandibular second premolar is similar to the mesial aspect except that more of the occlusal surface may be seen. This is possible, since the distal marginal ridge is at a lower level than the mesial marginal ridge when one is posing the tooth vertically. The crowns of all posterior teeth are tipped distally to the long axes of the roots, so that when the specimen tooth is held vertically more of the occlusal surface may be seen from the distal aspect than from the mesial aspect. This is a characteristic possessed by all posterior teeth, mandibular and maxillary. This is an important observation to remember, not only in the study of individual tooth forms but later on in the study of alignment and occlusion.

Occlusal Aspect (Figs. 239 and 242)

As mentioned before, there are two common forms of this tooth. The outline form of each type shows some variation from the occlusal aspect. The two types are similar in that portion which is buccal to the mesiobuccal and distobuccal cusp ridges.

The three-cusp type appears square lingual to the buccal cusp ridges when highly developed (Fig. 242, specimen 8). The round, or two-cusp, type appears round lingual to the buccal cusp ridges (Fig. 242, specimen 3).

The square type (specimen 8), has three cusps that are distinct; the buccal cusp

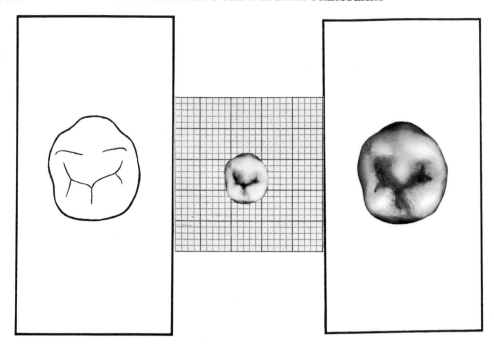

Figure 239. Mandibular left second premolar—occlusal aspect.

is the largest, the mesiolingual cusp is next, and the distolingual cusp is the smallest.

Each cusp has well-formed triangular ridges separated by deep developmental grooves. These grooves converge in a *central pit* and form a Y on the occlusal surface. The central pit is located midway between the buccal cusp ridge and the lingual margin of the occlusal surface and slightly distal to the central point between mesial and distal marginal ridges.

Starting at the central pit, the *mesial developmental groove* travels in a mesiobuccal direction and ends in the *mesial triangular fossa* just distal to the mesial marginal ridge. The *distal developmental groove* travels in a distobuccal direction, is somewhat shorter than the mesial groove, and ends in the *distal triangular fossa* mesial to the distal marginal ridge. The lingual developmental groove extends lingually between the two lingual cusps and ends on the lingual surface of the crown just below the convergence of the lingual cusp ridges. The mesiolingual cusp is wider mesiodistally than the distolingual cusp. This arrangement places the lingual developmental groove distal to center on the crown.

Supplemental grooves and depressions are often seen, radiating from the developmental grooves. Occasionally a groove crosses one or both of the marginal ridges. On a tooth of this type the point angles are distinct. Developmental grooves are often deep.

Specimen 8 (Fig. 242) is a usual form. Variations of this development may be seen in specimens 4, 5, 6 and 9.

The round, or two-cusp, type (specimen 3) differs considerably from the three-cusp type when viewed from the occlusal aspect. Specimen 3 is a true typal form of the two-cusp type. Variations may be seen in specimens 1, 2, 7 and 10.

The *occlusal* characteristics of the two-cusp type are as follows:

1. The outline of the crown is rounded lingual to the buccal cusp ridges.

2. There is some lingual convergence of mesial and distal sides, although no more than is found in some variations of the square type.

3. The mesiolingual and distolingual line angles are rounded.

4. There is one well-developed lingual cusp directly opposite the buccal cusp in a lingual direction.

A *central developmental groove* on the occlusal surface travels in a mesiodistal direction. This groove may be straight (Fig. 242, specimen 3), but it is most often crescent-shaped (specimens 1, 7 and 10). The central groove has its terminals centered in *mesial* and *distal fossae,* which are roughly circular depressions having supplemental grooves and depressions radiating from the central groove and its terminals. The enamel surface inside these fossae and around their peripheries is very irregular, acting as a contrast to the smoothness of cusp ridges, marginal ridges and the transverse ridge from buccal cusp to lingual cusp.

Some of these teeth show *mesial* and *distal developmental pits* centered in the mesial and distal fossae instead of an unbroken central groove (Fig. 242, specimen 2).

Although photographs do not demonstrate it very well, most of these two-cusp specimens show a developmental depression crossing the distolingual cusp ridge.

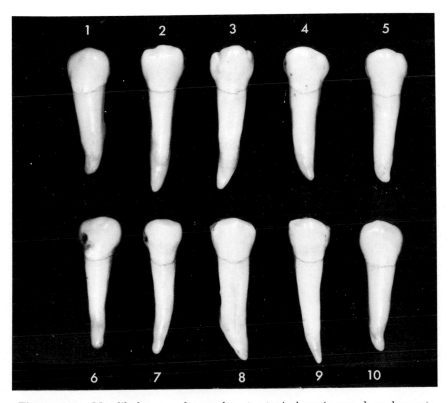

Figure 240.   Mandibular second premolar – ten typical specimens – buccal aspect.

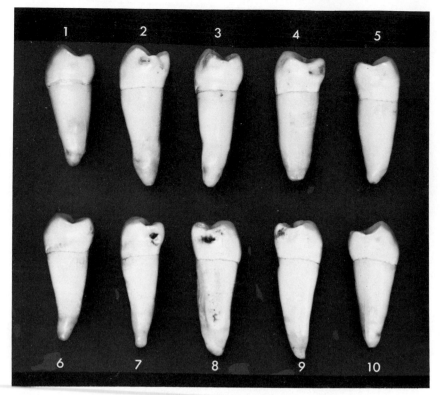

Figure 241. Mandibular second premolar—ten typical specimens—mesial aspect.

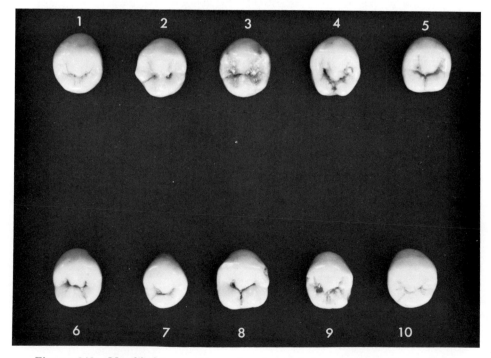

Figure 242. Mandibular second premolar—ten typical specimens—occlusal aspect.

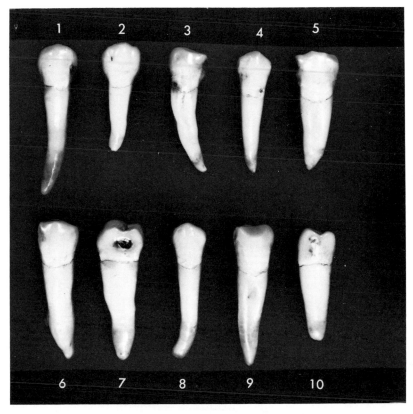

Figure 243. Mandibular second premolar—ten specimens showing uncommon variations. 1, Root extremely long. 2, Root dwarfed. 3, Malformed root, developmental groove on buccal surface. 4, Contact areas on crown high and constricted. 5, Crown oversize, developmental groove buccally on root. 6, Root oversize. 7, Root malformed and of extra length. 8, Root very long with blunt apex, extreme curvature at apical third. 9, Crown and root oversize, developmental groove buccally on root. 10, Crown narrow buccolingually, very little curvature buccally and lingually.

Chapter XI

THE PERMANENT
MAXILLARY MOLARS

THE MAXILLARY molars differ in design from any of the teeth previously described. These teeth assist the mandibular molars in performing the major portion of the work in the mastication and comminution of food. They are the largest and strongest maxillary teeth, by virtue both of their bulk and of their anchorage in the jaws. Although the crowns on the molars may be somewhat shorter than the premolars, their dimensions are greater in every other respect. The root portion may be no longer than that of the premolars, but instead of one root or a root bifurcated, the maxillary molar root is broader at the base in all directions and is trifurcated into three well-developed prongs which are actually three full-sized roots emanating from a common broad base above the crown.

Generally speaking, the maxillary molars have large crowns with four well-formed cusps. They have three roots, two buccal and one lingual. The lingual root is the largest. The crowns have two buccal cusps and two lingual cusps. The outlines and curvatures of all the maxillary molars are similar. Developmental variations will be set forth under descriptions of the separate molars.

Before a detailed description of the maxillary first molar is begun, some statements must be made which are applicable to all first molars, mandibular as well as maxillary:

The permanent first molars usually appear in the oral cavity when the child is six years old. The mandibular molars precede the maxillary molars. The first permanent molar (maxillary or mandibular) erupts posterior to the second deciduous molar, taking up a position in contact with it. Therefore, the first molar is not a succedaneous tooth, since it has no predecessor. The deciduous teeth are all still in position and functioning when the first molar takes its place. Because the development of the bones of the face is downward and forward, sufficient space has been created normally at the age of six for the accommodation of this tooth.

The normal location of the first permanent molar is at the center of the fully developed adult jaw anteroposteriorly. As a consequence of the significance of their positions and the circumstances surrounding their eruption, the first molars are considered the "cornerstones" of the dental arches. A full realization of the significance of these teeth as units in the arches—their function and their positions relative to the other teeth—will be thoroughly understood when the student has had an opportunity to study the arrangement of the teeth with their occlusion and the temporomandibular articulation of the jaws. Subsequent chapters cover those phases. The mandibular first molars will be described in Chapter XII.

MAXILLARY FIRST MOLAR

Maxillary First Molar

First evidence of calcification .... At birth
Enamel completed .... 3 to 4 years
Eruption .... 6 years
Root completed .... 9 to 10 years

Measurement Table

	Cervico-occlusal Length of Crown	Length of Root		Mesio-distal Diameter of Crown	Mesio-distal Diameter of Crown at Cervix	Labio- or Bucco-lingual Diameter of Crown	Labio- or Bucco-lingual Diameter at Cervix	Curvature of Cervical Line—Mesial	Curvature of Cervical Line—Distal
		b	l						
Dimensions suggested for carving technic	7.5*	12	13	10.0	8.0	11.0	10.0	1.0	0.0

* Millimeters.

The crown of this tooth is wider buccolingually than mesiodistally. Usually the extra dimension buccolingually is about 1 mm. (see table). This, however, varies in individuals (see Fig. 260, specimens 1, 5, 7 and 9). From the occlusal aspect the inequality of the measurements in the two directions appears slight. Although the crown is relatively short, it is broad mesiodistally and buccolingually, which results in a large occlusal surface.

The maxillary first molar is normally the largest tooth in the maxillary arch. It has four well-developed functioning cusps and one supplemental cusp of little practical use. The four large cusps of most physiologic significance are the mesiobuccal, the distobuccal, the mesiolingual and the distolingual. The fifth, or supplemental,

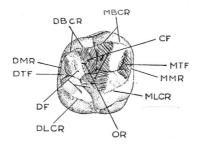

Figure 244. Maxillary right first molar—occlusal landmarks. *MBCR*, mesiobuccal cusp ridge; *CF*, central fossa (shaded area); *MTF*, mesial triangular fossa (shaded area); *MMR*, mesial marginal ridge; *MLCR*, mesiolingual cusp ridge; *OR*, oblique ridge; *DLCR*, distolingual cusp ridge; *DF*, distal fossa; *DTF*, distal triangular fossa (shaded area); *DMR*, distal marginal ridge; *DBCR*, distobuccal cusp ridge.

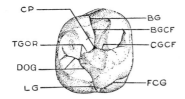

Figure 245. Maxillary right first molar—occlusal aspect—developmental grooves. *BG*, buccal groove; *BGCF*, buccal groove of central fossa; *CGCF*, central groove of central fossa; *FCG*, fifth cusp groove; *LG*, lingual groove; *DOG*, distal oblique groove; *TGOR*, transverse groove of oblique ridge; *CP*, central pit.

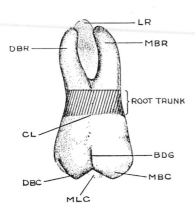

Figure 246. Maxillary right first molar—buccal aspect. *DBR*, distobuccal root; *LR*, lingual root; *MBR*, mesiobuccal root; *CL*, cervical line; *DBC*, distobuccal cusp; *MLC*, mesiolingual cusp; *BDG*, buccal development groove; *MBC*, mesiobuccal cusp.

cusp is also called the *cusp* or *tubercle of Carabelli*. The simple term "fifth cusp" will be used here. This cusp is found lingual to the mesiolingual cusp, which is the largest of the well-developed cusps. Often the fifth cusp is so poorly developed that it is scarcely distinguishable. Usually a developmental groove is found, leaving a record of cusp development unless it has been erased by frictional wear. The fifth cusp or a developmental trace at its usual site serves to identify the maxillary first molar. A specimen of this tooth showing no trace of its typical characteristic would be rare.

There are three *roots* of generous proportions: the mesiobuccal, distobuccal and lingual. These roots are well separated and well developed, and their placement gives this tooth maximum anchorage against forces which would tend to unseat it. The roots have their greatest spread parallel to the line of greatest force brought to bear against the crown—diagonally in a buccolingual direction. The lingual root is the longest root. It is tapered and smoothly rounded. The mesiobuccal root is not so long, and it is broader buccolingually and shaped (in cross section) so that its resistance to torsion is greater than that of the lingual root. The distobuccal root is the smallest of the three and smoothly rounded.

Detailed Description of the Maxillary First Molar
from All Aspects

Buccal Aspect (Figs. 247, 256, 257 and 258)

The crown is roughly trapezoidal, with cervical and occlusal outlines representing the uneven sides. The cervical line is the shorter of the uneven sides.

When looking at the buccal aspect of this tooth with the line of vision at right angles to the buccal developmental groove of the crown, one sees the distal side of the crown in perspective. This is caused by the obtuse character of the distobuccal line angle (see "Occlusal Aspect"). Parts of four cusps are seen, the mesiobuccal, distobuccal, mesiolingual and distolingual.

The mesiobuccal cusp is broader than the distobuccal cusp, and its mesial slope meets its distal slope at an obtuse angle. The mesial slope of the distobuccal cusp meets its distal slope at approximately a right angle. The distobuccal cusp is therefore sharper than the mesiobuccal cusp, and it is at least as long and often longer (Fig. 258, specimens 4, 6, 7, 8 and 9).

The buccal developmental groove which divides the two buccal cusps is approximately equidistant between the mesiobuccal and distolingual line angles.

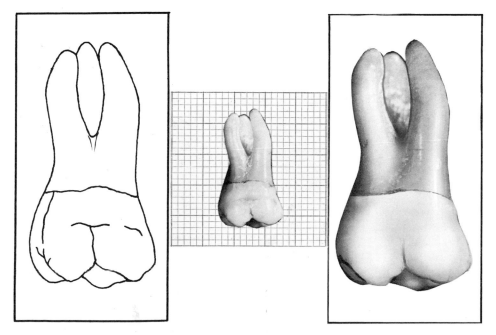

Figure 247. Maxillary right first molar – buccal aspect.

The groove slants occluso-apically in a line of direction parallel to the long axis of the distobuccal root. It terminates at a point approximately half the distance from its origin occlusally to the cervical line of the crown. Although the groove is not deep at any point, it becomes more shallow toward its termination, gradually fading out. Lateral to its terminus there is a dip in the enamel of the crown which is developmental in character and which extends for some distance mesially and distally.

The cervical line of the crown does not have much curvature from mesial to distal; however, it is not so smooth and regular as that found on some of the other teeth. The line is generally convex with the convexity toward the roots.

The mesial outline of the crown from this aspect follows a nearly straight path downward and mesially, curving occlusally as it reaches the crest of contour of the mesial surface which is the contact area. This crest is approximately two-thirds the distance from cervical line to tip of mesiobuccal cusp. The mesial outline continues downward and distally and becomes congruent with the outline of the mesial slope of the mesiobuccal cusp.

The distal outline of the crown is convex; the distal surface is spheroidal. The crest of curvature on the distal side of the crown is located at a level approximately half the distance from cervical line to tip of cusp. The distal contact area is in the middle of the middle third.

Often from this aspect a flattened area or a concave area is seen on the distal surface immediately above the distobuccal cusp at the cervical third of the crown.

All three of the roots may be seen from the buccal aspect. The axes of the roots are inclined distally. The roots are not straight, however, the buccal roots showing an inclination to curvature halfway between the point of bifurcation and the apices. The mesiobuccal root curves distally, starting at the middle third. Its axis usually is at right angles to the cervical line. The distal root is straighter, with its long axis at an acute angle distally with the cervical line. It has a tendency toward curvature mesially at its middle third.

The point of bifurcation of the two buccal roots is located approximately 4 mm. above the cervical line. This measurement varies somewhat, of course. Nevertheless, the point is much farther removed from the cervical line than in the deciduous molars. This relation is typical when all permanent molars are compared with all deciduous molars.

There is a deep developmental groove buccally on the root trunk of the maxillary first molar which starts at the bifurcation and progresses downward, becoming more shallow until it terminates in a shallow depression at the cervical line. Sometimes this depression extends slightly onto the enamel at the cervix.

The reader must keep in mind the fact that molar roots originate as a single root on the base of the crown. They then are divided into three roots, as in the maxillary molars, or into two roots, as in the mandibular molars. The common root base is called the *root trunk* (Figs. 246 and 251).

In judging the length of the roots and the direction of their axes, the part of the root trunk which is congruent with each root must be included as part of it, since it functions as an entity. Usually the lingual root is the longest and the two buccal roots are approximately equal in length. There is considerable variance in this, although the difference is a matter of a millimeter or so only in the average first molars with normal development.

From the buccal aspect, a measurement of the roots inclusively at their greatest extremities mesiodistally is less than a calibration of the diameter of the crown mesiodistally.

There is no invariable rule covering the relative length of crown and root when describing the upper first molar. On the average, the roots are about twice as long as the crown.

Lingual Aspect (Figs. 248, 249, 256 and 257)

From the lingual aspect the gross outline of the maxillary first molar is the reverse of that from the buccal aspect. Photographs or drawings show this only approximately because all teeth have breadth and thickness; consequently, perspective of two dimensions plus the human element (which enters into the technique of posing specimens and the making of drawings and photographs) are bound to result in some error in graphic interpretation.

The variation between the outline of the mesial surface and that of the distal surface is apparent. Because of the roundness of the distolingual cusp, the smooth curvature of the distal outline of the crown becoming confluent with the curvature of the cusp creates an arc which is almost a semicircle. The line which describes the lingual developmental groove is also confluent with the outline of the distolingual cusp, progressing mesially and cervically and ending at a point at the approximate center of the lingual surface of the crown. A shallow depression in the surface extends from the terminus of the lingual groove to the center of the lingual surface of the lingual root at the cervical line and then continues in an apical direction on the lingual root, fading out at the middle third of the root.

The lingual cusps are the only ones to be seen from the lingual aspect. The mesiolingual cusp is much the larger, and before occlusal wear it is always the longest cusp the tooth possesses. Its mesiodistal width is about three-fifths of the mesiodistal crown diameter, the distolingual cusp making up the remaining two-fifths. The angle formed by the mesial outline of the crown and the mesial slope of the mesiolingual cusp is almost 90 degrees. An obtuse angle describes the junction of the mesial and distal slopes of this cusp.

Figure 248. Maxillary right first molar—lingual aspect. *MBR*, mesiobuccal root; *DBR*, distobuccal root; *CL*, cervical line; *FC*, fifth cusp; *MLC*, mesiolingual cusp; *LDG*, lingual development groove; *DLC*, distolingual cusp.

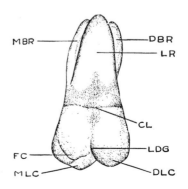

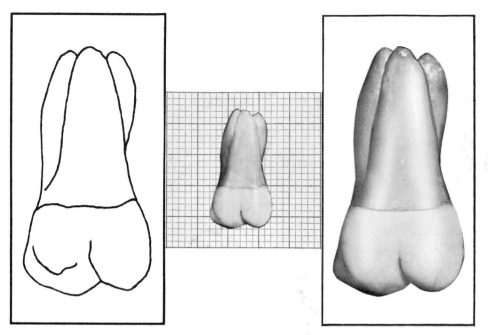

Figure 249.   Maxillary right first molar—lingual aspect.

The distolingual cusp is so spheroidal and smooth that it is difficult to describe any angulation on the mesial and distal slopes.

The lingual developmental groove starts approximately in the center of the lingual surface mesiodistally, curves sharply to the distal as it crosses between the cusps and continues on to the occlusal surface.

The fifth cusp appears attached to the mesiolingual surface of the mesiolingual cusp. It is outlined occlusally by an irregular developmental groove, which may be described as starting in a depression of the mesiolingual line angle of the crown, extending occlusally toward the point of the mesiolingual cusp, then making an obtuse angle turn toward the terminus of the lingual groove and fading out near the lingual groove terminus. If the fifth cusp is well developed, its cusp angle will be sharper and less obtuse than that of the mesiolingual cusp. The cusp ridge of the fifth cusp is approximately 2 mm. cervical to the cusp ridge of the mesiolingual cusp.

All three of the roots are visible from the lingual aspect, the large lingual root making up most of the foreground. The lingual portion of the root trunk is continuous with the entire cervical portion of the crown lingually. The lingual root is conical, terminating in a bluntly rounded apex.

All of the mesial outline of the mesiobuccal root may be seen from this angle, and part of its apex.

The distal outline of the distobuccal root is seen above its middle third, including all of its apical outline.

Mesial Aspect (Figs. 250, 251, 256 and 257)

From this aspect can be seen the increased buccolingual dimensions, cervical curvatures of the crown outlines at the cervical third buccally and lingually, and the difference in dimensions between the crown at its greatest measurement and the distance between the cusp tips in a buccolingual direction.

Starting at the cervical line buccally, the outline of the crown makes a short arc buccally to its crest of curvature within the cervical third of the crown. The extent of this curvature is about 0.5 mm. The line of the buccal surface then describes a shallow concavity immediately occlusal to the crest of curvature (see "Buccal Aspect"). The outline then becomes slightly convex as it progresses downward and inward to circumscribe the mesiobuccal cusp, ending at the tip of the cusp well within projected outlines of the root base.

If the tooth is posed so that the line of vision is at right angles to the mesial contact area, the only cusps in sight are the mesiobuccal, the mesiolingual and the fifth cusps. The distobuccal root is hidden by the mesiobuccal root.

The lingual outline of the crown curves outward and lingually approximately to the same extent as on the buccal side. The level of the crest of curvature is near the middle third of the crown rather than a point within the cervical third, as it is buccally.

If the fifth cusp is well developed, the lingual outline dips inward to illustrate it. If it is undeveloped the lingual outline continues from the crest of curvature as a smoothly curved arc to the tip of the mesiolingual cusp. The point of the cusp is more nearly centered within projected outlines of the root base than the tip of the

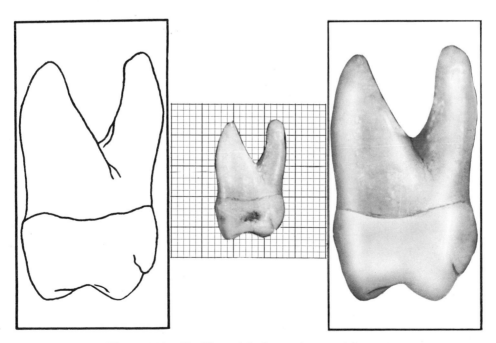

Figure 250. Maxillary right first molar—mesial aspect.

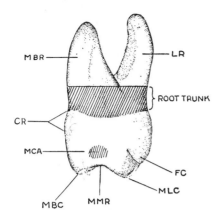

Figure 251. Maxillary right first molar— mesial aspect, *LR*, lingual root; *FC*, fifth cusp; *MLC*, mesiolingual cusp; *MMR*, mesial marginal ridge; *MBC*, mesiobuccal cusp; *MCA*, mesial contact area; *CR*, cervical ridge; *MBR*, mesiobuccal root.

mesiobuccal cusp. The mesiolingual cusp is on a line with the long axis of the lingual root.

The mesial marginal ridge, which is confluent with the mesiobuccal and mesiolingual cusp ridges, is irregular, the outline curving cervically about one-fifth the crown length and centering its curvature below the center of the crown buccolingually.

The cervical line of the crown is irregular, curving occlusally, but as a rule not more than 1 mm. at any one point. If there is definite curvature it reaches its maximum immediately above the contact area.

The mesial contact area is above the marginal ridge but closer to it than to the cervical line, approximately at the junction of the middle and occlusal thirds of the crown (see Fig. 251). It is also somewhat buccal to the center of the crown buccolingually. A shallow concavity is usually found just above the contact area on the mesial surface of the maxillary first molar. This concavity may be continued to the mesial surface of the root trunk at its cervical third.

The mesiobuccal root is broad and flattened on its mesial surface, this flattened surface often exhibiting smooth flutings for part of its length. The width of this root near the crown from the buccal surface to the point of bifurcation on the root trunk is approximately two-thirds of the crown measurement buccolingually at the cervical line. The buccal outline of the root extends upward and outward from the crown, ending at the blunt apex. The greatest projection on this root is usually buccal to the greatest projection of the crown. The lingual outline of the root is relatively straight from the bluntly rounded apex down to the bifurcation with the lingual root.

The level of the bifurcation is a little closer to the cervical line than is found between the roots buccally. A smooth depression congruent with the bifurcation extends occlusally and lingually almost to the cervical line directly above the mesiolingual line angle of the crown.

The lingual root is longer than the mesial root but is narrower from this aspect. It is banana-shaped, extending lingually with its convex outline to the lingual and its concave outline to the buccal. At its middle and apical thirds it is outside of the confines of the greatest crown projection. Although its apex is rounded, the root appears more pointed toward the end than the mesiobuccal root.

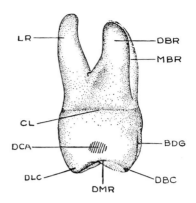

Figure 252. Maxillary right first molar—distal aspect. *DBR*, distobuccal root; *MBR*, mesiobuccal root; *BDG*, buccal developmental groove; *DBC*, distobuccal cusp; *DMR*, distal marginal ridge; *DLC*, distolingual cusp; *DCA*, distal contact area; *CL*, cervical line; *LR*, lingual root.

Distal Aspect (Figs. 253, 256 and 257)

The gross outline of this aspect is similar to that of the mesial aspect. Certain variations must be noted when the tooth is viewed from the distal aspect.

Because of the tendency of the crown to taper distally on the buccal surface, most of the buccal surface of the crown may be seen in perspective from the distal aspect. This is because the buccolingual measurement of the crown mesially is greater than the same measurement distally. All of the decrease in measurement distally is due to the slant of the buccal side of the crown.

The distal marginal ridge dips sharply in a cervical direction, exposing triangular ridges on the distal portion of the occlusal surface of the crown.

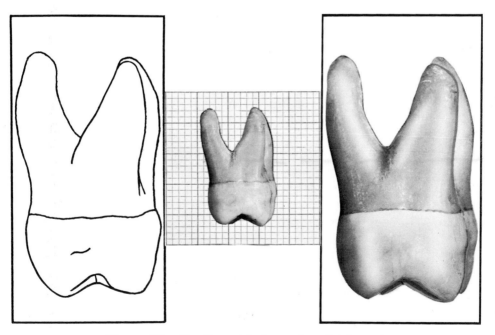

Figure 253. Maxillary right first molar—distal aspect.

The cervical line is almost straight across from buccal to lingual. Occasionally it curves apically 0.5 mm. or so.

The distal surface of the crown is generally convex, with a smoothly rounded surface except for a small area near the distobuccal root at the cervical third. This concavity continues on to the distal surface of the distobuccal root, from the cervical line to the area of the root which is on a level with the bifurcation separating the distobuccal and lingual roots.

The distobuccal root is narrower at its base than either of the others. An outline of this root, when one views the tooth from the distal aspect, starts buccally at a point immediately above the distobuccal cusp, follows a concave path inward for a short distance, then outward in a buccal direction, completing a graceful convex arc from the concavity to the rounded apex. This line lies entirely within the confines of the outline of the mesiobuccal root. The lingual outline of the root from the apex to the bifurcation is slightly concave. There is no concavity between the bifurcation of the roots and the cervical line. If anything, the surface at this point on the root trunk has a tendency toward convexity.

The bifurcation here is more apical than either of the other two areas on this tooth. The area from cervical line to bifurcation is 5 mm. or more in extent.

Occlusal Aspect (Figs. 244, 245, 255, 256, 257 and 260)

The maxillary first molar is somewhat rhomboidal from the occlusal aspect. An outline following the four major cusp ridges and the marginal ridges is especially so.

A measurement of the crown buccolingually and mesial to the buccal and lingual grooves will be greater than the measurement on that portion of the crown which is distal to these developmental grooves. Also, a measurement of the crown immediately lingual to contact areas mesiodistally is greater than the measurement immediately buccal to the contact areas. Thus it is apparent that the maxillary first molar crown is wider mesially than distally, and wider lingually than buccally.

The four major cusps are well developed, with the small minor, or fifth, cusp appearing on the lingual surface of the mesiolingual cusp near the mesiolingual line angle of the crown. The fifth cusp may be indistinct, or all the cusp form may be absent. At this site, however, there will be nearly always traces of developmental lines in the enamel.

The mesiolingual cusp is the largest cusp; it is followed in point of size by the mesiobuccal, distolingual, distobuccal and fifth cusps.

If reduced to a geometric schematic figure, the occlusal aspect of this molar locates the various angles of the rhomboidal figure as follows: acute angles, mesiobuccal and distolingual; obtuse angles, mesiolingual and distobuccal.

An analysis of the occlusal design of all of the maxillary molars brings out the following observations: Developmentally there are only three major cusps which are primary, the two buccal cusps and the mesiolingual cusp. The distolingual and fifth cusps must be secondary. The three cusps named as primary are more nearly centered over the root base, with its three divisions. The triangular outline formed by the three primary cusps is reflected in the triangular form of the crown and root when sectioned near the cervical line (see root sections, Chapter XIII).

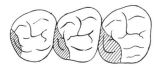

Figure 254. Maxillary molar primary cusp triangle. The distolingual lobe, represented by shaded areas, becomes progressively smaller on maxillary molars, starting with the first molar, which presents the greatest development of the lobe. The plain areas, roughly triangular in outline, represent the "maxillary molar primary cusp triangles."

Another observation which bears out this theory is that the distolingual cusp becomes progressively smaller on second and third maxillary molars, often disappearing as a major cusp (Fig. 254).

The triangular form of the three most important cusps developmentally might be called the *"maxillary molar primary cusp triangle."* The characteristic triangular figure, made by tracing the cusp outlines of these cusps, the mesial marginal ridge and the oblique ridge of the occlusal surface, is representative of all maxillary molars.

The occlusal surface of the maxillary first molar is within the confines of the cusp ridges and marginal ridges. It may be described as follows:

There are two major fossae and two minor fossae. The major fossae are the *central fossa*, which is roughly triangular and mesial to the oblique ridge, and the *distal fossa*, which is roughly linear and distal to the oblique ridge. The two minor fossae are the *mesial triangular fossa*, immediately distal to the mesial marginal ridge, and the *distal triangular fossa*, immediately mesial to the distal marginal ridge (Fig. 244).

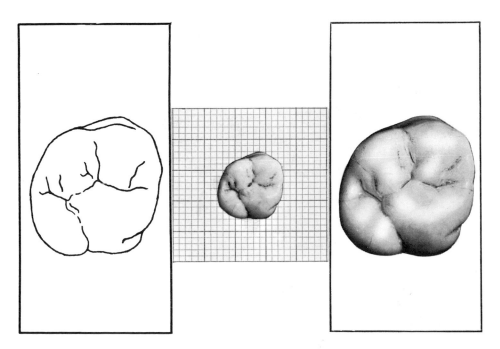

Figure 255.   Maxillary right first molar — occlusal aspect.

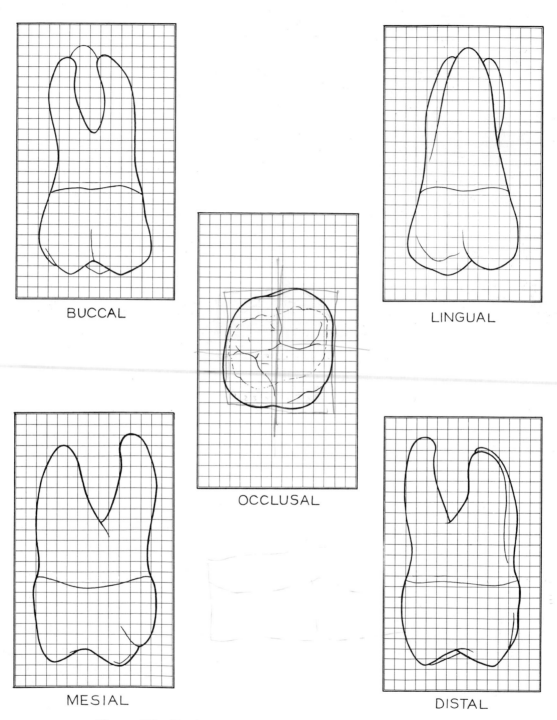

BUCCAL

LINGUAL

OCCLUSAL

MESIAL

DISTAL

Figure 256. Maxillary right first molar. Graph outlines of five aspects.

shaded in:
Grooves

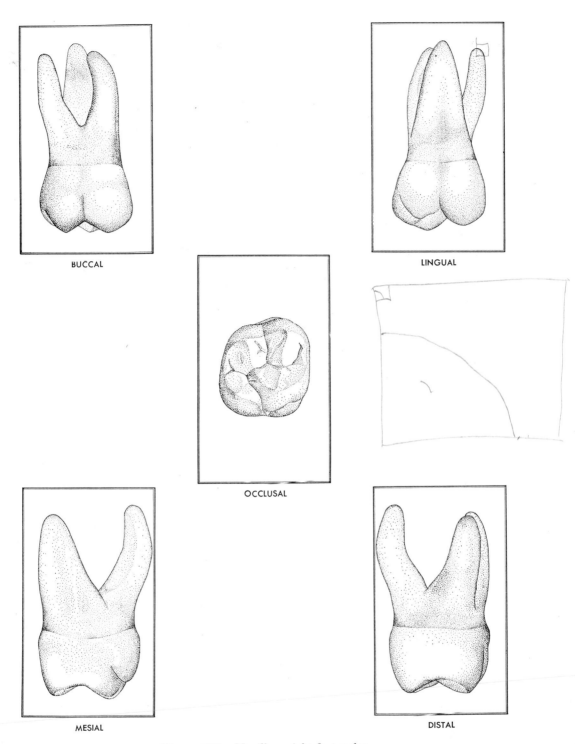

Figure 257. Maxillary right first molar.

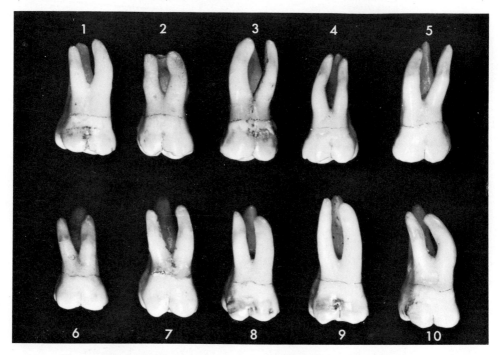

Figure 258.   Maxillary first molars — ten typical specimens — buccal aspect.

The *oblique ridge* is a triangular ridge which traverses the occlusal surface of this tooth in an oblique direction from the tip of the mesiolingual cusp to the tip of the distobuccal cusp. This ridge is reduced in height in the center of the occlusal surface, being about on a level with the marginal ridges of the occlusal surface. Sometimes it is crossed by a developmental groove which partially joins the two major fossae by means of its shallow sulcate groove.

The *mesial marginal ridge* and the *distal marginal ridge* are irregular ridges confluent with the mesial and distal cusp ridges of the mesial and distal major cusps.

The *central fossa* of the occlusal surface is a concave area bounded by the distal slope of the mesiobuccal cusp, the mesial slope of the distobuccal cusp, the crest of the oblique ridge, and the crests of the two triangular ridges of the mesiobuccal and mesiolingual cusps. The central fossa has connecting sulci within its boundaries, with developmental grooves at the deepest portions of these sulci (sulcate grooves). In addition, it contains supplemental grooves, short grooves which are disconnected, and also the central developmental pit. A worn specimen may show developmental or sulcate grooves only.

In the center of the central fossa the central developmental pit has sulcate developmental grooves, radiating from it at obtuse angles to each other. This pit is located in the approximate center of that portion of the occlusal surface which is circumscribed by cusp ridges and marginal ridges (Fig. 244). From this pit the *buccal developmental groove* radiates buccally at the bottom of the buccal sulcus of the central fossa, continuing on to the buccal surface of the crown between the buccal cusps.

Starting again at the central pit, the *central developmental groove* is seen to progress in a mesial direction at an obtuse angle to the buccal sulcate groove. The central groove at the bottom of the sulcus of the central fossa usually terminates at the apex of the *mesial triangular fossa*. Here it is joined by short supplemental grooves which radiate from its terminus into the triangular fossa. These supplemental grooves often appear as branches of the central groove. Occasionally one or more supplemental grooves cross the mesial marginal ridge of the crown.

The *mesial triangular fossa* is rather indistinct in outline, but it is generally triangular in shape with its base at the mesial marginal ridge and its apex at the point where the supplemental grooves join the central groove.

An additional short developmental groove radiates from the central pit of the central fossa at an obtuse angulation to the buccal and central developmental grooves. Usually it is considered a projection of one of these, since it is very short and usually fades out before reaching the crest of the oblique ridge. When it crosses the oblique ridge transversely, however, as it sometimes does, joining the central and distal fossae with a shallow groove, it is called the *transverse groove of the oblique ridge* (Fig. 260, specimens 3, 4 and 5).

The *distal fossa* of the maxillary first molar is roughly linear in form and is located immediately distal to the oblique ridge. An irregular developmental groove traverses its deepest portion. This developmental groove is called the *distal oblique groove*. It connects with the *lingual developmental groove* at the junction of the cusp ridges of the mesiolingual and distolingual cusps. These two grooves travel in the

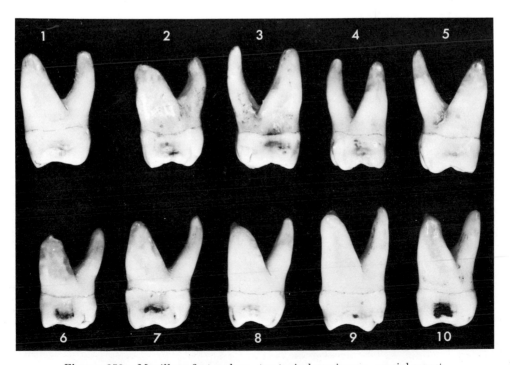

Figure 259. Maxillary first molars—ten typical specimens—mesial aspect.

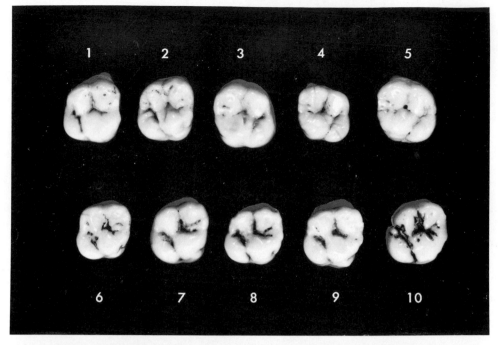

Figure 260.   Maxillary first molars—ten typical specimens—occlusal aspect.

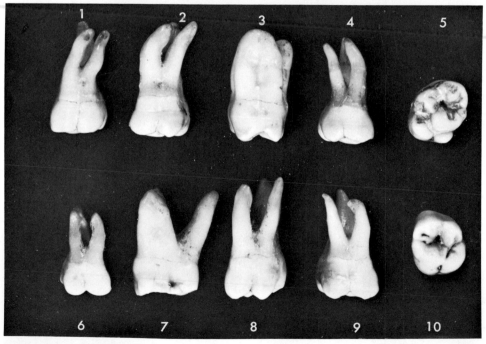

Figure 261.   Maxillary first molars—ten specimens showing uncommon variations. 1, Unusual curvature of buccal roots. 2, Roots abnormally long with extreme curvature. 3, Lingual and distobuccal roots fused. 4, Mesiodistal measurement of root trunk smaller than usual. 5, Extreme rhomboidal development of crown, fifth cusp with maximum development. 6, Tooth well developed but much smaller than usual. 7, Extreme buccolingual measurement. 8, Extreme length, especially of the distobuccal root; buccal cusps narrow mesiodistally. 9, Well-developed crown, roots poorly developed. 10, Extreme development of lingual portion of the crown when compared with the buccal development.

same oblique direction to the terminus of the lingual groove, which is centered below the lingual root at the approximate center of the crown lingually. If the fifth cusp development is distinct, a developmental groove outlining it joins the lingual groove near its terminus. Any part of the developmental groove which outlines a fifth cusp is called the *fifth cusp groove*.

The distal oblique groove in most cases shows several supplemental grooves. Two terminal branches usually appear, forming two sides of the triangular depression immediately mesial to the distal marginal ridge. These two sides, in combination with the slope mesial to the distal marginal ridge, form the *distal triangular fossa*. The distal outline of the distal marginal ridge of the crown shows a slight concavity.

The distolingual cusp is smooth and rounded from the occlusal aspect, and an outline of it, from the distal concavity of the distal marginal ridge to the lingual groove of the crown, describes an arc of an ellipse.

The lingual outline of the distolingual cusp is straight with the lingual outline of the fifth cusp, unless the fifth cusp is unusually large. In the latter case the lingual outline of the fifth cusp is more prominent lingually (see specimen 9, Fig. 260). The cusp ridge of the distolingual cusp always extends lingually farther than the cusp ridge of the mesiolingual cusp.

MAXILLARY SECOND MOLAR

Maxillary Second Molar

First evidence of calcification .... 2½ to 3 years
Enamel completed .... 7 to 8 years
Eruption .... 12 to 13 years
Root completed .... 14 to 16 years

Measurement Table

	Cervico-occlusal Length of Crown	Length of Root	Mesio-distal Diam-eter of Crown	Mesio-distal Diam-eter of Crown at Cervix	Labio- or Bucco-lingual Diameter of Crown	Labio- or Bucco-lingual Diameter at Cervix	Curvature of Cervical Line—Mesial	Curvature of Cervical Line—Distal
Dimensions suggested for carving technic	7.0*	b 11 112	9.0	7.0	11.0	10.0	1.0	0.0

* Millimeters.

The maxillary second molar supplements the first molar in function. In describing this tooth, direct comparisons will be made with the first molar both in form and development.

Generally speaking, the roots of this tooth are as long as, if not somewhat longer than, those of the first molar. The distobuccal cusp is not so large or so well developed, and the distolingual cusp is smaller. No fifth cusp is evident.

The crown of the maxillary second molar is 0.5 mm. or so shorter cervico-occlusally than that of the first molar, but the measurement of the crown buccolingually is about the same. *Two types* of maxillary second molars are found when one is viewing the occlusal aspect: (1) The type that is seen most has an occlusal form which resembles the first molar, although the rhomboidal outline is more extreme. This is accentuated by the lesser measurement mesiodistally. (2) This type bears more resemblance to a typical third molar form. The distolingual cusp is poorly developed and makes the development of the other three cusps predominate. This results in a heart-shaped form from the occlusal aspect that is typical of the maxillary *third* molar (Fig. 269, specimens 1 and 7).

Detailed Description of the Maxillary Second Molar from All Aspects

Buccal Aspect (Figs. 262 and 267)

The crown is a little shorter cervico-occlusally and narrower mesiodistally than the maxillary first molar. The distobuccal cusp is smaller and allows part of the distal marginal ridge and part of the distolingual cusp to be seen.

2 buccal & 1 lingual root

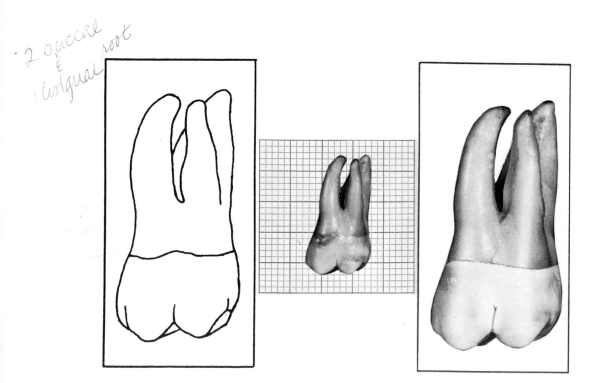

Figure 262.   Maxillary left second molar—buccal aspect.

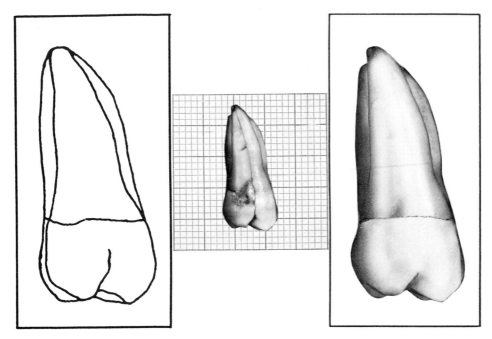

Figure 263. Maxillary left second molar – lingual aspect.

The buccal roots are about the same length. These roots are more nearly parallel and are inclined distally more than those of the maxillary first molar, so that the end of the distobuccal root is slightly distal to the distal extremity of the crown. The apex of the mesiobuccal root is on a line with the buccal groove of the crown instead of the tip of the mesiobuccal cusp as was found on the first molar.

Lingual Aspect (Fig. 263)

Differences between the second and first molars to be noted here in addition to those mentioned before are these: (1) The distolingual cusp of the crown is smaller; (2) the distobuccal cusp may be seen through the sulcus between the mesiolingual and distolingual cusp, and (3) no fifth cusp is evident.

The apex of the lingual root is in line with the distolingual cusp tip instead of the lingual groove as was found on the first molar.

Mesial Aspect (Figs. 264 and 268)

The buccolingual dimension is about the same as that of the first molar, but the crown length is less. The roots do not spread so far buccolingually, being within the confines of the buccolingual crown outline.

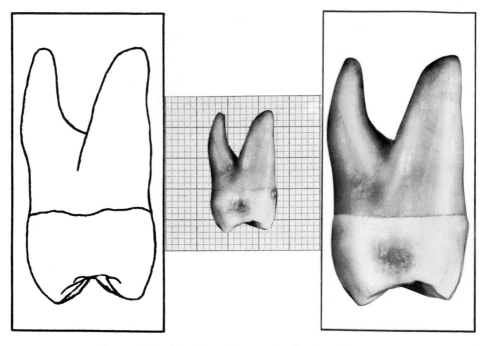

Figure 264.   Maxillary left second molar—mesial aspect.

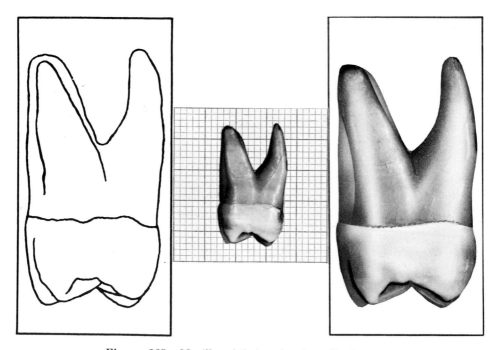

Figure 265.   Maxillary left second molar—distal aspect.

Distal Aspect (Fig. 265)

Because the distobuccal cusp is smaller than in the maxillary first molar, more of the mesiobuccal cusp may be seen from this angle. The mesiolingual cusp cannot be seen. The apex of the lingual root is in line with the distolingual cusp.

Occlusal Aspect (Figs. 266 and 269)

The rhomboidal type of second maxillary molar is most frequent, although in comparison with the first molar the acute angles of the rhomboid are less and the obtuse angles greater. The buccolingual diameter of the crown is about equal, but the mesiodistal diameter is approximately 1 mm. less. The mesiobuccal and mesiolingual cusps are just as large and well developed as in the first molar, but the distobuccal and distolingual cusps are smaller and less well developed. Usually a calibration made of the crown at the greatest diameter buccally and lingually of the distal portion is considerably less than one made at the greatest diameter buccally and lingually of the mesial portion, showing more convergence distally than the maxillary first molar.

It is not uncommon to find more supplemental grooves as well as accidental grooves and pits on the occlusal surface of a maxillary second molar than are usually found on a maxillary first molar.

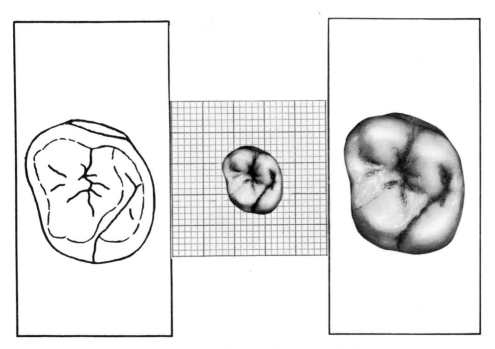

Figure 266.   Maxillary left second molar—occlusal aspect.

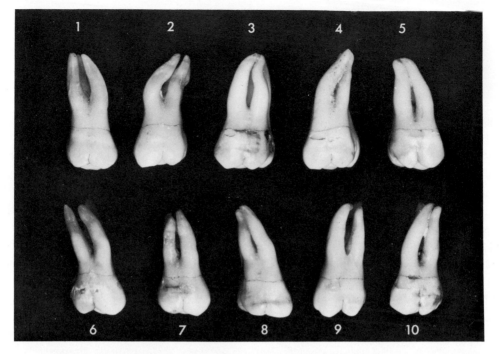

Figure 267. Maxillary second molars — ten typical specimens — buccal aspect.

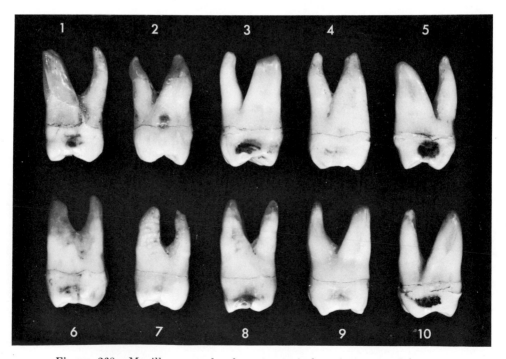

Figure 268. Maxillary second molars — ten typical specimens — mesial aspect.

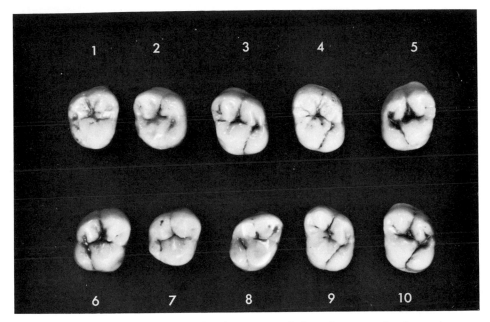

Figure 269. Maxillary second molars — ten typical specimens — occlusal aspect.

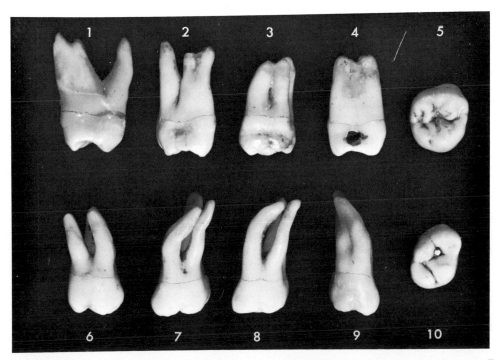

Figure 270. Maxillary second molars — ten specimens showing uncommon variations. 1, Roots spread similar to first molar. 2, Bifurcated mesiobuccal root. 3, Roots very short and fused. 4, Mesiobuccal and lingual roots with complete fusion. 5, Crown similar to the typical third molar form. 6, Short roots with spread similar to first molar. 7, Roots extra long with abnormal curvatures. 8, Another variation similar to specimen 7. 9, Very long roots fused. 10, Crown with extreme rhomboidal form.

MAXILLARY THIRD MOLAR

Maxillary Third Molar

First evidence of calcification .... 7 to 9 years
Enamel completed .... 12 to 16 years
Eruption .... 17 to 21 years
Root completed .... 18 to 25 years

Measurement Table

	Cervico-occlusal Length of Crown	Length of Root	Mesio-distal Diameter of Crown	Mesio-distal Diameter of Crown at Cervix	Labio- or Bucco-lingual Diameter of Crown	Labio- or Bucco-lingual Diameter at Cervix	Curvature of Cervical Line— Mesial	Curvature of Cervical Line— Distal
Dimensions suggested for carving technic	6.5*	11.0	8.5	6.5	10.0	9.5	1.0	0.0

* Millimeters.

The maxillary third molar often appears as a developmental anomaly. It varies considerably in size, contour and relative position to the other teeth. It is seldom so well developed as the maxillary second molar, to which it bears some resemblance. The third molar supplements the second molar in function, and its fundamental design is similar. The crown is smaller and the roots are, as a rule, shorter with the inclination toward fusion with the resultant anchorage of one tapered root.

The predominating third molar design, when one views the occlusal surface, is that of the heart-shaped type of second molar. The distolingual cusp is very small and poorly developed in most cases and it may be absent entirely.

All third molars, mandibular and maxillary, show more variation in development than any of the other teeth in the mouth. Occasionally they appear as anomalies bearing little or no resemblance to neighboring teeth. A few of the variations in form are shown in Figure 279.

For the purposes at hand it is necessary to give a short description of the third molar that is considered average in its development and one that would be in good proportion to the other maxillary molars and with an occlusal form considered normal. In describing the normal maxillary third molar, direct comparisons will be made with the maxillary second molar.

Detailed Description of the Maxillary Third Molar from all Aspects

Buccal Aspect (Figs. 271 and 276)

The crown is shorter cervico-occlusally and narrower mesiodistally than that of the second molar. The roots are usually fused, functioning as one large root, and they

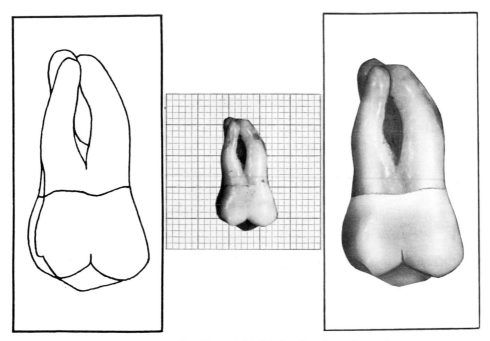

Figure 271.   Maxillary right third molar – buccal aspect.

are shorter cervicoapically. The fused roots end in a taper at the apex. The roots have a distinct slant to the distal, giving the apices of the fused root a more distal relation to the center of the crown.

Lingual Aspect (Fig. 272)

In addition to the differences mentioned above, in comparison with the maxillary second molar, there is usually just one large lingual cusp and therefore no lingual

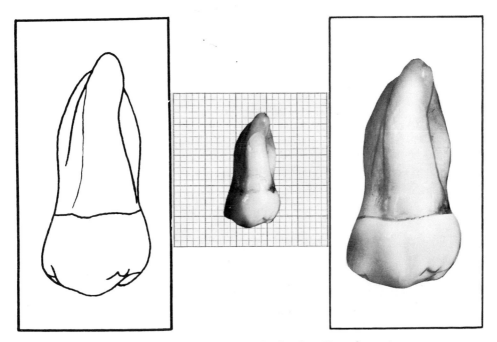

Figure 272.   Maxillary right third molar – lingual aspect.

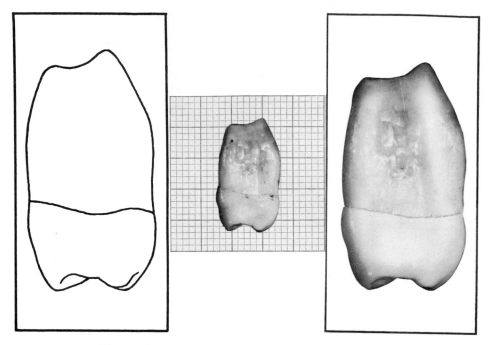

Figure 273.   Maxillary right third molar — mesial aspect.

groove. However, in many cases, a third molar with the same essential features has a poorly developed distolingual cusp with a developmental groove lingually. (Fig. 278, specimen 2.)

Mesial Aspect (Figs. 273 and 277)

Here, aside from the differences in measurement, the main feature is the taper to the fused roots and a bifurcation, usually in the region of the apical third. (Fig. 273 does not show a bifurcation. See specimens 1, 2 and 3 in Fig. 277.) The root portion is considerably shorter in relation to the crown length. Both the crown and the root portions are inclined to be poorly developed, with irregular outlines.

Distal Aspect (Fig. 274)

From this aspect most of the buccal surface of the crown is in view. More of the occlusal surface may be seen than can be seen on the second molar from this aspect because of the more acute angulation of the occlusal surface in relation to the long axis of the root. The measurement from the cervical line to the marginal ridge is short.

Occlusal Aspect (Figs. 275 and 278)

The occlusal aspect of a typical maxillary third molar presents a heart-shaped outline. The lingual cusp is large and well developed and there is little or no distolingual cusp — which gives a semicircular outline to the tooth from one contact area to

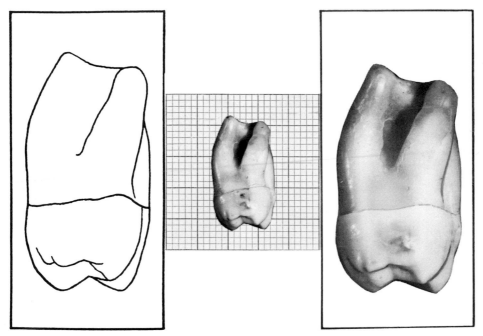

Figure 274. Maxillary right third molar—distal aspect.

the other. On this type of tooth there are *three* functioning cusps: two buccal and one lingual.

The occlusal aspect of this tooth usually presents many supplemental grooves and many accidental grooves unless the tooth is very much worn.

The third molar may show four distinct cusps. This type may have a strong oblique ridge, a central fossa and a distal fossa, with a lingual developmental groove

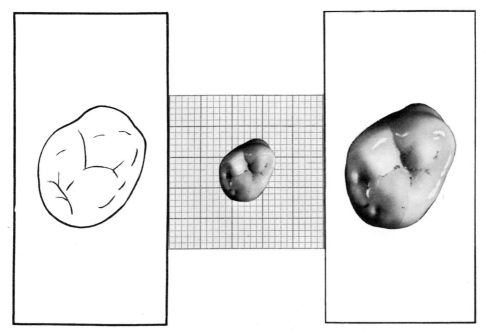

Figure 275. Maxillary right third molar—occlusal aspect.

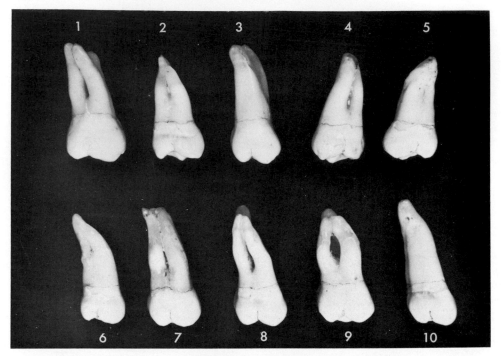

Figure 276. Maxillary third molars—ten typical specimens—buccal aspect.

similar to that of the rhomboidal type of second molar. In most instances, the crown converges more lingually from the buccal areas than the second molar does, losing its rhomboidal outline. This is not, however, always true (compare specimens 1 and 3 in Fig. 278).

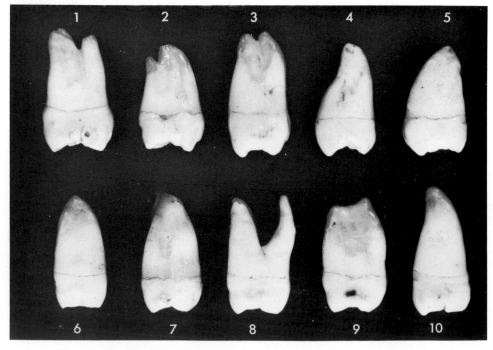

Figure 277. Maxillary third molars—ten typical specimens—mesial aspect.

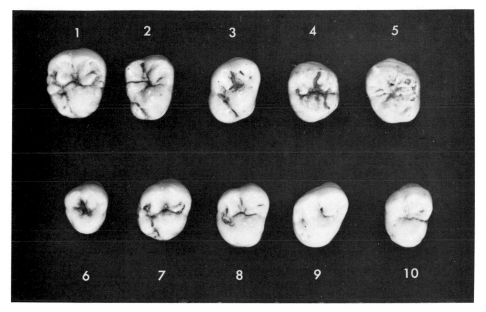

Figure 278. Maxillary third molars—ten typical specimens—occlusal aspect.

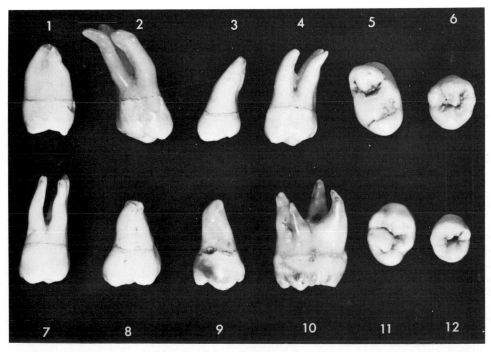

Figure 279. Maxillary third molars—twelve specimens showing uncommon variations. 1, Very short fused root form. 2, Extremely long roots with extreme distal angulation. 3, Complete fusion of roots with extreme distal angulation. 4, Three roots well separated, crown very wide at cervix. 5, Extreme rhomboidal outline to crown with developmental grooves oddly placed. 6, Overdeveloped mesiobuccal cusp. 7, Crown wide at cervix, with roots perpendicular. 8, Very large crown, poorly developed root form. 9, Complete absence of typical design. 10, Specimen abnormally large, with four roots well separated. 11, Five well-developed cusps, atypical in form. 12, Small specimen, atypical cusp form.

Chapter XII

THE PERMANENT
MANDIBULAR MOLARS

THE MANDIBULAR molars are larger than any other mandibular teeth. They are three in number on each side of the mandible: the first, second and third mandibular molars. They resemble each other in form, although comparison of one with another shows variations in the number of cusps and variations in size, occlusal design and the relative length and positions of the roots.

The crown outlines exhibit similarities of outline from all aspects, and each mandibular molar has two roots, one mesial and one distal. Third molars and some second molars may show a fusion of these roots. All mandibular molars have crowns that are roughly quadrilateral, being somewhat longer mesiodistally than buccolingually. Maxillary molar crowns have their widest measurement buccolingually.

The mandibular molars help to perform the major portion of the work in the mastication and comminution of food. They are the largest and strongest mandibular teeth, both because of their bulk and because of their anchorage in the mandible.

The crowns of the molars are shorter cervico-occlusally than those of the teeth anterior to them, but their dimensions are greater in every other respect. The root portions are not so long as those of some of the other mandibular teeth, but the combined measurements of the multiple roots, with their broad bifurcated root trunks, result in superior anchorage and greater efficiency.

Usually the sum of the mesiodistal measurements of mandibular molars is equal to, or greater than, the combined mesiodistal measurements of all the teeth anterior to the first molar and up to the median line.

The crowns of these molars are wider mesiodistally than buccolingually. The opposite arrangement is true of maxillary molars.

258

MANDIBULAR FIRST MOLAR

Normally the mandibular first molar is the largest tooth in the mandibular arch. It has five well-developed cusps: two buccal, two lingual and a distal cusp (Fig. 281). It has two well-developed roots, one mesial and one distal, which are very broad buccolingually. These roots are widely separated at the apices.

The dimension of the crown mesiodistally is greater by about 1 mm. than the dimension buccolingually. Although the crown is relatively short cervico-occlusally, it has mesiodistal and buccolingual measurements which provide a broad occlusal form.

Mandibular First Molar

First evidence of calcification .... At birth
Enamel completed .... 2½ to 3 years
Eruption 6   to 7 years
Root completed 9   to 10 years

Measurement Table

	Cervico-occlusal Length of Crown	Length of Root	Mesio-distal Diam-eter of Crown	Mesio-distal Diam-eter of Crown at Cervix	Labio- or Bucco-lingual Diameter of Crown	Labio- or Bucco-lingual Diameter of Crown at Cervix	Curvature of Cervical Line— Mesial	Curvature of Cervical Line— Distal
Dimensions suggested for carving technic	7.5*	14.0	11.0	9.0	10.5	9.0	1.0	0.0

* Millimeters.

Figure 280. Mandibular right first molar —occlusal aspect. *DBCR*, distobuccal cusp ridge; *DBDG*, distobuccal developmental groove; *DCR*, distal cusp ridge; *DTF*, distal triangular fossa (shaded area); *DLCR*, distolingual cusp ridge; *LDG*, lingual developmental groove; *MLCR*, mesiolingual cusp ridge; *MTF*, mesial triangular fossa (shaded area); *SG*, a supplemental groove; *MBCR*, mesiobuccal cusp ridge; *MBDG*, mesiobuccal developmental groove.

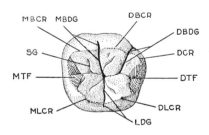

The mesial root is broad and curved distally, with mesial and distal fluting which provides the anchorage of two roots (Fig. 338, D). The distal root is rounder, broad at the cervical portion, and pointed in a distal direction. The formation of these roots and their positions in the mandible serve to brace the crown of the tooth against the lines of force brought to bear against it.

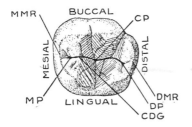

Figure 281. Mandibular right first molar—occlusal aspect. Shaded area—central fossa; *CP*, central pit; *DMR*, distal marginal ridge; *DP*, distal pit; *CDG*, central developmental groove; *MP*, mesial pit; *MMR*, mesial marginal ridge.

Detailed Description of the Mandibular First Molar from All Aspects

Buccal Aspect (Figs. 282, 283, 291, 292 and 293)

From the buccal aspect the crown of the mandibular first molar is roughly trapezoidal, with cervical and occlusal outlines representing the uneven sides of the trapezoid. The occlusal side is the longer.

If this tooth is posed vertically, all five of its cusps are in view. The two buccal cusps and the buccal portion of the distal cusp are in the foreground, with the tips of the lingual cusps in the background. The lingual cusps may be seen because they are higher than the others.

Two developmental grooves appear on the crown portion. These grooves are called the *mesiobuccal developmental groove* and the *distobuccal developmental groove*. The first-named groove acts as a line of demarcation between the mesiobuccal lobe and the distobuccal lobe. The latter groove separates the distobuccal lobe from the distal lobe (Fig. 282).

The mesiobuccal, distobuccal and distal cusps are relatively flat. These cusp ridges show less curvature than those of any of the teeth described so far. The distal cusp, which is small, is more pointed than either of the buccal cusps. Flattened buccal cusps are typical of all mandibular molars. Most first molar specimens have their buccal cusps worn considerably, showing the buccal cusp ridges almost at the same

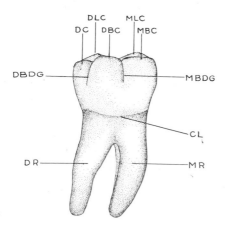

Figure 282. Mandibular right first molar—buccal aspect. *MBDG*, mesiobuccal developmental groove; *CL*, cervical line; *MR*, mesial root; *DR*, distal root; *DBDG*, distobuccal developmental groove; *DC*, distal cusp; *DLC*, distolingual cusp; *DBC*, distobuccal cusp; *MLC*, mesiolingual cusp; *MBC*, mesiobuccal cusp.

level. Before they are worn, the buccal cusps and the distal cusp have curvatures that are characteristic of each one (Figs. 283 and 293, specimen 1).

The mesiobuccal cusp is usually the widest mesiodistally of the three cusps. This cusp has some curvature but is relatively flat. The distobuccal cusp is almost as wide, with a cusp ridge of somewhat greater curvature. The two buccal cusps make up the major portion of the buccal surface of the crown. The distal cusp provides a very small part of the buccal surface, since the major portion of the cusp makes up the distal portion of the crown, providing the distal contact area on the center of the distal surface of the distal cusp. The distal cusp ridge is very round occlusally, being sharper than either of the two buccal cusps.

These three cusps have the mesiobuccal and distobuccal grooves as lines of demarcation. The mesiobuccal groove is the shorter of the two, having its terminus centrally located cervico-occlusally. This groove is situated a little mesial to the root bifurcation buccally. The distobuccal groove has its terminus near the distobuccal line angle at the cervical third of the crown. It travels occlusally and somewhat mesially, parallel with the axis of the distal root.

The cervical line of the mandibular first molar is commonly regular in outline, dipping apically toward the root bifurcation.

The mesial outline of the crown is somewhat concave at the cervical third up to its junction with the convex outline of the broad contact area. The distal outline of the crown is straight above the cervical line to its junction with the convex outline of the distal contact area, which is also the outline of the distal portion of the distal cusp.

The measurement of this tooth at the cervical line is 1.5 to 2 mm. less

5 cusps → 5 pulpal horns

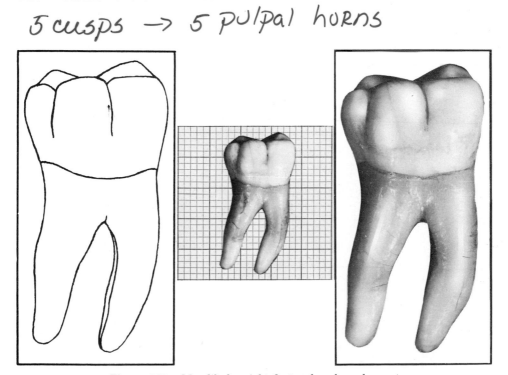

Figure 283. Mandibular right first molar — buccal aspect.

mesiodistally than the mesiodistal measurement at the contact areas, which of course represents the greatest mesiodistal measurement of the crown.

The surface of the buccal portion of the crown is smoothly convex at the cusp portions with developmental grooves between the cusps. Approximately at the level of the ends of the developmental grooves, in the middle third, a developmental depression is noticeable. It runs in a mesiodistal direction just above the cervical ridge of the buccal surface (Fig. 293, specimens 1 and 2). This cervical ridge may show a smooth depression in it which progresses cervically, joining with the developmental concavity just below the cervical line which is congruent with the root bifurcation buccally (Fig. 293, specimen 8).

The roots of this tooth are, in most instances, well formed and constant in development.

When the tooth is posed so that the mesiobuccal groove is directly in the line of vision, part of the distal surface of the root trunk may be seen and, in addition, one may see part of the distal area of the mesial root because the lingual portion of the root is turned distally. These areas may be seen in addition to the buccal areas of the roots and root trunk.

The mesial root is curved mesially from a point shortly below the cervical line to the middle third portion. From this point it curves distally to the tapered apex, which is located directly below the mesiobuccal cusp. The crest of curvature of the root mesially is mesial to the crown cervix. The distal outline of the mesial root is concave from the bifurcation of the root trunk to the apex. The distal area of the mesial root is concave (Fig. 293, specimen 5).

The distal root is less curved than the mesial root, and its axis is in a distal direction from cervix to apex. The root may show some curvature at its apical third in either a mesial or a distal direction (Fig. 293, specimens 1 and 8). The apex is usually more pointed than that of the mesial root and is located below or distal to the distal contact area of the crown. There is considerable variation in the comparative lengths of mesial and distal roots (Fig. 293).

Both roots are wider mesiodistally at the buccal areas than they are elsewhere. Developmental depressions are present on the mesial and distal sides of both roots— a fact which lessens the mesiodistal measurement at those points. They are somewhat thicker at the lingual borders. This arrangement provides a secure anchorage for the mandibular first molar, since rotation is prevented. This I-beam principle increases the anchorage of each root (Chapter XIII, Fig. 338).

The point of bifurcation of the two roots is located approximately 3 mm. below the cervical line. There is a deep developmental depression buccally on the root trunk which starts at the bifurcation and progresses cervically, becoming more shallow until it terminates at or immediately above the cervical line. This depression is smooth with no developmental groove or fold.

Lingual Aspect (Figs. 284, 285, 291 and 292)

From the lingual aspect, three cusps may be seen: two lingual cusps and the lingual portion of the distal cusp (Fig. 284). The two lingual cusps are pointed, and

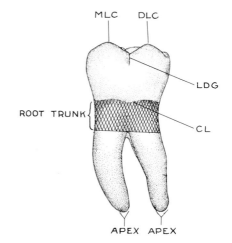

Figure 284. Mandibular right first molar —lingual aspect. *MLC*, mesiolingual cusp; *DLC*, distolingual cusp; *LDG*, lingual developmental groove; *CL*, cervical line.

the cusp ridges are high enough to hide the two buccal cusps from view. The mesiolingual cusp is the widest mesiodistally, with its cusp tip somewhat higher than the distolingual cusp. The distolingual cusp is almost as wide mesiodistally as the mesiolingual cusp. The mesiolingual and distolingual cusp ridges are inclined at angles that are similar on both lingual cusps. These cusp ridges form obtuse angles at the cusp tips of approximately 100 degrees.

The *lingual developmental groove* serves as a line of demarcation between the lingual cusps, extending downward on the lingual surface of the crown for a short distance only. Some mandibular first molars show no groove on the lingual surface but show a depression lingual to the cusp ridges. The angle formed by the distolingual cusp ridge of the mesiolingual cusp and the mesiolingual cusp ridge of the distolingual cusp is more obtuse than the angulation of the cusp ridges at the tips of the lingual cusps.

The distal cusp is at a lower level than either of the lingual cusps.

The mesial outline of the crown from this aspect is convex from the cervical line to the marginal ridge. The crest of contour, which represents the contact area, is somewhat higher than the crest of contour of the distal outline of the crown.

The distal outline of the crown is straight immediately above the cervical line to a point immediately below the distal contact area; this area is represented by a convex curvature which also outlines the distal surface of the distal cusp. The junction of the distolingual cusp ridge of the distolingual cusp with the distal marginal ridge is abrupt; it gives the impression of a groove at this site from the lingual aspect. Sometimes there is a shallow developmental groove at this point (Fig. 289). Part of the mesial and distal surfaces of the crown and root trunk may be seen from this aspect because the mesial and distal sides converge lingually.

The cervical line lingually is irregular and tends to point sharply toward the root bifurcation and immediately above it.

The surface of the crown lingually is smooth and spheroidal on each of the lingual lobes. The surface is concave at the side of the lingual groove above the center of the crown lingually. Below this point the surface of the crown becomes almost flat as it approaches the cervical line.

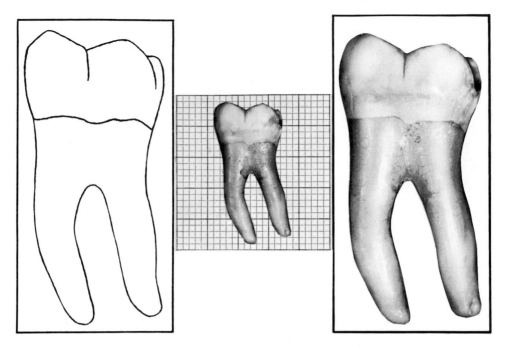

Figure 285. Mandibular right first molar—lingual aspect.

The roots of the mandibular first molar appear somewhat different from the lingual aspect. They measure about 1 mm. longer lingually than buccally, but the length *seems* more extreme (Fig. 285). This impression is derived from the fact that the cusp ridges and cervical line are at a higher level (about 1 mm.). This arrangement adds a millimeter to the distance from root bifurcation to cervical line. In addition, the mesiodistal measurement of the root trunk is less toward the lingual surface than toward the buccal surface. Consequently this slenderness lingually, in addition to the added length, makes the roots appear longer than they are from the lingual aspect (Fig. 288).

As was mentioned, the root bifurcation lingually starts at a point approximately 4 mm. below the cervical line. This developmental depression is quite deep at this point, although it is smooth throughout and progresses cervically and becomes more shallow until it fades out entirely immediately below the cervical line. The depression is rarely reflected in the cervical line or the enamel of the lingual surface of the crown as is found in many cases on the buccal surface of this tooth.

This bifurcation groove of the root trunk is located directly in line with the lingual developmental groove of the crown.

Mesial Aspect (Figs. 286, 291, 292 and 294)

When the mandibular first molar is viewed from the mesial aspect, the specimen being held with its mesial surface at right angles to the line of vision, two cusps and one root only are to be seen: the mesiobuccal and mesiolingual cusps and the mesial root (Fig. 286).

The buccolingual measurement of the crown is greater at the mesial portion

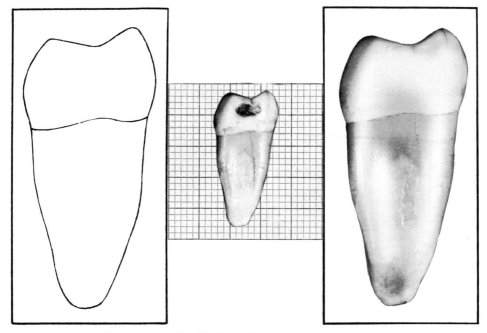

Figure 286.   Mandibular right first molar – mesial aspect.

than it is at the distal portion. The buccolingual measurement of the mesial root is also greater than the same measurement of the distal root. Therefore, since the mesial portions of the tooth are broader and the mesial cusps are higher, the distal portions of the tooth cannot be seen from this angle.

As mentioned before, all of the posterior mandibular teeth have crown outlines from the mesial aspect which show a characteristic relation between crown and root. The crown from the mesial or distal aspect is roughly rhomboidal and the entire crown has a lingual tilt in relation to the root axis. It should be remembered that the crowns of maxillary posterior teeth have the center of the occlusal surfaces between the cusps in line with the root axis (Fig. 102E, F).

It is interesting to note the difference between the *outline form of the mandibular first molar and the mandibular second premolar from the mesial aspect.* The first molar compares as follows:

1. The crown is a fraction of a millimeter to a millimeter shorter in the first molar.

2. The root is usually that much shorter also.

3. The buccolingual measurement of crown and root is 2 mm. or more greater.

4. The lingual cusp is longer than the buccal cusp. (The opposite is true of the second premolar.)

Regardless of these differences, *the two teeth have the same functional form except for the added reinforcement given to the molar lingually.* Because of the added root width buccolingually, the buccal cusps of the first molar do not approach the center axis of the root as closely as does the second premolar, and the lingual cusp tips are within the lingual outline of the roots instead of being on a line with them.

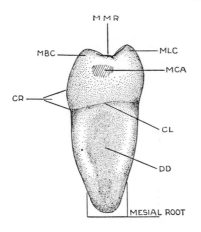

Figure 287. Mandibular right first molar — mesial aspect. *MMR*, mesial marginal ridge; *MLC*, mesiolingual cusp; *MCA*, mesial contact area; *CL*, cervical line; *DD*, developmental depression; *CR*, cervical ridge; *MBC*, mesiobuccal cusp.

From the mesial aspect, the buccal outline of the crown of the mandibular first molar is convex immediately above the cervical line. Before occlusal wear has shortened the buccal cusps, this curvature is over the cervical third of the crown buccally, outlining the *buccal cervical ridge* (Fig. 287). This ridge is more prominent on some first molars than on others (Fig. 294). Just as on mandibular premolars, this ridge curvature does not exceed similar contours on other teeth as a rule when the mandibular first molar is posed in the position it assumes in the mandibular arch (Fig. 286 and Fig. 294, specimens 1 and 2).

Above the buccal cervical ridge, the outline of the buccal contour may be slightly concave on some specimens (Fig. 294, specimens 1 and 2); or the outline may become much less convex or even straight as it continues occlusally outlining the contour of the mesiobuccal cusp. The mesiobuccal cusp is located directly above the buccal third of the mesial root.

The lingual outline of the crown is straight in a lingual direction, starting at the cervical line and joining the lingual curvature at the middle third, the lingual curvature being pronounced between this point and the tip of the mesiolingual cusp. The crest of the lingual contour is located at the center of the middle third of the crown. The tip of the mesiolingual cusp is in a position directly above the lingual third of the mesial root.

The mesial marginal ridge is confluent with the mesial ridges of the mesiobuccal and mesiolingual cusps. The marginal ridge is placed about 1 mm. below the level of the cusp tips.

The cervical line mesially is rather irregular and tends to curve occlusally about 1 mm. toward the center of the mesial surface of the tooth (Fig. 294, specimens 1, 4, 9 and 10). The cervical line may assume a relatively straight line buccolingually (specimens 3, 6 and 8).

In all instances the cervical line is at a higher level lingually than buccally, usually about 1 mm. higher. The difference in level may be greater. This relation depends upon the assumption that the tooth is posed vertically. When the first molar is in its normal position in the lower jaw, leaning to the lingual, the cervical line is nearly level buccolingually.

The surface of the crown is convex and smooth over the mesial contours of the

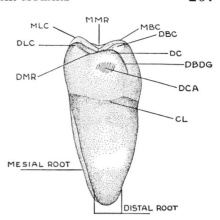

Figure 288. Mandibular right first molar —distal aspect. *MMR*, mesial marginal ridge; *MBC*, mesiobuccal cusp; *DBC*, distobuccal cusp; *DC*, distal cusp; *DBDG*, distobuccal developmental groove; *DCA*, distal contact area; *CL*, cervical line; *DMR*, distal marginal ridge; *DLC*, distolingual cusp; *MLC*, mesiolingual cusp.

mesiolingual and mesiobuccal lobes. A flattened or slightly concave area exists at the cervical line immediately above the center of the mesial root. This area is right below the contact area and joins the concavity of the central portion of the root at the cervix. The contact area is almost centered buccolingually on the mesial surface of the crown, and it is placed below the crest of the marginal ridge about one third the distance from marginal ridge to cervical line. (See stained contact area on specimen, Fig. 288. Before contact wear has occurred, the contact area is not so broad. Refer also to Fig. 283.)

The buccal outline of the mesial root drops straight down from the cervical line buccally to a point near the junction of cervical and middle thirds of the root. There is a gentle curve lingually from this point to the apex, which is located directly below the mesiobuccal cusp.

The lingual outline of the mesial root is slanted in a buccal direction, although the outline is nearly straight from the cervical line lingually to the point of junction of middle and apical thirds of the root. From this point the curvature is sharply buccal to the bluntly tapered apex. On those specimens which show a short bifurcation at the mesial root end, the curvature at the apical third lingually is slight (Fig. 294, specimens 2 and 10).

The mesial surface of the mesial root is convex at the buccal and lingual borders, with a broad concavity between these convexities the full length of the root from cervical line to apex. If a specimen tooth is held in front of a strong light so that one may see the distal side of the mesial root from the apical aspect, it is noted that the same contours exist on the root distally as are found mesially, and the root is very thin where the concavities are superimposed. The root form appears to be two narrow roots fused together with thin hard tissue between.

The mesial surface of the distal root is smooth, with no deep developmental depressions.

Distal Aspect (Figs. 289, 291 and 292)

Since the gross outline of the distal aspect of crown and root of the mandibular first molar is similar to the mesial aspect, the description of outline form will not be repeated. When considering this aspect from the standpoint of a three-dimensional figure, however, one sees more of the tooth from the distal aspect because the crown is shorter distally than mesially, and the buccal and lingual surfaces of the crown converge distally. The buccal surface shows more convergence than the lingual surface. The distal root is narrower buccolingually than the mesial root.

If a specimen of the first molar is held with the distal surface of the crown at right angles to the line of vision, a great part of the occlusal surface may be seen and some part of each of the five cusps also, as was the case in the mandibular second premolar. This is caused in part by the placement of the crown on the roots with a distal inclination to the long axes. The slight variation in crown length distally does not provide this view of the occlusal surface (Fig. 288).

From the distal aspect, the distal cusp is in the foreground on the crown portion. The distal cusp is placed a little buccal to center buccolingually, the distal contact area appearing on its distal contour.

The distal contact area is placed just below the distal cusp ridge of the distal cusp and at a slightly higher level above the cervical line than was found mesially when considering the location of the mesial contact area.

The distal marginal ridge is short and is made up of the distal cusp ridge of the distal cusp and the distolingual cusp ridge of the distolingual cusp. These cusp ridges dip sharply in a cervical direction, meeting at an obtuse angle. Often a developmental groove or depression is found crossing the marginal ridge at this point. The point of this angle is above the lingual third of the distal root instead of being centered over the root as is true of the center of the mesial marginal ridge.

The distal contact area is centered over the distal root, which arrangement places it buccal to the center point of the distal marginal ridge.

The surface of the distal portion of the crown is convex on the distal cusp and the distolingual cusp. Contact wear may produce a flattened area at the point of contact on the distal surface of the distal cusp. Just above the cervical line, the enamel surface is flat where it joins the flattened surface of the root trunk distally.

The cervical line distally usually extends straight across buccolingually. It may be irregular, dipping root-wise just below the distal contact area (Fig. 289).

The end of the distobuccal developmental groove is located on the distal surface and forms a concavity at the cervical portion of the distobuccal line angle of the crown. The distal portion of the crown extends out over the root trunk distally at quite an angle (Fig. 283). The smooth flat surface below the contact area remains fairly constant to the apical third of the distal root. Sometimes a developmental depression is found here. The apical third portion of the root is more rounded as it tapers to a sharper apex than is found on the mesial root.

The lingual border of the mesial root may be seen from the distal aspect.

Occlusal Aspect (Figs. 280, 281, 290, 291, 292 and 295)

The mandibular first molar is somewhat hexagonal from the occlusal aspect (Fig. 281). The dimension of the crown is 1 mm. or more greater mesiodistally than

(Text continued on page 272.)

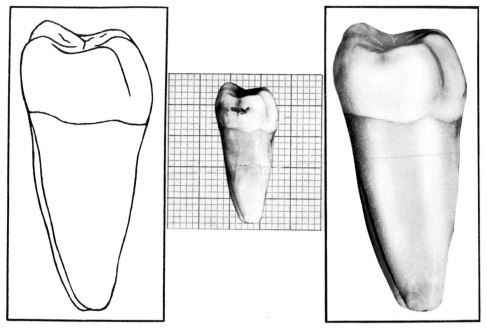

Figure 289. Mandibular right first molar—distal aspect.

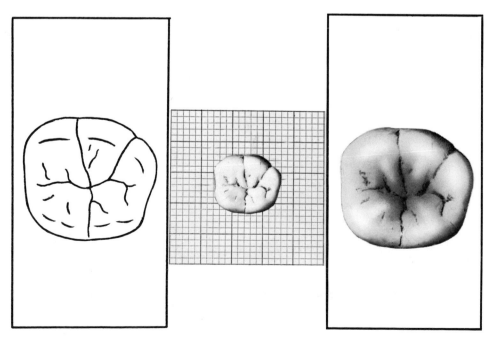

Figure 290. Mandibular right first molar—occlusal aspect.

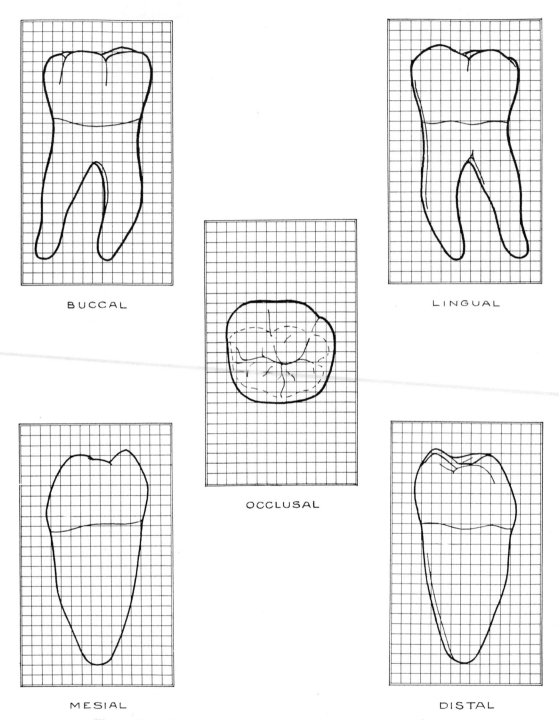

BUCCAL

LINGUAL

OCCLUSAL

MESIAL

DISTAL

Figure 291. Mandibular right first molar. Graph outlines from five aspects.

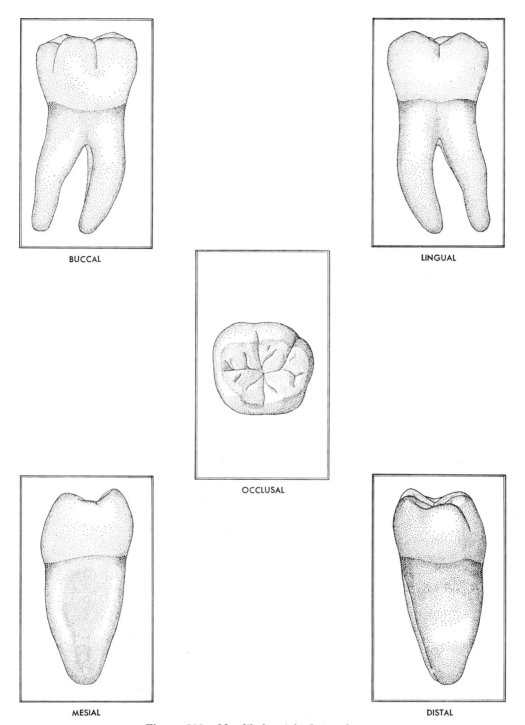

BUCCAL

LINGUAL

OCCLUSAL

MESIAL

DISTAL

Figure 292. Mandibular right first molar.

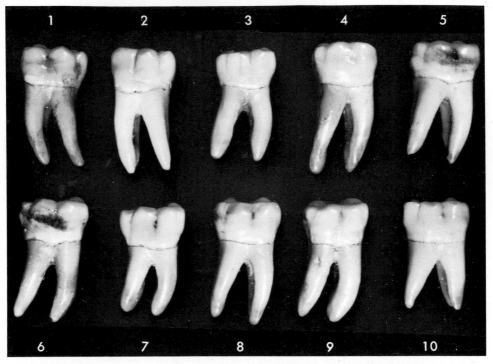

Figure 293.   Mandibular first molars — ten typical specimens — buccal aspect.

buccolingually. It must be remembered that the opposite arrangement is true of the maxillary first molar.

The buccolingual measurement of the crown is greater on the mesial than on the distal. Also, a measurement of the crown at the contact areas, which includes the two buccal cusps and the distal cusp, shows greater measurement than the mesiodistal measurement of the two lingual cusps. In other words, the crown converges lingually from the contact areas. This convergence varies in individual specimens (Fig. 295, specimens 1 and 4).

It is interesting to note the degree of development of the individual cusps from the occlusal aspect. The mesiobuccal cusp is slightly larger than either of the two lingual cusps, which are almost equal to each other in size; the distobuccal cusp is smaller than any one of the other three mentioned, and the distal cusp is in most cases much the smallest of all.

There is more variance in the development of the distobuccal and distal lobes than in any of the others (Fig. 295, specimens 4, 8 and 9).

When the tooth is posed so that the line of vision is parallel with the long axis, a great part of the buccal surface may be seen, whereas only a small portion of the lingual surface may be seen lingual to the lingual cusp ridges. No part of the mesial or distal surfaces is in view below the outline of the mesial and distal marginal ridges. (Compare tooth outlines from the other aspects.)

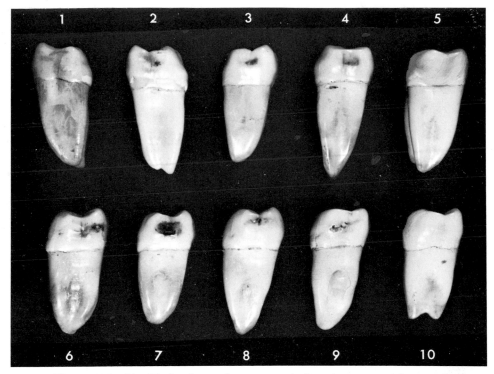

Figure 294. Mandibular first molars—ten typical specimens—mesial aspect.

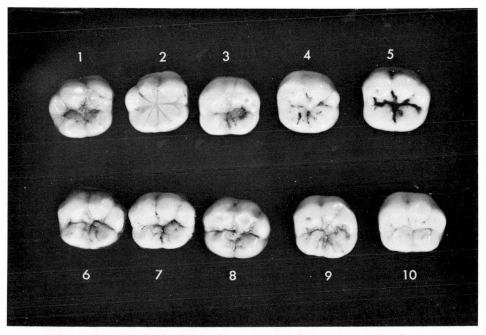

Figure 295. Mandibular first molars—ten typical specimens—occlusal aspect.

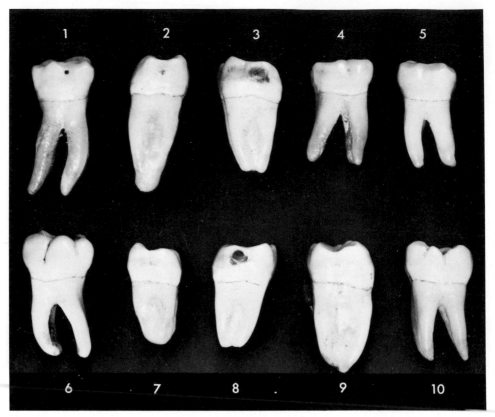

Figure 296. Mandibular first molars — ten specimens showing uncommon variations. 1, Roots extremely long, crown small. 2, Mesial root longer than average with rounded apex. 3, Crown very wide buccolingually, roots short. 4, Roots short. 5, Crown has no buccal developmental grooves. 6, Crown and roots poorly formed. 7, Roots dwarfed. 8, Short roots, crown wide buccolingually. 9, Crown and root oversize buccolingually. 10, Extra tubercle or cusp attached to mesiolingual lobe.

All mandibular molars, including the first molar, are essentially quadrilateral in form. The mandibular first molar, in most instances, has a functioning distal cusp, although this is small in comparison with the other cusps. Occasionally four-cusp first molars are found, and more often one discovers first molars with distobuccal and distal cusps showing fusion with little or no trace of a distobuccal developmental groove between them (Fig. 295, specimen 3; Fig. 296, specimens 4 and 5). *From a developmental viewpoint all mandibular molars have four major cusps, whereas maxillary molars have only three major cusps* (Fig. 254).

The *occlusal* surface of the mandibular first molar may be described as follows: There is a major fossa and there are two minor fossae. The major fossa is the *central fossa* (Fig. 281). It is roughly circular, and it is centrally placed on the occlusal surface between buccal and lingual cusp ridges. The two minor fossae are the *mesial triangular fossa,* immediately distal to the mesial marginal ridge, and the *distal triangular fossa,* placed immediately mesial to the distal marginal ridge (Fig. 280).

The developmental grooves on the occlusal surface are the *central developmental groove*, the *mesiobuccal developmental groove*, the *distobuccal developmental groove* and the *lingual developmental groove*. Supplemental grooves, accidental short grooves and developmental pits are also found. Most of the supplemental grooves are tributary to the developmental grooves within the bounds of cusp ridges.

The *central fossa* of the occlusal surface is a concave area bounded by the distal slope of the mesiobuccal cusp, both mesial and distal slopes of the distobuccal cusp, the mesial slope of the distal cusp, the distal slope of the mesiolingual cusp and the mesial slope of the distolingual cusp.

All of the developmental grooves converge in the center of the central fossa at the *central pit*.

The *mesial triangular fossa* of the occlusal surface is a smaller concave area than the central fossa, and it is bounded by the mesial slope of the mesiobuccal cusp, the mesial marginal ridge and the mesial slope of the mesiolingual cusp. The mesial portion of the central developmental groove terminates in this fossa. Usually a buccal and a lingual supplemental groove join it at a *mesial pit* within the boundary of the mesial marginal ridge. Sometimes a supplemental groove crosses the mesial marginal ridge lingual to the contact area (Fig. 295, specimens 2, 8, 9 and 10).

The *distal triangular fossa* is in most instances less distinct than the mesial fossa. It is bounded by the distal slope of the distal cusp, the distal marginal ridge and the distal slope of the distolingual cusp. The central groove has its other terminal in this fossa. Buccal and lingual supplemental grooves are less common here. An extension of the central groove quite often crosses the distal marginal ridge, however, lingual to the distal contact area.

Starting at the central pit in the central fossa, the central developmental groove travels an irregular course mesially, terminating in the mesial triangular fossa. A short distance mesially from the central pit, it joins the mesiobuccal developmental groove. The latter groove courses in a mesiobuccal direction at the bottom of a sulcate groove separating the mesiobuccal and distobuccal cusps. At the junction of the cusp ridges of those cusps, the mesiobuccal groove of the occlusal surface is confluent with the mesiobuccal groove of the buccal surface of the crown. The lingual developmental groove of the occlusal surface is an irregular groove coursing in a lingual direction at the bottom of the lingual sulcate groove to the junction of lingual cusp ridges, where it is confluent with the lingual extension of the same groove. Again starting at the central pit, the central groove may be followed in a distobuccal direction to a point where it is joined by the distobuccal developmental groove of the occlusal surface. From this point the central groove courses in a distolingual direction, terminating in the distal triangular fossa. The distobuccal groove passes from its junction with the central groove in a distobuccal course, joining its buccal extension on the buccal surface of the crown at the junction of the cusp ridges of the distobuccal and distal cusps.

The central developmental groove seems to be centrally located in relation to the buccolingual crown dimension. This arrangement makes the triangular ridges of lingual cusps longer than the triangular ridges of buccal cusps.

Students should note the relative position and relative size of the distal cusp from the occlusal aspect. The distal portion of it joins the distal contact area of the crown.

MANDIBULAR SECOND MOLAR

Mandibular Second Molar

First evidence of calcification .... 2½ to 3 years
Enamel completed .... 7 to 8 years
Eruption .... 11 to 13 years
Root completed .... 14 to 15 years

Measurement Table

	Cervico-occlusal Length of Crown	Length of Root	Mesio distal Diameter of Crown	Mesio-distal Diam eter of Crown at Cervix	Labio- or Bucco-lingual Diameter of Crown	Labio- or Bucco-lingual Diameter of Crown at Cervix	Curvature of Cervical Line— Mesial	Curvature of Cervical Line— Distal
Dimensions suggested for carving technic	7.0*	13.0	10.5	8.0	10.0	9.0	1.0	0.0

* Millimeters.

The mandibular second molar supplements the first molar in function. Its anatomy differs in some details.

Normally, the second molar is smaller than the first molar by a fraction of a millimeter in all dimensions. It does not, however, run true to form. It is not uncommon to find mandibular second molar crowns somewhat larger than first molars, and although the roots are not so well formed, they may be longer.

The crown has four well-developed cusps: two buccal and two lingual, of nearly equal development. There is neither a distal nor a fifth cusp, but the distobuccal cusp is larger than that found on the first molar.

The tooth has two well-developed roots, one mesial and one distal. These roots are broad buccolingually, but they are not so broad as those of the first molar, nor are they so widely separated.

Detailed Description of the Mandibular Second Molar from All Aspects

In describing this tooth, direct comparisons will be made with the first mandibular molar.

Buccal Aspect (Figs. 297 and 302)

The crown is somewhat shorter cervico-occlusally and narrower mesiodistally than in the first molar. The crown and root show a tendency toward greater over-all length, but are not always longer (Fig. 302, specimens 4, 7 and 9).

There is but one developmental groove buccally, the *buccal developmental*

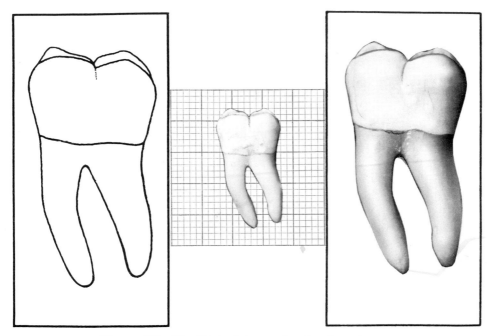

Figure 297. Mandibular left second molar – buccal aspect.

groove. This groove acts as a line of demarcation between the mesiobuccal and the distobuccal cusps, which are about equal in their mesiodistal measurements.

The cervical line buccally in many instances points sharply toward the root bifurcation (Fig. 302, specimens 1, 2, 3, 5, 7, 9 and 10).

The roots may be shorter than those of the first molar, but they vary considerably in this as well as in their development generally. The roots are usually closer together, and their axes are nearly parallel. They may spread as much as those of the first molar (Fig. 302, specimen 5), or they may be fused for all or part of their length (specimens 8 and 9).

The roots are inclined distally in relation to the occlusal plane of the crown, their axes forming more of an acute angle with the occlusal plane than is found on the first molar. When one compares all of the mandibular molars, it may seem that the first molar shows one angulation of roots to occlusal plane, the second molar a more acute angle and the third molar an angle which is more acute still. (See Chapter XVI on Occlusion.)

Lingual Aspect (Fig. 298)

Differences in detail between the mandibular second molar and the mandibular first molar, to be noted from the lingual aspect, are these:

1. The crown and root of the mandibular second molar converge lingually but to a slight degree; little of the mesial or distal surfaces may therefore be seen from this aspect.

2. The mesiodistal calibration at the cervix lingually is always greater than that of the first molar.

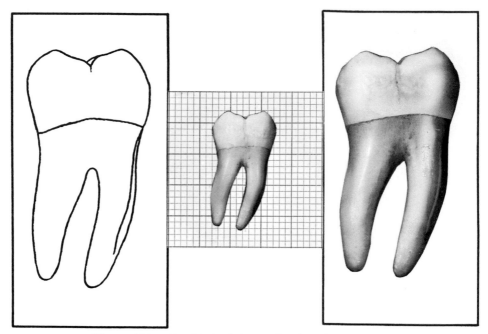

Figure 298. Mandibular left second molar — lingual aspect.

3. The curvatures mesially and distally on the crown which describe the contact areas are more noticeable from the lingual aspect. They prove to be at a slightly lower level, especially in the distal area, than those of the first molar.

Mesial Aspect (Figs. 299 and 303)

Except for the differences in measurement from the mesial aspect, the second molar differs little from the first molar.

The cervical ridge buccally on the crown portion is in most instances less pronounced, and the occlusal surface may be more constricted buccolingually (Fig. 303, specimens 2, 5, 6, 7, 8 and 10).

The cervical line shows less curvature, being straight and regular in outline buccolingually.

The mesial root is somewhat pointed apically. If part of the distal root is in sight, it is seen buccally. In the first molar, when the distal root is in sight from the mesial aspect, it is in view lingually.

Distal Aspect (Fig. 300)

From the distal aspect, the second molar is similar in form to the first molar except for the absence of a distal cusp and a distobuccal groove. The contact area is centered on the distal surface buccolingually and is placed equidistant from cervical line and marginal ridge.

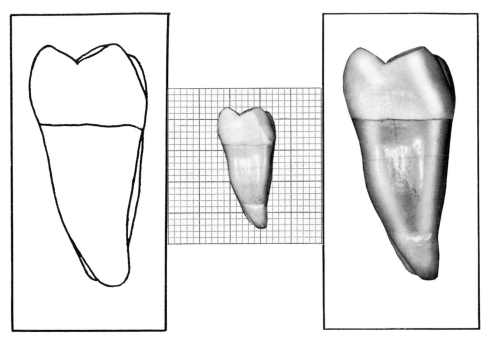

Figure 299. Mandibular left second molar — mesial aspect.

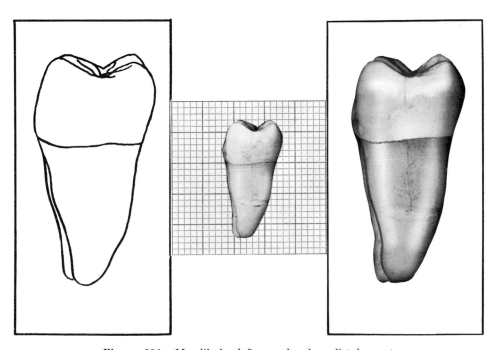

Figure 300. Mandibular left second molar — distal aspect.

Occlusal Aspect (Figs. 301 and 304)

The occlusal aspect of the mandibular second molar has outstanding variations from the first molar. These variations serve as marks of identity.The small distal cusp of the first molar is not present, and the distobuccal lobe development is just as pronounced as that of the mesiobuccal lobe. There is no distobuccal developmental groove occlusally or buccally. The buccal and lingual developmental grooves meet the central developmental groove at right angles at the central pit on the occlusal surface. These grooves form a cross, dividing the occlusal portion of the crown into four parts which are nearly equal.

In general, the cusp slopes on the occlusal surface are not so smooth as those found on first molars, since they are roughened by many supplemental grooves radiating from the developmental grooves.

The following characteristics of mandibular second molars from the occlusal aspect should be observed and noted:

1. Many of them are rectangular from the occlusal aspect (Fig. 304, specimens 7 and 9).

2. Many show considerable prominence cervically on the mesiobuccal lobe only (Fig. 304, specimens 1, 3, 5, 6 and 10).

3. Most second molars exhibit more curvature of the outline of the crown distally than mesially, showing a semicircular outline to the disto-occlusal surface in comparison with a square outline mesially (Fig. 304).

4. The cusp ridge of the distobuccal cusp lies buccal to the cusp ridge of the mesiobuccal cusp (Fig. 304, specimens 2, 3, 8 and 10; Fig. 301).

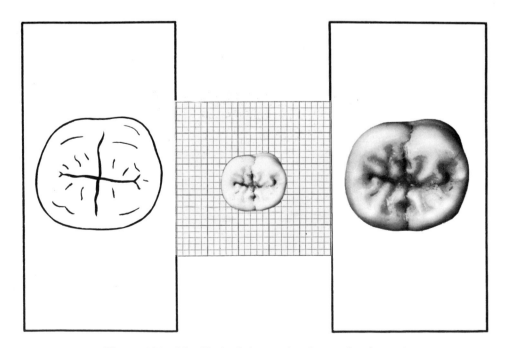

Figure 301. Mandibular left second molar—occlusal aspect.

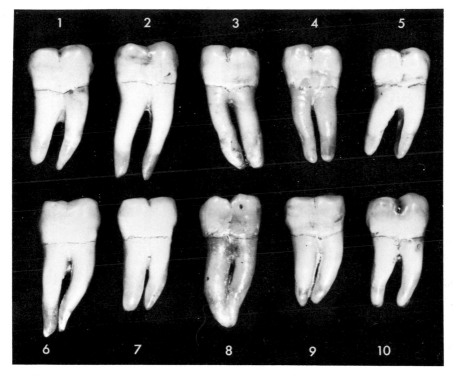

Figure 302. Mandibular second molars—ten typical specimens—buccal aspect.

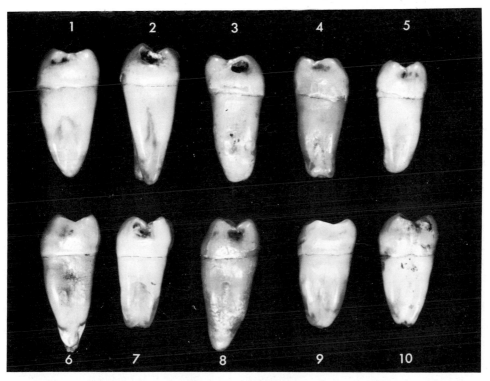

Figure 303. Mandibular second molars—ten typical specimens—mesial aspect.

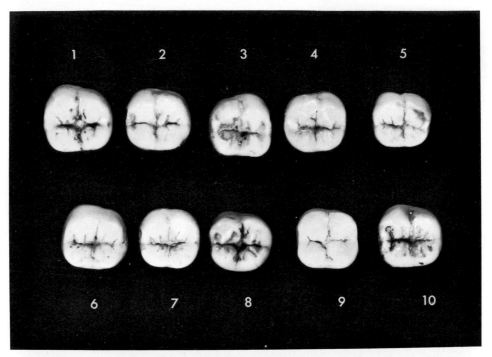

Figure 304. Mandibular second molars—ten typical specimens—occlusal aspect.

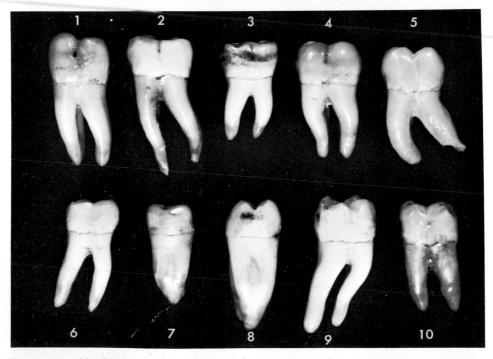

Figure 305. Mandibular second molars—ten specimens showing uncommon variations. 1, Mesio-distal measurements at contact areas and cervix almost equal. 2, Roots twisted and of extra length. 3, Very small specimen, short roots. 4, Roots short for such a large crown. 5, Roots thick and malformed generally. 6, Dwarfed crown, roots extra long. 7, Mesial aspect, protective curvature buccally and lingually is absent. 8, Roots of extra size, occlusal surface constricted buccolingually. 9, Roots malformed. 10, Crown wide mesiodistally at the cervix, roots short.

MANDIBULAR THIRD MOLAR

Mandibular Third Molar

First evidence of calcification .... 8 to 10 years
Enamel completed .... 12 to 16 years
Eruption .... 17 to 21 years
Root completed .... 18 to 25 years

Measurement Table

	Cervico-occlusal Length of Crown	Length of Root	Mesio-distal Diameter of Crown	Mesio-distal Diameter of Crown at Cervix	Labio- or Bucco-lingual Diameter of Crown	Labio- or Bucco-lingual Diameter of Crown at Cervix	Curvature of Cervical Line—Mesial	Curvature of Cervical Line—Distal
Dimensions suggested for carving technic	7.0*	11.0	10.0	7.5	9.5	9.0	1.0	0.0

* Millimeters.

The mandibular third molar varies considerably in different individuals and presents many anomalies both in form and in position. It supplements the second molar in function, although the tooth is seldom so well developed, the average mandibular third molar showing irregular development of the crown portion, with undersized roots, more or less malformed. Generally speaking, however, its design conforms to the general plan of all mandibular molars, conforming more closely to that of the second mandibular molar in the number of cusps and occlusal design than it does to the mandibular first molar. Occasionally, mandibular third molars are seen that are well formed and comparable in size and development to the mandibular first molar.

Many instances of mandibular third molars with five or more cusps are found, with the crown portions larger than those of the second molar. In these cases the alignment and occlusion with other teeth is not normal, because insufficient room is available in the alveolar process of the mandible for the accommodation of such a large tooth and the occlusal form is improper.

Although it is possible to find dwarfed specimens of mandibular third molars (Fig. 314, specimen 2), most of them which are not normal in size are larger than normal in the crown portion particularly. Roots of these oversize third molars may be short and poorly formed.

The opposite situation is true in maxillary third molars. Most of the anomalies are undersized. Mandibular third molars are the most likely to be impacted, wholly or partially, in the jaw. The lack of space accommodation may be the chief cause.

Detailed Description of the Mandibular Third Molar
from All Aspects

Buccal Aspects (Figs. 306 and 311)

From the buccal aspect, mandibular third molars vary considerably in outline. At the same time, they all have certain characteristics in common.

The outline of the crowns from this aspect is in a general way that of all mandibular molars. The crown is wider at contact areas mesiodistally than at the cervix, the buccal cusps are short and rounded, and the crest of contour mesially and distally is located a little more than half the distance from cervical line to tips of cusps. The type of third molar which is more likely to be in fair alignment and in good occlusion with other teeth is the four-cusp type; this is smaller and shows two buccal cusps only from this aspect (Fig. 311, specimens 1, 4, 5, 8, 9 and 10).

The average third molar also shows two roots, one mesial and one distal. These roots are usually shorter, with a poorer development generally, than the roots of first or second molars, and their distal inclination in relation to the occlusal plane of the crown is greater. The roots may be separated with a definite point of bifurcation, or they may be fused for all or part of their length (Fig. 311).

Lingual Aspect (Fig. 307)

Observations from the lingual aspect add little to those already made from the buccal aspect. The mandibular third molar, when well developed, corresponds closely to the form of the second molar except for size and root development.

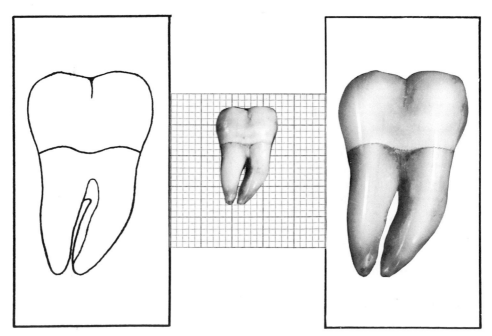

Figure 306. Mandibular right third molar—buccal aspect.

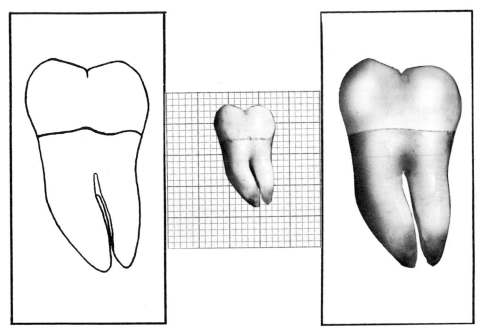

Figure 307. Mandibular right third molar—lingual aspect.

Mesial Aspect (Figs. 308 and 312)

From the mesial aspect, this tooth resembles the mandibular second molar except in dimensions. The roots, of course, are shorter, with the mesial root tapering more from cervix to apex. The apex of the mesial root is usually more pointed.

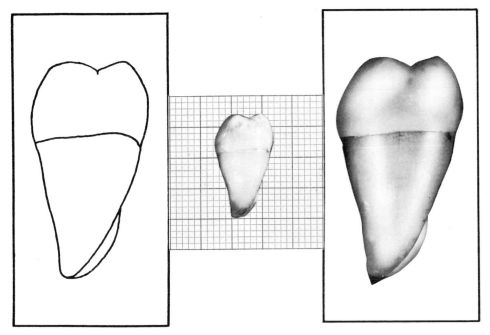

Figure 308. Mandibular right third molar—mesial aspect.

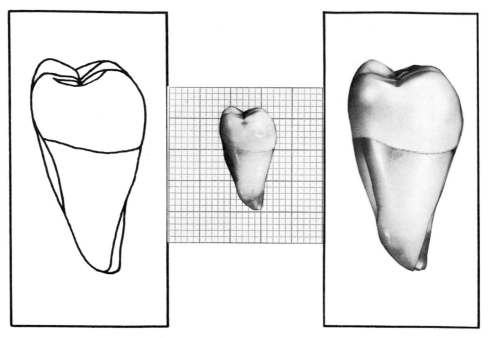

Figure 309.   Mandibular right third molar—distal aspect.

Distal Aspect (Fig. 309)

The anatomic appearance of the distal portion of this tooth is much like that of the second molar except for size.

Those specimens which have oversize crown portions are much more spheroidal above the cervical line. The distal root appears small, both in length and in buccolingual measurement, when compared with the large crown portion.

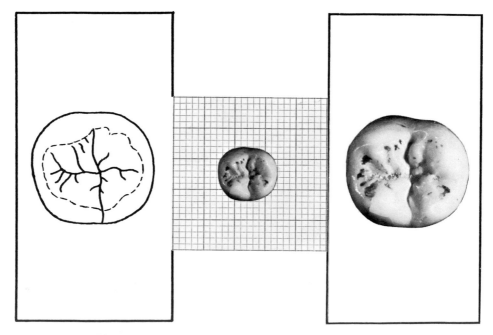

Figure 310.   Mandibular right third molar—occlusal aspect.

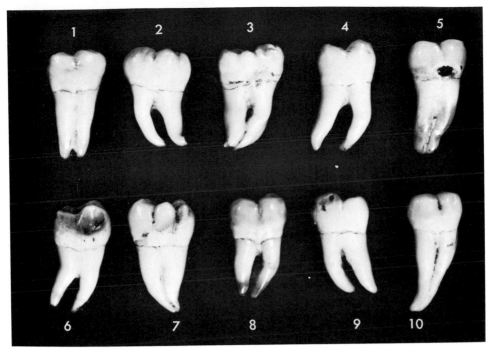

Figure 311. Mandibular third molars—ten typical specimens—buccal aspect.

Occlusal Aspect (Figs. 310 and 313)

The occlusal aspect is quite similar to that of the second mandibular molar when the development is such as to facilitate good alignment and occlusion (Fig. 313, specimens 2, 3, 4, 6, 7, 8 and 9).

The tendency is toward a more rounded outline and a smaller buccolingual measurement distally.

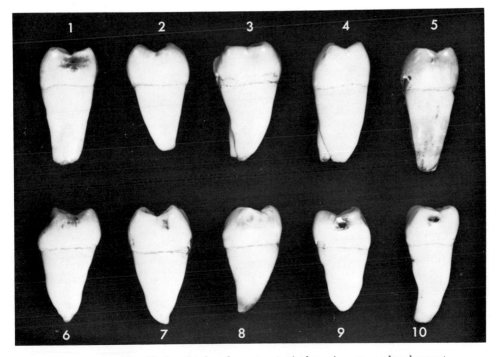

Figure 312. Mandibular third molars—ten typical specimens—occlusal aspect.

287

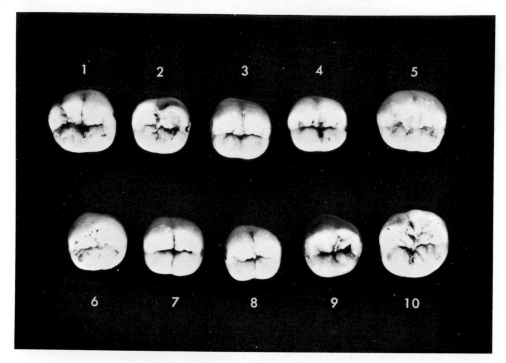

Figure 313. Mandibular third molars—ten typical specimens—occlusal aspect.

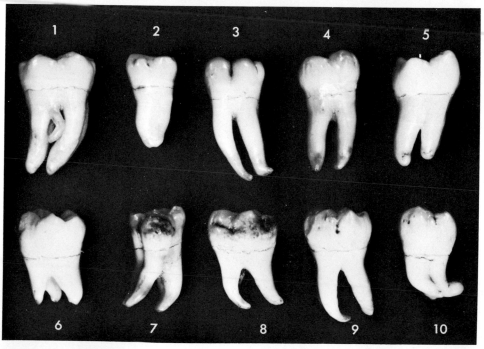

Figure 314. Mandibular third molars—ten specimens showing uncommon variations. 1, Oversize generally, extra root lingually. 2, Dwarfed specimen, odd extra cusp, fused roots. 3, Crown resembling first molar, long slender roots. 4, Formation closely resembling second molar. 5, Large crown, malformed roots. 6, Multicusp crown, dwarfed roots. 7, No resemblance to typical functional form. 8, Large crown, dwarfed roots. 9, Odd crown form and root form. 10, Crown long cervico-occlusally, roots fused and malformed.

Chapter XIII

THE PULP CAVITIES
OF THE PERMANENT TEETH

For study of the anatomy of pulp cavities in teeth, longitudinal sections of each tooth, labio- or buccolingually and also mesiodistally, must be made. In addition, transverse sections should be prepared with cuts through the crowns or roots at various levels. These dissections expose to view a central cavity with an outline corresponding in general to that of the tooth itself. This space is called the *pulp cavity,* and in life it contains the dental pulp (Figs. 315 and 316). That portion of the pulp cavity found mainly within the coronal portion of the tooth is called the *pulp chamber,* while the remainder, found within the root, is called the *pulp canal.* The constricted opening of the pulp canal at the root end is called the *apical foramen.* It is possible for any tooth root to have more than one foramen; in such cases, the canals have two or more branches which make their exits at or near the apical end of the root. These may be called *multiple foramina* or *supplementary canals* (Figs. 317, 318 and 320).

The *pulp chamber* is in the center of the crown and is always a single cavity. The pulp canals of roots are continuous with this cavity. Many roots are found with more than one canal. The mesial root of the mandibular first molar, for instance, usually contains two pulp canals; these two canals, however, may end in a common foramen (Fig. 338, *A-3*).

The shape of the pulp chambers varies with the shape of the crown. Usually, when the roots are much wider in one direction than in another, the pulp canal forms vary accordingly. Since the crowns of the teeth generally have the largest diameter and the roots taper from the cervices to the apices, the pulp cavities of the teeth have the same proportions. The pulp cavities taper from the largest outline at the crown to

(Text continued on page 292.)

289

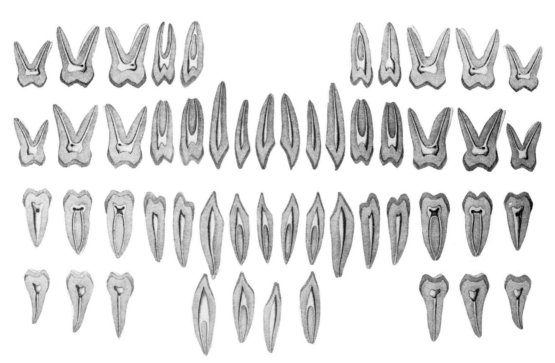

Figure 315.   A comparison of pulp cavity outlines with tooth outlines—mesiodistal sections. (Taken from original engravings, *Anatomie des Mundes,* Carabelli, 1843.)

Figure 316.   A comparison of pulp cavity outlines with tooth outlines—faciolingual sections. Although we are not in complete agreement today with either tooth form or pulp cavity design as shown in some instances in this illustration, nevertheless it serves very well as an over-all picture of all the teeth from the aspects portrayed. (Taken from original engravings, *Anatomie des Mundes,* Carabelli, 1843.)

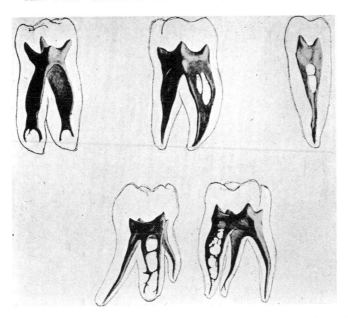

Figure 317. Molar pulp canal filling. Note the formation in the pulp chambers of the original pulp horns. (Prepared by Dr. Richard H. Riethmüller.)

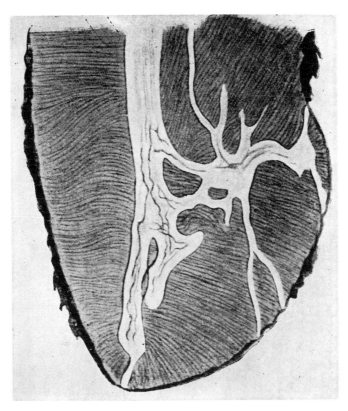

Figure 318. Apical end of root showing branching pulp canals. (Prepared by Dr. Richard H. Riethmüller.)

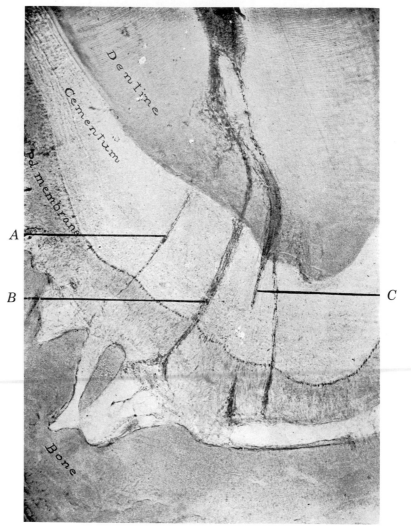

Figure 319. A section through the apex of a root showing three foramina, *A, B* and *C* (Talbot).

an extremely constricted outline at the apical foramen. Sometimes the canals are so constricted as they approach the apical foramen that it is very difficult to follow them in making cross sections.

The size of the pulp cavity is influenced by the age of the tooth, its functional activity and its history. The dental pulp decreases in size gradually as the tooth ages. The youngest teeth are provided, therefore, with the largest pulp cavities (Fig. 320).

Throughout its life the *dental pulp* retains its ability to deposit what is called *secondary dentin,* a deposit which reduces the pulp cavity in size. Sometimes in old age or as a result of pathologic changes, the pulp cavity may become partially or entirely obliterated.

During the period of root development the diameter of the root canal is greatest at the free, or apical, end of the root, at which point it presents a funnel-shaped opening (Figs. 37 and 320). As the root continues to develop, this funnel-shaped

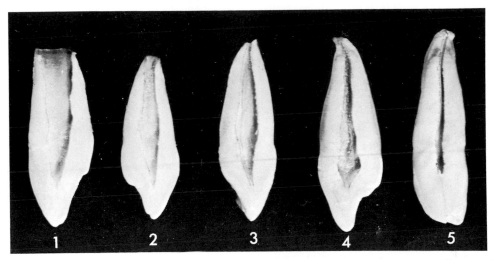

Figure 320.   Labiolingual sections showing various stages of development of the maxillary canine. 1, Crown complete, root partially completed with large pulp cavity, wide open at the apical end. 2, Tooth almost complete except for constriction of apical foramen. 3, Canine of young individual with large pulp cavity and complete root tip with generous foramen. 4, Typical average canine in adult stage with constricted apical foramen. 5, Canine of an old individual with constricted pulp chamber and canal; it will be noted that this specimen has lost its original crown form through wear and erosion.

opening is reduced in size, and finally, as the formative process nears completion, the opening becomes more constricted until the apex of the root is completed with a small apical foramen.

There are prolongations or domes in the pulp chamber which correspond to the various cusps of the crown. The projections of pulp tissue occupying these spaces are called *pulp horns* (Fig. 317). If the cusp form of the crown of a tooth is well developed, the horns of the pulp chamber will correspond; but if the cusps are small the pulp horns will be short or missing entirely. Posterior teeth have well-accented pulp horns. When anterior teeth, in young persons, have well-marked developmental lobes, accented pulp horns may be expected, especially in the labial portion, as extensions into the three labial lobes. These are always most marked in young teeth and they usually disappear as age advances. (Compare *B*-1 with *B*-5, Fig. 321.)

The entire pulp cavity tends to become smaller with age, owing to the development of secondary dentin. Several things may contribute to this activity — malocclusion, thermal shock, occlusal trauma, abrasion, etc. Cross sections of teeth with considerable secondary dentin are easy to obtain. Often it is possible, when studying such sections, to see the original outline of the pulp chamber because of the translucency and color variation between the secondary dentin and the primary dentin (Fig. 321, *B*-3).

When studying teeth in cross section it is important to observe the labio- or buccolingual sections, for it is in this direction that the pulp cavities show the greatest number of variations. Students and practitioners are apt to be less familiar with the root canal anatomy from the mesial and distal aspects. *Routine radiographs*

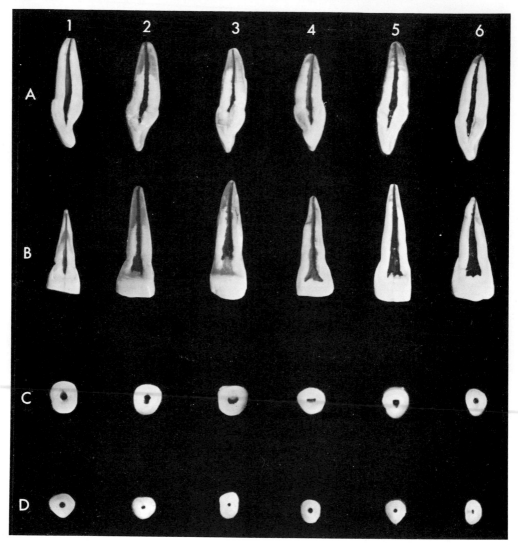

Figure 321. Maxillary central incisor – cross sections of natural specimens. *A,* 1 to 6, Labiolingual sections. This aspect does not show in radiographs. *B,* 1 to 6, Mesiodistal sections. *C,* 1 to 6, Cervical sections of root. *D,* 1 to 6, Mid-root sections.

of the teeth show the cross-sectional anatomy well from the labial and buccal aspects only. The outlines of the pulp cavities vary little from those aspects, since they tend to conform generally to the crown and root outlines. Because of technical difficulties it is impossible to get radiographs of the teeth in situ showing the cross-sectional anatomy mesially or distally (Fig. 321, *A*). Often single-rooted teeth may have more than one canal, or teeth which are ordinarily single-rooted may show bifurcation or multiple roots without this being discovered by means of radiographs. The practitioner must be aware of these variations, and he must be continuously on the alert when making a diagnosis.

THE PULP CAVITIES OF MAXILLARY TEETH

Maxillary Incisors (Figs. 321 and 322)

The pulp cavities of the central and lateral maxillary incisors are similar. This is to be expected, since the form of these two teeth is similar. There are, of course, variations in size. The labiolingual section of the central incisor shows the pulp chamber to be pointed near the incisal edge. It increases in size labiolingually, as does the crown, as it approaches the cervical line. From a point on a level with the cervical line labially and lingually, the pulp canal starts to taper in proportion to the root taper as it approaches the apical foramen. It narrows with the root taper. The apical foramen in the adult tooth is quite constricted.

The pulp chamber, as seen in the mesiodistal section, differs in outline from the labiolingual section. Since the outline of the crown is different from this aspect, the outline of the pulp chamber differs also. In young individuals, the pulp chamber incisally is wide and shows three pulp horns which correspond to the three develop-

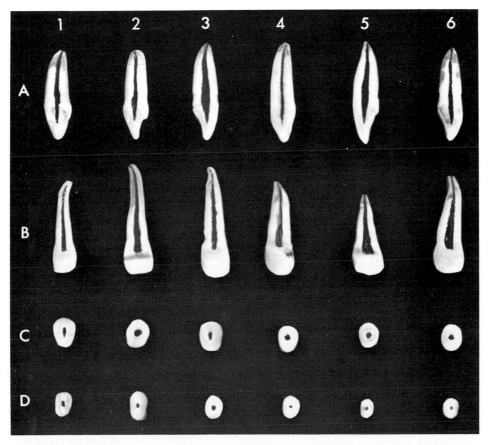

Figure 322.   Maxillary lateral incisor—cross sections of natural specimens. *A,* 1 to 6, Labiolingual sections. This aspect does not show in radiographs. *B,* 1 to 6, Mesiodistal sections. *C,* 1 to 6, Cervical sections of root. *D,* 1 to 6, Mid-root sections.

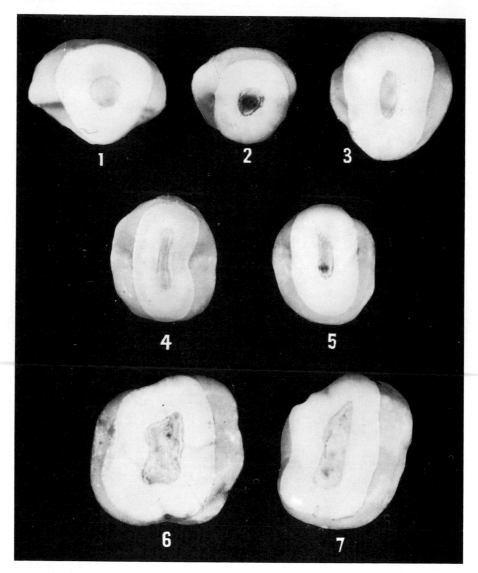

Figure 323. Maxillary permanent teeth. 1, Central incisor. 2, Lateral incisor. 3, Canine. 4, First premolar. 5, Second premolar. 6, First molar. 7, Second molar.

Interesting photographs of natural teeth made by a process of double exposure. Tooth specimens were sawed through at the cervical line, an exposure was made with the sections placed together and an exposure made of occlusal and incisal views. Then the crown was removed and another exposure made of the cross section at the cervix on the same film.

The result is shown above, and the proportion of crown outline to cervical outline is accurately portrayed. The angulation of the field when such small specimens were posed, and the possibility of movement, made standardization too difficult; consequently, some of the pictures do not have the crown and cervices centered in line with the long axis. Nevertheless, from an operative point of view, a comparison of the above photos makes an interesting study. (Made and submitted by Dr. John T. Bird, Washington University School of Dentistry.)

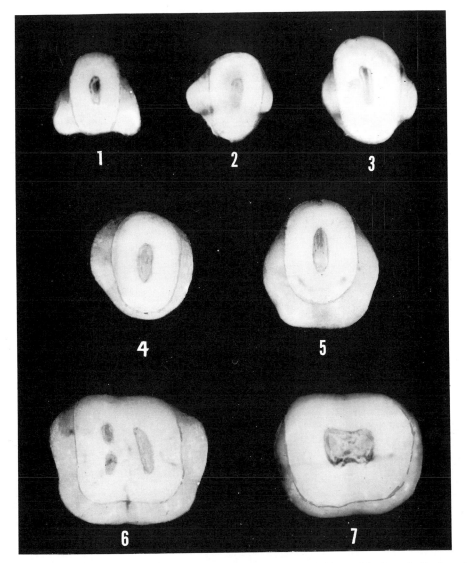

Figure 324. Mandibular Permanent Teeth. 1, Central incisor. 2, Lateral incisor. 3, Canine. 4, First premolar. 5, Second premolar. 6, First molar. 7, Second molar.
Double-exposure photos of mandibular teeth to be compared with Fig. 323.

mental lobes (Fig. 321, *B*-5 and *B*-6). The pulp cavity tapers apically from this point, but it is still wide as far as the cervix of the crown. It then tapers in direct proportion to the root taper as it approaches the apical foramen.

The pulp canal in the central incisor is usually uniform and readily accessible. A transverse section at the cervix shows the pulp canal almost perfectly centered in the root. In very young individuals it is somewhat triangular in form (Fig. 321, *C*-5), corresponding with the outline of the root at this level. In older individuals the canal becomes round or crescent-shaped as it becomes more constricted.

A cross section of this canal at the mid-root level is about half the circumference of the canal at the cervical level.

The foregoing material serves as a description of the pulp chamber and canal in the *lateral* incisor also. Since the crown of this tooth is smaller than that of the central incisor, the mesiodistal section does not show the same width to the pulp chamber. Rarely does this tooth show more than two pulp horns, of varying degrees in length. In the adult stage, the periphery of the pulp chamber is rounded incisally.

Maxillary Canine (Fig. 325)

The labiolingual section of the maxillary canine shows the pulp chamber to be narrow and pointed incisally. This point disappears in older individuals, and the pulp chamber has a rounded appearance and recedes considerably toward the root.

Since the root of this tooth is wide labiolingually, the canal is wide also. The canal is usually consistent in this width until it approaches the apical third of the

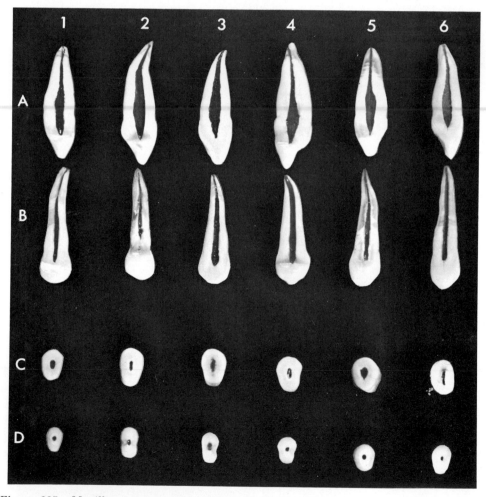

Figure 325. Maxillary canine—cross sections of natural specimens. *A,* 1 to 6, Labiolingual sections. This aspect does not show in radiographs. *B,* 1 to 6, Mesiodistal sections. *C,* 1 to 6, Cervical sections of root. *D,* 1 to 6, Mid-root sections.

root. The canal near the apex is much more constricted, although the apical foramen on this tooth tends to be larger than the foramina of incisor teeth.

The mesiodistal section presents a different outline entirely from the labiolingual section: The pulp chamber is pointed incisally, and the pulp canal is narrow for its entire length.

The transverse section at the cervical line of the tooth shows a canal that is oblong, with the measurement labiolingually much greater than the measurement mesiodistally. As the mid-root section is approached, the labiolingual measurement becomes less in relation to the mesiodistal measurement; the cross section of the canal is rounder and less elliptical.

Maxillary First Premolar (Fig. 326)

The maxillary first premolar may have two well-developed, fully formed roots or, as is more often the case, two root projections from the middle third of the root to the

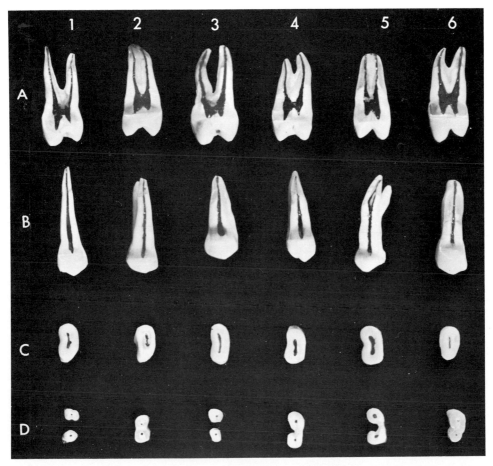

Figure 326.   Maxillary first premolar—cross sections of natural specimens. *A,* 1 to 6, Buccolingual sections. This aspect does not show in radiographs. *B,* 1 to 6, Mesiodistal sections. *C,* 1 to 6, Cervical sections of root, *D,* 1 to 6, Mid-root sections.

apices. It is not uncommon for this tooth to have one broad root for its entire length. *Rarely, however, does it have less than two fully formed canals.*

The pulp chamber is wide buccolingually, in accordance with the crown form, and two distinct pulp horns are usually present. The pulp chamber floor is round apically, with smooth funnel-like openings to the root canals. The pulp chamber floor is usually within the confines of the root portion apical to the cervix of the crown.

The root canals taper evenly with the roots when two roots are present. The lingual root canal tends to be larger and more accessible than the buccal canal. Even when this tooth has one large oval root instead of two well-separated roots, it does not seem to make much difference in the outline of the root canals. The canals may be more nearly parallel to each other, tending to follow the outlines of the side of the root instead of separating from each other as they follow the direction of separated roots.

The shape of the pulp cavity in the mesiodistal section is similar to the shape found in the canine, except that the pulp canal is more constricted and shorter, since the root or roots of this tooth are narrower mesiodistally and shorter. The pulp chamber is narrow from this aspect. On cross section at the cervical line, the canal is long buccolingually and narrow mesiodistally. The root at this point is rather kidney-shaped, and the canal corresponds to this outline. From the mid-root section on to the apex the two canals are round and constricted. The lingual canal is usually somewhat the larger.

Maxillary Second Premolar (Fig. 327)

The majority of maxillary second premolars have only one root canal. The pulp chamber is wide buccolingually and has two well-defined pulp horns. The pulp chamber extends apical to cervical line, and although a constriction at this point usually shows the termination of the pulp chamber, the canal is still wide. It tapers, of course, as it approaches the apical foramen, but since this root is wide buccolingually, the canal is relatively large and accessible. It is not uncommon for this tooth to show two canals for part of the root length. Quite often, this is merely a branching arrangement continuing for a short distance only, the two branches joining at the apical third with a relatively large foramen (Fig. 327, A-3).

Sometimes the pulp canal branches at the apical third with two foramina (Fig. 327, A-2, 6).

The pulp chamber and canal as seen in the mesiodistal section are similar to those found in the first premolar. Cross section at the cervical line differs somewhat, since the root at this point is oval rather than kidney-shaped. Usually there is only one canal showing at the mid-root section, and although it is rather small, it is wider buccolingually than mesiodistally.

Maxillary First Molar (Fig. 328)

The buccolingual section of the maxillary first molar shows only the mesial and lingual roots, but since the pulp canal in the distal root is usually rounded and

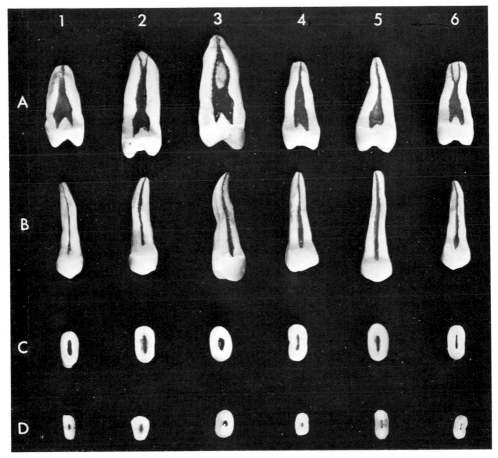

Figure 327. Maxillary second premolar—cross sections of natural specimens. *A*, 1 to 6, Buccolingual sections. This aspect does not show in radiographs. *B*, 1 to 6, Mesiodistal sections. *C*, 1 to 6, Cervical sections of root. *D*, 1 to 6, Mid-root sections.

uniform in a buccolingual section, the buccolingual section of the distobuccal root will not be described. There is apt to be greater variance in the canal form in the mesiobuccal root, and the buccolingual section of this tooth will show this from the mesial aspect.

The distobuccal root is relatively small and round, and its canal has a similar form.

The pulp chamber in a buccolingual section appears broad and generous, in direct proportion to the crown from this aspect. The pulp chamber horns, extending toward the mesiobuccal cusp and mesiolingual cusp, are distinct. The pulp chamber floor is smooth and regular, and the canal openings into the pulp chamber widen out as they enter the pulp chamber.

The pulp canal of the lingual root is relatively large and easily accessible. The mesiobuccal root canal is small in comparison with the canal of the lingual root, and it is shorter. The mesiobuccal canal often has supplementary branches and multiple foramina, or it may be wide and flat (Fig. 328, *A*-2 and *A*-4). It is not uncommon for this root to have a supplementary canal which branches off above the pulp chamber

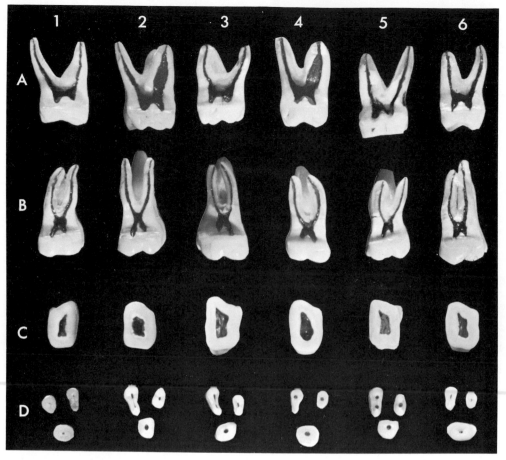

Figure 328. Maxillary first molar—cross sections of natural specimens. *A*, 1 to 6, Buccolingual sections. This aspect does not show in radiographs. *B*, 1 to 6, Mesiodistal sections. *C*, 1 to 6, Cervical sections of root. *D*, 1 to 6, Mid-root sections.

(Fig. 328, *D*-5). The supplementary branch may turn crownwise, with a blind terminal which is inaccessible from the pulp chamber. (Fig. 317.)

The pulp chamber does not appear so wide in the mesiodistal section as in the buccolingual section. Two horns are usually visible, corresponding to the mesiobuccal cusp and the distobuccal cusp. The floor of the pulp chamber is apical to the cervical level of the crown.

Comparisons show that it is necessary in operative procedures to penetrate the crown of this tooth at or above the normal gum line before reaching the pulp chamber. The mesiobuccal and distobuccal root canals are narrow and taper with the outlines of the root. Root canals generally tend to follow the direction of the curvature of the root.

The cervical cross section of the maxillary first molar serves to designate the relative positions of the root canals. Since the mesiobuccal root of this tooth is placed farther buccally than the distobuccal root, the relative positions of the two canals must be in accordance with this arrangement. A straight line may be drawn from the mesiobuccal aperture of the root canal to the aperture of the lingual canal. The opening from the pulp chamber into the distobuccal root canal lies distal to this line and is of course lingual to the mesiobuccal canal (Fig. 328, C-3).

Since pulp therapy is needed for all first molars more often than for any of the other teeth, the dentist must become familiar with the arrangement of these canals in relation to one another.

Mid-root sections give an interesting comparison in relative sizes and shapes of the canals. The lingual root canal appears round and relatively large in comparison with the round constricted canal of the distobuccal root. The mesiobuccal canal often appears as a narrow slit; it is exceedingly constricted mesiodistally but wide buccolingually in comparison with the other two roots.

Maxillary Second Molar (Fig. 329)

The buccolingual and mesiodistal sections of the maxillary second molar are similar to those of the maxillary first molar. The roots do not spread so wide,

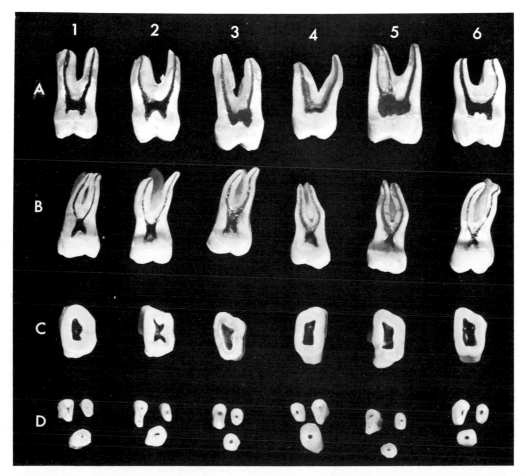

Figure 329. Maxillary second molar—cross sections of natural specimens. *A*, 1 to 6, Buccolingual sections. This aspect does not show in radiographs. *B*, 1 to 6, Mesiodistal sections. *C*, 1 to 6, Cervical sections of root. *D*, 1 to 6, Mid-root sections.

however, and since the roots are straighter and closer together, the direction of the canals varies accordingly. Instead of the distobuccal canal extending distally in its entirety, as happens in the first molar, the distobuccal canal may turn mesially at the apical third (Fig. 329 *B*-1, 4).

A cross section of this tooth at the cervical line shows some variation when compared with that of the first molar. Although the mesiobuccal and lingual canals have the same relative positions, the distobuccal root canal is placed differently. It approaches the halfway point between the mesiobuccal and lingual canals and is not placed so far distally. This is caused by the extreme rhomboidal form of the tooth section at this level.

Mid-root sections are very similar to the corresponding sections of the first molar.

Maxillary Third Molar (Fig. 330)

The development of the maxillary third molar varies so much in different individuals that a description of a pulp cavity taken from a single tooth would be

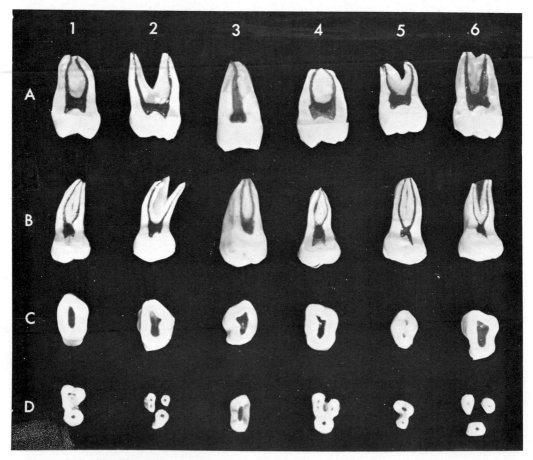

Figure 330. Maxillary third molar—cross sections of natural specimens. *A*, 1 to 6, Buccolingual sections. This aspect does not show in radiographs. *B*, 1 to 6, Mesiodistal sections. *C*, 1 to 6, Cervical sections of root. *D*, 1 to 6, Mid-root sections.

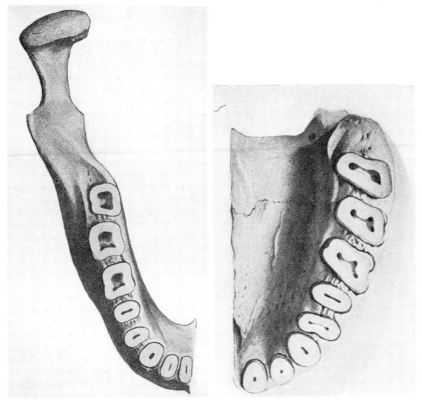

Figure 331   Figure 332

Figure 331. Horizontal sections through the cervical portions of the teeth of the right mandible in situ. Note the relative positions of root canals. (Sicher, *Oral Anatomy,* C. V. Mosby Company.)

Figure 332. Horizontal sections through the cervical portions of the teeth of the right maxilla in situ. Note the relative positions of root canals. (Sicher, *Oral Anatomy,* C. V. Mosby Company.)

inadequate. In the majority of instances, this tooth crown is more triangular than quadrilateral in form, and the pulp chamber varies accordingly.

The roots of this tooth are often fused, and the number of root canals may be greater or less than the usual number for maxillary molars. In general, the pulp chamber and root canals of this tooth resemble those of the second molar when the form of the tooth happens to be similar (Fig. 330, *A*-2 and *B*-2).

PULP CAVITIES OF THE MANDIBULAR TEETH

The outlines of the pulp cavities of the mandibular teeth, like those of the maxillary, correspond in general to the gross outlines of the crown and roots.

Mandibular Incisors (Figs. 333 and 334)

The pulp cavities of the mandibular central and lateral incisors are so nearly alike that they will be described together:

A view of the labiolingual section shows that the pulp chamber is pointed incisally, taking on the general shape of the crown from this aspect and being wide labiolingually at the level which is even with the cervical line.

The root canal remains wide as it follows the root apically and does not show any reduction in labiolingual width until the middle third of the root is passed. Then it starts to taper to the apical foramen. Sometimes the mesial or distal view will show branching of the canal with an island in the center (Fig. 333, A-4) or a branching with two separate canals for the entire length, either with one common foramen or with two separate ones (Fig. 316).

The mesiodistal section shows a pulp chamber and canal which is narrow, although it follows the general outline of the crown. At the cervical line the canal becomes more constricted and is very narrow near the apex. The canal and root usually curve toward the distal at the apical third. Since this root is thin mesiodistally and since the amount of tooth structure is limited between the pulp canal and the

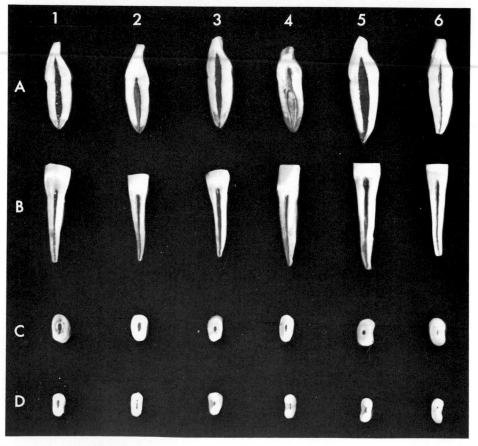

Figure 333. Mandibular central incisor—cross sections of natural specimens. *A*, 1 to 6, Labiolingual sections. This aspect does not show in radiographs. *B*, 1 to 6, Mesiodistal sections. *C*, 1 to 6, Cervical sections of root. *D*, 1 to 6, Mid-root sections.

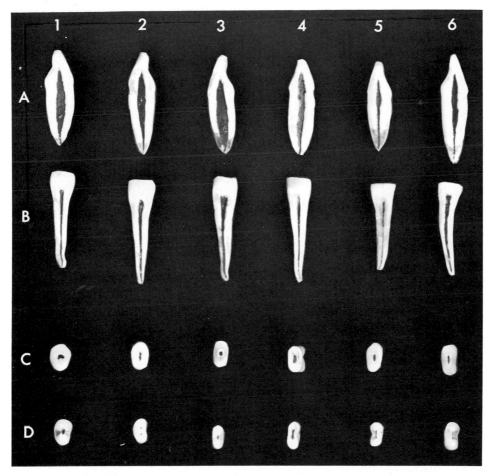

Figure 334. Mandibular lateral incisor—cross sections of natural specimens. *A*, 1 to 6, Labiolingual sections. This aspect does not show in radiographs. *B*, 1 to 6, Mesiodistal sections. *C*, 1 to 6, Cervical sections of root. *D*, 1 to 6, Mid-root sections.

periphery of the root mesially at the apical third, it is relatively easy to cause a perforation of this root during operative procedures unless great care is taken.

A cross section of the root at the cervical line demonstrates an oval canal usually constricted mesiodistally and wider labiolingually.

The mid-root section shows the canal more constricted and narrower labiolingually. Note the proximity of the outside surfaces of this root mesiodistally to the canal at the mid-root section.

The *lateral* incisor has pulp canals and pulp chambers similar in outline to those of the central incisor. The root is usually somewhat longer and tends to curve more sharply at the apical third (Fig. 334 B-1 and 3).

Mandibular Canine (Fig. 335)

Generally speaking, the pulp cavity in the mandibular canine tooth is similar to that in the maxillary canine. The root is usually not quite so large on cross sections,

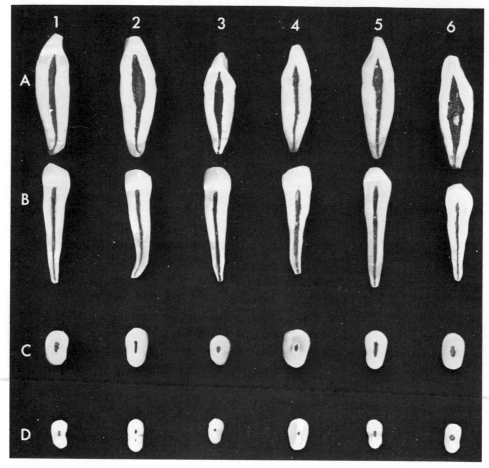

Figure 335. Mandibular canine—cross sections of natural specimens. *A*, 1 to 6, Labiolingual sections. This aspect does not show in radiographs. *B*, 1 to 6, Mesiodistal sections. *C*, 1 to 6, Cervical sections of root. *D*, 1 to 6, Mid-root sections.

and therefore the pulp canal is not so large. This is relative, however, and depends upon the size of the tooth. The mandibular canine is usually not so wide mesiodistally and also not so thick labiolingually as the maxillary canine. However, the root is often just as long and occasionally longer. There is one outstanding anatomic variation in the mandibular canine; it is not uncommon to find this tooth with two roots, one labial and one lingual, or two fused roots with two pulp canals, one labial and one lingual. These anomalies do not always show on radiographs; consequently, great care must be used in searching for two canals when the mandibular canine is under treatment (Fig. 198, specimens 1, 2, 5 and 6).

Mandibular Premolars (Figs. 336 and 337)

The pulp cavities of the mandibular premolars may best be described together, the description thereby affording an opportunity for comparison. The pulp chamber is

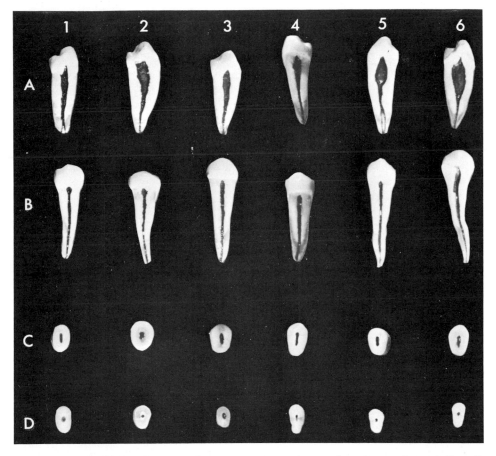

Figure 336.   Mandibular first premolar—cross sections of natural specimens. *A,* 1 to 6, Buccolingual sections. This aspect does not show in radiographs. *B,* 1 to 6, Mesiodistal sections. *C,* 1 to 6, Cervical sections of root. *D,* 1 to 6, Mid-root sections.

wide in the buccolingual section of both teeth, with the pulp horn corresponding to the buccal cusp well accented. The pulp horn, which extends toward the lingual cusp on the lower first premolar, is slight; it is somewhat larger on the second premolar, which has a better-developed lingual cusp or cusps. The pulp canals are wide until they reach the middle third of the root, where they become more restricted in buccolingual width and terminate in small foramina.

The mesiodistal sections show pulp chambers and pulp canals somewhat similar to those found in the mandibular canine, both in design and proportion, except for the variation in root length. The second premolar root is usually longer than the first premolar root. Either of the premolar roots may be curved at the apical third, usually but not always, in a distal direction.

Buccolingual sections of the mandibular premolars may show islands near the apical third of the root; these create temporarily two canals before they join again into one canal near the apical foramen (Fig. 336, *A*-5, and Fig. 337, *D*-4 and *D*-5).

A comparison of cross sections of the first and second premolars at the cervical

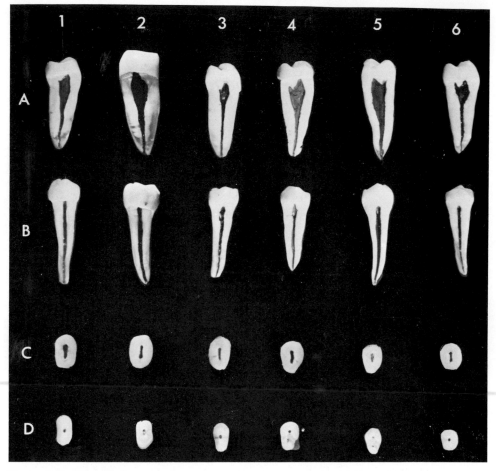

Figure 337. Mandibular second premolar—cross sections of natural specimens. *A*, 1 to 6, Buccolingual sections. This aspect does not show in radiographs. *B*, 1 to 6, Mesiodistal sections. *C*, 1 to 6, Cervical sections of root. *D*, 1 to 6, Mid-root sections.

line brings out the fact that the first premolar root is rounder on the average than the second premolar root. The second premolar root is wider buccolingually in comparison with its mesiodistal width than the first premolar root. This proportion affects the shape of the canal near the cervix. Both canals are similar at the mid-root section, being smaller than they are at the cervical line and having a tendency toward a round outline rather than an elliptical one.

Mandibular First and Second Molars (Figs. 338 and 339)

Since the pulp cavities of the mandibular first and second molars bear a close resemblance to each other, they will be described together. As might be expected, the forms of the pulp chambers of the lower molars correspond in general to the shapes of the crowns, and the form of the root canals resembles the general contours of the roots.

Since the buccolingual dimension of the lower first molar crown mesially is greater than the buccolingual dimension distally, the pulp chamber is wider mesially than distally. The same is true of the second molar.

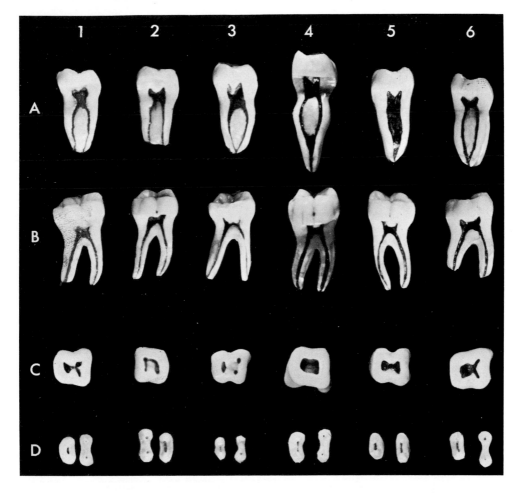

Figure 338. Mandibular first molar—cross sections of natural specimens. *A,* 1 to 6, Buccolingual sections. This aspect does not show in radiographs. *B,* 1 to 6, Mesiodistal sections. *C,* 1 to 6, Cervical sections of root. *D,* 1 to 6, Mid-root sections.

Buccolingual sections show large pulp chambers, with pulp horns extending up toward the mesiobuccal cusps and the mesiolingual cusps. The lingual horns are longer and more pointed than the buccal horns.

The mesial root of the lower molars is very wide, especially in the lower first molar. In the majority of cases there are two root canals in the mesial root, one buccal and one lingual. These root canals join the pulp chamber considerably below the cervical line; they are constricted as they follow the root toward the apex and in many cases join together into a common canal at the apical third, with a common foramen. However, the two canals in the mandibular molars, mesial root, do not always join together at the apical third. Sometimes they remain separate for the full length of the root, with separate foramina at the apex. It should be emphasized, at this point, that a single canal may be encountered in the mesial root which is quite wide buccolingually and narrow mesiodistally (Fig. 338, *A*-5, and Fig. 339, *A*-2 and *A*-6).

Buccolingual sections of the *mandibular second molar* may show the same arrangement. Sometimes they show one large canal for the greater part of the mesial root length, this canal being wide buccolingually but being very constricted

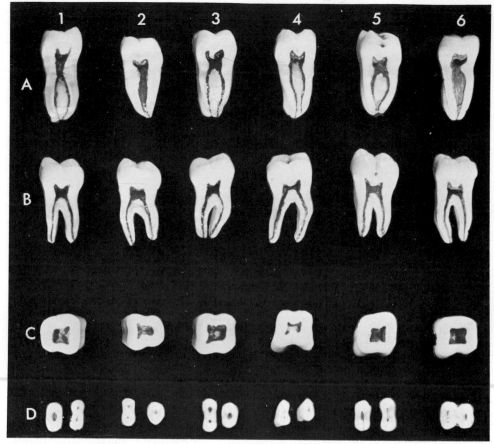

Figure 339. Mandibular second molar—cross sections of natural specimens. *A*, 1 to 6, Buccolingual sections. This aspect does not show in radiographs. *B*, 1 to 6, Mesiodistal sections. *C*, 1 to 6, Cervical sections of root. *D*, 1 to 6, Mid-root sections.

mesiodistally. They may show one canal branching into two for a short distance before continuing on at the apical third as a constricted single canal.

The mesiodistal sections of the lower molars show a relatively large pulp chamber, most of which is apical to the cervical line. They show two short pulp horn extensions and two canals, of which one is the buccal canal in the mesial root and the other a single canal in the distal root. The distal canal is almost straight and corresponds to the shape of the distal root. The mesial canal takes a gradual curve distally in line with the mesial root. The distal root canal is nearly always larger and more accessible than the mesial canals.

The pulp chambers, when viewed from cross sections of the teeth at the cervical line, are wide buccolingually toward the mesial and narrower buccolingually toward the distal. There is considerable separation between the entrances of two mesial canals, the funnel-like openings appearing constricted in comparison with the larger opening of the distal canal.

The pulp chamber of the second molar is not so large as that of the first molar, and it has the mesial root canals, if there are two of them, closer together, since the mesial root of the second molar is narrower than the mesial root of the first molar. Occasionally, the second molar has one mesial root canal also, which is wide buccolingually and constricted mesiodistally.

The mid-root section of the mesial root of the first molar nearly always shows two distinct canals in a kidney-shaped root. The canals at this point are small. The distal root is not so broad buccolingually and the canal at the mid-section is much larger than either of the two mesial canals. The mid-root section of the second molar roots shows canals of almost the same size and shape except in the type of tooth which has one mesial canal. In this case the one canal is narrow mesiodistally and flattened in the buccolingual direction.

Mandibular Third Molar (Fig. 340)

The mandibular third molar is so often malformed and poorly developed that it is impossible to outline any design for pulp cavities which may be taken as a general

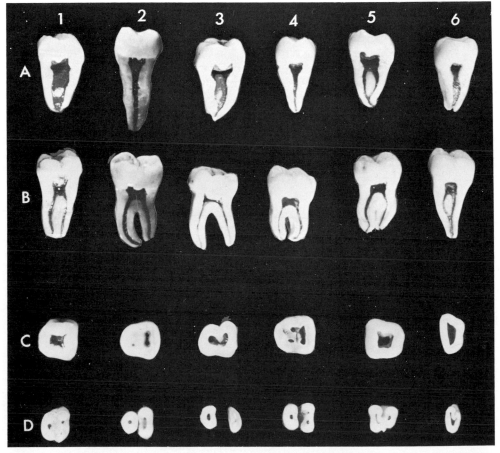

Figure 340. Mandibular third molar—cross sections of natural specimens. *A,* 1 to 6, Buccolingual sections. This aspect does not show in radiographs. *B,* 1 to 6, Mesiodistal sections. *C,* 1 to 6, Cervical sections of root. *D,* 1 to 6, Mid-root sections.

description. If the development of the tooth is normal, it has many characteristics of the mandibular second molar and of course has a pulp cavity which conforms in a general way to that tooth.

The mandibular third molar may have numerous cusps and numerous roots. In that case it may have as many pulp horns as cusps, and as many canals as roots. Since this tooth develops later in life than the other teeth, the canals and pulp chambers are relatively large when compared with those of the other two molars. The roots are usually short, with root canals in proportion. In the single-root type, made by the fusion of more than one root developmentally, it is possible that the tooth may have one canal only, of an odd shape (Fig. 340, C-6 and D-6).

Because of the possibility of malformations, usually this tooth does not lend itself well to root canal therapy. However, under certain conditions and circumstances the patient's welfare may demand retention of this tooth for successful rehabilitation.

Chapter *XIV*

DENTO-OSSEOUS STRUCTURES

T<small>HE OSSEOUS</small> structures which support the teeth are the maxilla and the mandible. The maxilla, or upper jaw, consists of two bones: a *right maxilla* and a *left maxilla* sutured together at the median line. Both maxillae in turn are joined to other bones of the head. The *mandible*, or lower jaw, has no osseous union with the skull and is movable.

A description of the maxilla and the mandible must include the normally developed framework encompassing the teeth in complete dental arches. *This establishes the teeth as foundation tissues to be included with the bones for jaw support and as a part of the framework for the mobile portion of the face. The root forms with their size and angulation will govern the shape of the alveoli in the jaw bones, and this in turn shapes the contour of the dento-osseous portions facially.*

The loss of teeth brings about an atrophic reduction of valuable portions of the maxilla and mandible, adding disfigurement and psychological injury to the more obvious one of masticatory malfunction.

THE MAXILLAE

The maxillae make up a large part of the bony framework of the facial portion of the skull. They form the major portion of the roof of the mouth, or hard palate, and assist in the formation of the floor of the orbit and the sides and base of the nasal cavity. They bear the sixteen maxillary teeth.

Each maxilla is an irregular bone somewhat cuboidal in shape which consists of a body and four processes: the *zygomatic, nasal* or *frontal, palatine* and *alveolar processes*. It is hollow and contains the *maxillary sinus* air space, also called the *antrum of Highmore*. From the dental viewpoint, in addition to its general shape and

315

the processes mentioned, the following landmarks on this bone are among those most important:

1. Incisive fossa
2. Canine fossa
3. Canine eminence
4. Infra-orbital foramen

5. Posterior alveolar foramina
6. Maxillary tuberosity
7. Pterygopalatine sulcus
8. Incisive canal

The *body* of the maxilla has four surfaces:

1. Anterior or facial surface
2. Posterior infratemporal surface
3. Orbital or superior surface
4. Medial or nasal surface

The maxilla has four *processes*:

1. Zygomatic process
2. Frontal process
3. Palatine process
4. Alveolar process

Anterior Surface

The *anterior* or *facial surface* is separated above from the orbital aspect by the *infra-orbital ridge*. Medially it is limited by the margin of the nasal notch, and posteriorly it is separated from the posterior surface by the anterior border of the zygomatic process, which has a confluent ridge directly over the roots of the first molar. The ridge corresponding to the root of the canine tooth is usually the most pronounced and is called the *canine eminence* (Figs. 341 and 342).

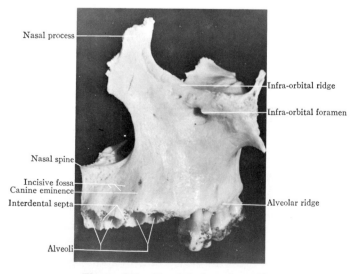

Figure 341.   Frontal view of maxilla.

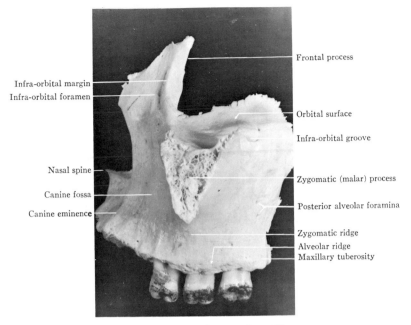

Figure 342. Lateral view of maxilla.

Mesial to the canine eminence, overlying the roots of the incisor teeth, is a shallow concavity known as the *incisive fossa*. Distal to the canine eminence on a higher level is a deeper concavity called the *canine fossa*. The floor of this canine fossa is formed in part by the projecting zygomatic process. Above this fossa and below the infra-orbital ridge is the *infra-orbital foramen*, the external opening of the infra-orbital canal. The major portion of the canine fossa is directly above the roots of the premolars.

Posterior Surface

The *posterior* or *infratemporal surface* is bounded above by the posterior edge of the orbital surface. Inferiorly and anteriorly it is separated from the anterolateral surface by the zygomatic process and its lower border. This surface is more or less convex and is pierced in a downward direction by the apertures of the *posterior alveolar foramina*, which are two or more in number (Figs. 342 and 345).

These two canals are on a level with the lower border of the zygomatic process and are somewhat distal to the roots of the last molar. The lower part of this area is slightly more prominent where it overhangs the root of the third molar and is called the *maxillary tuberosity*. Medially this tuberosity is limited by a sharp, irregular margin with which the palate bone articulates (see Fig. 345).

Orbital or Superolateral Surface

This surface is smooth and forms part of the floor of the orbit. The anterior edge of this surface corresponds to the infra-orbital margin or ridge as it travels up to become part of the nasal process. Its posterior border or edge coincides with the inferior boundary of the inferior orbital fissure.

Its thin medial edge is notched in front to form the *lacrimal groove*, behind which groove it articulates with the lacrimal bone for a short distance, then for a greater length with a thin portion of the ethmoid bone, and terminates posteriorly in a surface which articulates with the orbital process of the palate bone. Its lateral area is continuous with the base of the zygomatic process.

Traversing part of this area to the distal is the *infra-orbital canal*, the anterior opening of which is located directly below the infra-orbital ridge in the anterolateral area. Distally, however, owing to a deficiency of its covering, the canal forms a groove on the orbital surface toward the uppermost boundary of the posterolateral surface.

If the covered portion of this canal were to be laid open, the orifices of the middle and anterior alveolar canal would be seen transmitting the corresponding vessels and nerves to the premolars, canines and incisor teeth.

Nasal or Medial Surface

This surface is directed medially toward the nasal cavity. It is bordered below by the superior surface of the palatine process; anteriorly it is limited by the sharp edge of the nasal notch. Above and anteriorly it is continuous with the medial surface of the frontal process; behind this it is deeply channeled by the *lacrimal groove*, which is of course converted into a canal by articulation with the lacrimal and inferior turbinate bones.

Behind this groove the upper edge of this area corresponds to the medial margin of the orbital surface, and the maxilla articulates in this region with the lacrimal bone, a thin portion of the ethmoid bone and the orbital process of the palate bone.

The posterior border of the maxilla, which articulates with the palate bone, is traversed obliquely from above downward and slightly medially by a groove which, by articulation with the palate bone, is converted into the *posterior palatine canal*.

Toward the posterior and upper part of this nasal surface an irregular or angular opening of the *maxillary sinus* or *antrum of Highmore* may be seen. In front of the lacrimal groove the nasal surface is ridged for the attachment of the *inferior turbinate* bone. Below this the bone forms a lateral wall of the *inferior nasal meatus*. Above the ridge for some little distance on the medial side of the nasal process, the smooth lateral wall of the *middle meatus* appears.

Processes

The *zygomatic process* may be seen in the lateral views of the bone. Illustrations show it to be rough and spongelike in appearance where it has been disarticulated from the zygomatic or cheek bone (Fig. 342). The lower border of this process, directly over the first molar, is considered to be an important landmark.

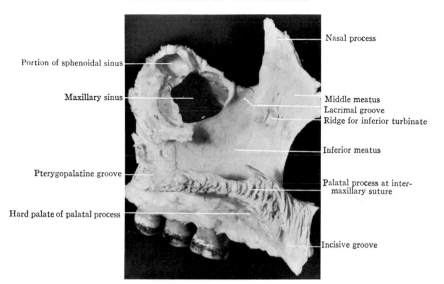

Portion of sphenoidal sinus

Maxillary sinus

Pterygopalatine groove

Hard palate of palatal process

Nasal process

Middle meatus
Lacrimal groove
Ridge for inferior turbinate

Inferior meatus

Palatal process at inter-
maxillary suture

Incisive groove

Figure 343.   Medial view of maxilla.

The *frontal process* arises from the upper and anterior part of the body of the maxilla. Part of this extension is the upward continuation of the infra-orbital margin laterally. Its anterior edge articulates with the nasal bone. Superiorly the summit of the process articulates with the frontal bone. The medial surface of the frontal process is directed toward the nasal cavity.

The *palatine process* has two surfaces, the superior and the inferior. Its superior surface helps form the floor of the nasal cavity. Its inferior surface when sutured with the maxilla of the opposite side forms the anterior three-fourths of the hard palate. The posterior portion of the hard palate is formed by the horizontal part of the palate bone (Fig. 351). The inferior surface of the palatine process is rough and pitted for the glands of the mucous membrane in the roof of the mouth and by small foramina for rich blood and nerve supply. As mentioned before, the posterior palatine canal makes its appearance where the palate bones have been disarticulated from the palatine process of the maxilla (Fig. 351).

The posterior edge of the palatine process becomes relatively thin where it joins the palatine bone at the point of the greater palatine foramen. The palatine process becomes progressively thicker anteriorly from the posterior border. Anteriorly it becomes quite thick, its thickness being measured from the alveolar border of the anterior teeth to the nasal sinus. This portion of the palatal process is confluent with the alveolar process surrounding the roots of the anterior teeth.

Immediately posterior to the central incisor alveolus, when looking at the medial aspect of the maxilla, one sees a smooth canal which is half of the *incisive canal*, when the two bones are joined together (Fig. 351). The *incisive fossa* into which the canals open may be seen immediately lingual to the central incisors at the median line or *intermaxillary suture*, when the maxillae are joined.

The posterior border of the palatine process, when observed from the inferior aspect, falls in line with the second molar and articulates with the horizontal part of

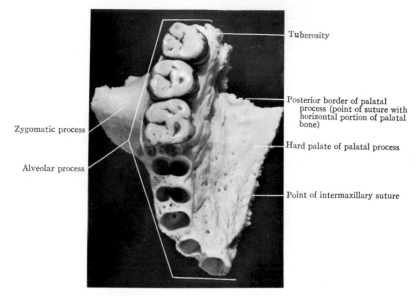

Figure 344. Palatal view of maxilla.

the palatal bone (see Figs. 344 and 351). The intermaxillary suture and the suture joining the palate bone to the palatal process of the maxilla (transverse palatine suture) are nearly at right angles.

The *alveolar process* makes up the inferior portion of the maxilla; it is that portion of the bone which surrounds the roots of the maxillary teeth and which gives them their osseous support. The process extends from the base of the tuberosity posterior to the last molar to the median line anteriorly, where it articulates with

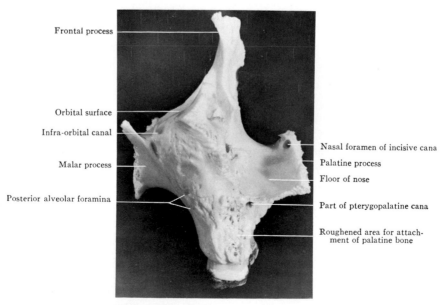

Figure 345. Posterior view of maxilla.

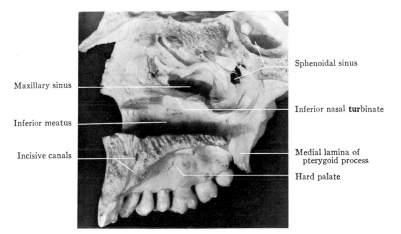

Sphenoidal sinus

Maxillary sinus

Inferior nasal turbinate

Inferior meatus

Incisive canals

Medial lamina of
pterygoid process

Hard palate

Figure 346. Medial view of maxilla. This specimen has not been disarticulated completely and has the maxillary teeth in situ.

the same process of the opposite maxilla (Figs. 344, 346 and 347). It merges with the palatine process medially and with the zygomatic process laterally (Fig. 347).

When one looks directly at the inferior aspect of the maxilla toward the alveoli with teeth removed, it is apparent that the alveolar process is curved to conform with the dental arch. It completes, with its fellow of the opposite side, the alveolar arch supporting the roots of the teeth of the maxilla.

The process has a facial (labial and buccal) surface and a lingual surface with ridges corresponding to the surfaces of the roots of the teeth invested in it. It is made up of labiobuccal and lingual plates of very dense but thin cortical bone separated by interdental septa of cancellous bone.

The facial plate is thin, and the positions of the alveoli are well marked on it by visible ridges as far posteriorly as the distobuccal root of the first molar (Fig. 341).

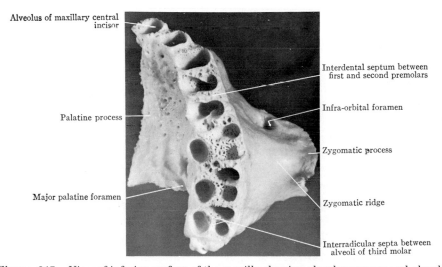

Alveolus of maxillary central
incisor

Interdental septum between
first and second premolars

Infra-orbital foramen

Palatine process

Zygomatic process

Major palatine foramen

Zygomatic ridge

Interradicular septa between
alveoli of third molar

Figure 347. View of inferior surface of the maxilla showing alveolar process and alveoli.

The margins of these alveoli are frail and their edges sharp and thin. The buccal plate over the second and third molars, including the alveolar margins, is thicker. Generally speaking, the lingual plate of the alveolar process is heavier than the facial plate. In addition, it is longer where it surrounds the anterior teeth, and sometimes this added coverage includes the premolars. In short, it extends farther down in covering the lingual portion of the roots.

The bone is very thick lingually, over the deeper portions of the alveoli of the anterior teeth and premolars. This formation is brought about by the merging of the alveolar process with the roof of the mouth. The lingual plate is paper thin over the lingual alveolus of the first molar, however, and rather thin over the lingual alveoli of the second and third molars. This thin lingual plate over the molar roots is part of the formation of the *major palatine canal* (Fig. 347).

The Alveoli, or Tooth Sockets

These cavities are formed by the facial and lingual plates of the alveolar process and by connecting septa of bone placed between the two plates. The form and depth of each alveolus is regulated by the form and length of the root it supports. (See table, "Measurements of the Teeth," Chapter I.)

The *alveolus* nearest the median line is that of the *central incisor*. The periphery is regular and round, and the interior of the alveolus is evenly cone-shaped.

The second *alveolus* in line is that of the *lateral incisor*. It is generally cone-shaped. It is narrower mesiodistally than labiolingually and is smaller on cross section, although it is often deeper than the central alveolus. Sometimes it is curved at the upper extremity.

The *canine alveolus* is third from the median line. It is much larger and deeper than those just described. The periphery is oval and regular in outline with the labial width greater than the lingual. The socket extends distally. It is flattened mesially and somewhat concave distally. The bone is so frail at the canine eminence on the facial surface of the alveolus that the root of the canine is often exposed on the labial surface near the middle third (Fig. 341).

The *first premolar alveolus* is kidney-shaped, with the cavity partially divided by a spine of bone which fits into the mesial developmental groove of the root of this tooth. This spine divides the cavity into a buccal and a lingual portion. If the tooth root is bifurcated for part of its length, as is often the case, the terminal portion of the cavity is separated into buccal and lingual alveoli. The socket is flattened distally and much wider buccolingually than mesiodistally. (See "Measurements of the Teeth," Chapter I.)

The *second premolar alveolus* is also kidney-shaped, but the curvatures are in reverse to those of the first premolar alveolus. The proportions and depth are almost the same. The septal spine is located on the distal side instead of the mesial, since the second premolar root is inclined to have a well-defined developmental groove distally. This tooth usually has one broad root with a blunt end, but it is occasionally bifurcated at the apical third.

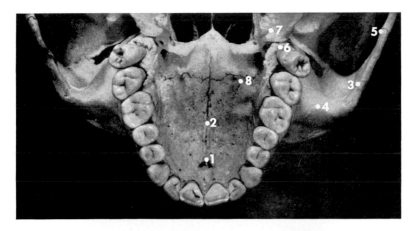

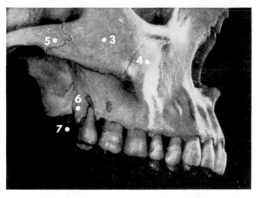

Figure 348. Photographs of dry specimen of maxilla, illustrating anatomic landmarks. (By H. Berton McCauley, D.D.S., in *Dental Radiography and Photography,* Eastman Kodak Co.)

1, Incisive fossa. 2, Median palatine suture. 3, Zygomatic (malar) bone. 4, Zygomatic process of maxilla. 5, Zygomaticotemporal suture. 6, Tuberosity of maxilla. 7, Hamular process of spheroid bone. 8, Major (or greater) palatine foramen.

The *first molar alveolus* is made up of three distinct alveoli widely separated. The *lingual alveolus* is the largest; it is round, regular and deep. The cavity extends in the direction of the hard palate, having a lingual plate over it which is very thin. The lingual periphery of this alveolus is extremely sharp and frail. This condition may contribute to tissue recession often seen at this site.

The *mesiobuccal* and *distobuccal alveoli* of the first molar have no outstanding characteristics except that the buccal plates are thin. The bone is somewhat thicker at the peripheries than that found on the lingual alveolus. Nevertheless it is thinner farther up on the buccal plate. It is not uncommon for one to find the roots uncovered by bone in spots when examining dry specimens.

The forms of the buccal alveoli resemble the forms of the roots they support. The mesiobuccal alveolus is broad buccolingually, with the mesial and distal walls flattened. The distobuccal alveolus is rounder and more conical.

The *septa* which separate the three alveoli (interradicular septa) are broad at the area which corresponds to the root bifurcation, and they become progressively thicker as the peripheries of the alveoli are approached. The bone septa are very cancellous, denoting a rich blood supply, as is true of all the septa, those separating the various teeth as well.

A general description of the alveoli of the *second molar* would coincide with that of the first molar; these alveoli are closer together, since the roots of this tooth do not spread as much. As a consequence, the septa separating the alveoli are not so heavy.

The *third molar alveolus* is similar to that of the second molar except that it is somewhat smaller in all dimensions. Figure 347 shows a third molar socket to accommodate a tooth with three well-defined roots, a rare occurrence. Usually the roots will be fused, the buccal roots at least, and often all three. The interradicular septum changes accordingly. If the roots of the tooth are fused, a septal spine will appear in the alveolus at the points of fusion on the roots marked by deep developmental grooves.

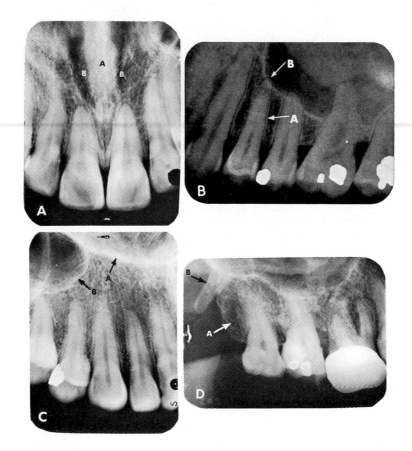

Figure 349, I. *A,* Radiograph of central incisor region that visualizes the nasal septum (A) and fossae (B).

B, Radiograph that demonstrates the normal appearance of (A) the lamina dura, (B) the periodontal membrane.

C, Radiograph that depicts the Y (inverted) formed by the junction of the lateral wall (A) of the nasal fossa and the antemedial wall (B) of the maxillary sinus.

D, Radiograph that visualizes (A) the tuberosity of the maxilla, (B) the hamular process of the sphenoid bone.

(By H. Berton McCauley, D.D.S., in *Dental Radiography and Photography,* Eastman Kodak Co.)

Maxillary Sinus

The maxillary sinus lies within the body of the bone and is of corresponding pyramidal form; the base is directed toward the nasal cavity. Its summit extends laterally into the root of the zygomatic process. It is closed in laterally and above by the thin walls which form the anterolateral, posterolateral and orbital surfaces of the body. The sinus overlies the alveolar process in which the molar teeth are implanted, more particularly the first and second molars, the alveoli of which are separated

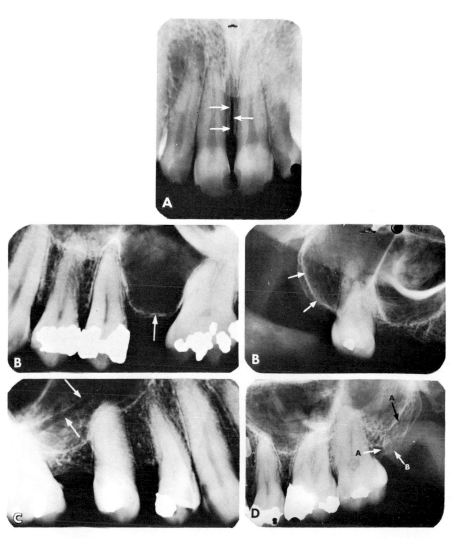

Figure 349, II. *A,* Radiograph of the medial palatine suture, the appearance of which might be interpreted as a fracture.

B, Radiographs that visualize various extensions of the maxillary sinus; left, alveolar extension; right, tuberosity extension.

C, Radiograph in which the canal for a superior alveolar artery is seen.

D, Radiograph showing typical superimposition of the coronoid process: (A) of the mandible on the tuberosity, (B) of the maxilla.

(By H. Berton McCauley, D.D.S., in *Dental Radiography and Photography,* Eastman Kodak Co.)

from the sinus by a thin layer of bone. Occasionally the maxillary sinus will extend forward far enough to overlie the premolars also. It is not uncommon to find the bone covering the alveoli of some of the posterior teeth extending above the floor of the cavity of the maxillary sinus, forming small hillocks.

Regardless of the irregularity and the extension of the alveoli into the maxillary sinus, there is always a layer of bone separating the roots of the teeth and the floor of the sinus in the absence of pathologic conditions. There is always, also, a layer of sinus mucosa between the root tips and the sinus cavity.

Maxillary Articulation

The maxilla articulates with the nasal, frontal, lacrimal and ethmoid bones, above, and laterally with the zygomatic bone and occasionally with the sphenoid bone (Fig. 343). Posteriorly and medially it articulates with the palate bone besides joining the maxilla on its medial side. In addition, it supports the inferior turbinate and the vomer medially. (See Figs. 350, 351, and 352.)

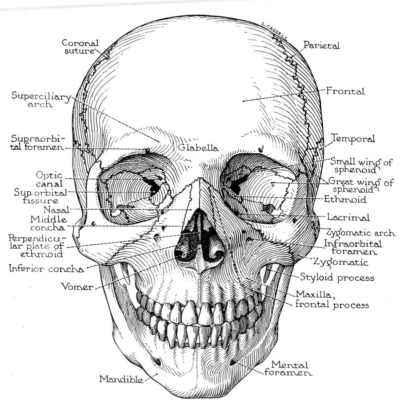

Figure 350. Anterior view of the skull. (King and Showers, Human Anatomy and Physiology, 5th Edition.)

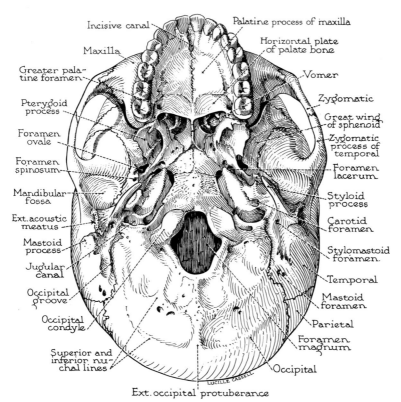

Figure 351. View of base of skull from below. (King and Showers, Human Anatomy and Physiology, 5th Edition.)

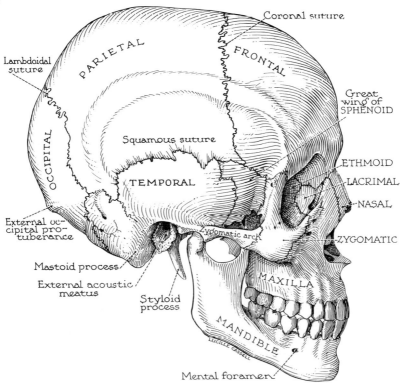

Figure 352. Lateral view of the skull. (King and Showers, Human Anatomy and Physiology, 5th Edition.)

THE MANDIBLE

The mandible is horseshoe-shaped and supports the teeth of the lower dental arch. This bone is movable and therefore has no bony attachment to the skull. It is the heaviest and strongest bone of the head and serves as a framework for the floor of the mouth. It is situated immediately below the maxillary and zygomatic bone, and its *condyles* rest in the *glenoid fossa* of the temporal bone, a formation which makes possible a movable articulation (Figs. 353 to 360).

The mandible has a horizontal portion or *body* and two vertical portions or *rami*. The rami join the body at an obtuse angle.

The *body* consists of two lateral halves, which are joined at the median line shortly after birth. The line of fusion, usually marked by a slight ridge, is called the symphysis. The body of the mandible has two surfaces, an external and an internal, and two borders, a superior and an inferior.

To the right and left of the symphysis, near the lower border of the mandible, are two prominences called *mental tubercles*. A prominent triangular surface made by the symphysis and these two tubercles is called the *mental protuberance* (Fig. 354).

Immediately posterior to the symphysis and immediately above the mental protuberance, there is a shallow depression called the *incisive fossa*. This fossa is immediately below the alveolar border of the central and lateral incisors and anterior to the canines. The alveolar portion of the mandible overlying the root of the canine is prominent and is called the *canine eminence* of the mandible. This eminence does not extend down very far toward the lower border of the mandible,

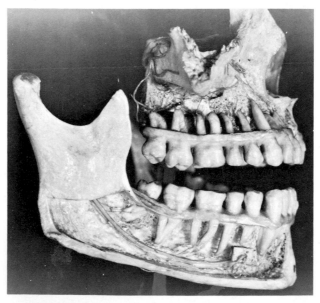

Figure 353. Dissected specimen of maxilla and mandible. This specimen illustrates the extent of the alveolar processes, the angulations of the long axes of the teeth, the relative lengths of the roots and the spacing of those roots, which of course governs the size, form and direction of the alveoli.

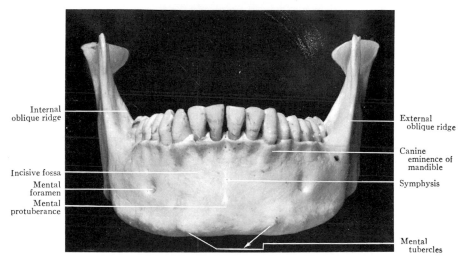

Figure 354. Frontal view of mandible.

however, before it is lost in the prominence of the mental protuberance and the lower border of the mandible in this area.

The external surface of the mandible from a lateral viewpoint presents a number of important areas for examination:

The *external oblique ridge* (external oblique line) extends obliquely across the external surface of the mandible from the mental tubercle to the anterior border of the ramus, with which it is continuous. It lies below the mental foramen. It is usually not prominent except in the molar area (Figs. 354 and 355).

This ridge thins out as it progresses upward and becomes the anterior border of the ramus and ends at the tip of the *coronoid process.* The coronoid process is one of two processes making up the superior border of the ramus. It is a pointed, smooth

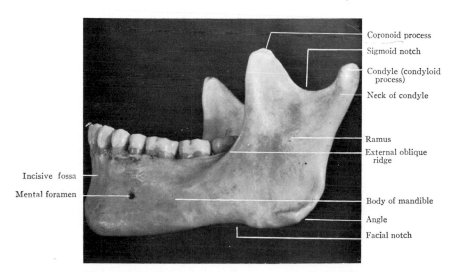

Figure 355. Lateral view of outer surface of mandible.

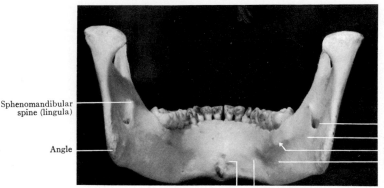

Figure 356. Posterior view of mandible.

projection flattened externally and internally, and it is roughened toward the tip to give attachment for a part of the temporal muscle.

The *condyle*, or *condyloid process*, on the posterior border of the ramus, is variable in form. It is divided into a superior or articular portion and an inferior portion or *neck*. Although the articular portion, the condyle, appears as a rounded knob when one sees the mandible from the side, exteriorly, from a *posterior* aspect the condyle is much wider and is oblong in outline (compare Figs. 355 and 356).

The condyle is convex above, fitting into the glenoid fossa of the temporal bone when the mandible is articulated to the skull, and forms, with the interarticular cartilage which lies between the two surfaces and with the tissue attachment, the *temporomandibular articulation*.

The neck of the condyle is a constricted portion immediately below the articular surface. It is flattened in front and presents a concave pit medially—the *pterygoid fossa*. A smooth semicircular notch, the *sigmoid notch*, forms the sharp upper border of the ramus between the condyle and coronoid process.

The distal border of the ramus is smooth and rounded and presents a concave outline from the neck of the condyle to the angle of the jaw, where the posterior border of the ramus and the inferior border of the body of the mandible join. The border of this angle is rough, being the attachment of the masseter muscle and the stylomandibular ligament.

An important landmark on the external aspect of the mandible is the *mental foramen*. It should be noted that this opening of the anterior end of the mandibular canal is directed upward and backward as well as laterally. The foramen is usually located midway between the superior and inferior border of the body of the mandible when the teeth are in position, and most often it is below the second premolar tooth, a little below the apex of the root. The position of this foramen is not constant and it may be between the first premolar and the second premolar tooth. After the teeth are lost and resorption of alveolar bone has taken place, the mental foramen may appear near the crest of the alveolar border. In childhood, before the first permanent molar has come into position, this foramen is usually immediately below the first deciduous molar and nearer the lower border.

It is interesting to note, when one observes the mandible from a point directly opposite the first molar, that most of the distal half of the third molar is hidden by the anterior border of the ramus. When looking at the mandible from in front, directly opposite the median line, the student sees the second and third molars located 5 to 7 mm. lingually to the anterior border of the ramus. (Compare Figs. 354 and 355.)

The Internal Surface of the Mandible

Observation of the mandible from the rear shows that the median line is marked by a slight vertical depression, representing the line of union of the right and left halves of the mandible, and immediately below this, at the lower third, that the bone is roughened by eminences called the *genial tubercles* (Fig. 356).

The internal surface of the body of the mandible is divided into two portions by a well-defined ridge, the *mylohyoid* or *internal oblique ridge*. It occupies a position closely corresponding to the external oblique ridge on the external surface. It starts at or near the lowest part of the genial tubercles and passes backward and upward, increasing in prominence until the anterior portion of the ramus is reached; there it smooths out and gradually disappears (Fig. 357).

This ridge is the point of origin of the mylohyoid muscle, which forms the central portion of the floor of the mouth. Immediately posterior to the median line and above the anterior part of the mylohyoid ridge a smooth depression, the *sublingual fossa*, may be seen. The sublingual gland lies in this area.

A small oval roughened depression, the *digastric fossa*, is found on each side of the symphysis immediately below the mylohyoid line and extending onto the lower border. Toward the center of the body of the mandible, between the mylohyoid ridge and the lower border of the bone, a smooth oblong depression is located, called the

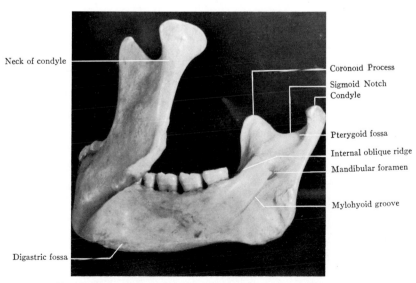

Figure 357.   Posterolateral view of inner surface of mandible.

submaxillary fossa. It continues back on the medial surface of the ramus to the attachment of the internal pterygoid muscle. The submaxillary gland lies within this fossa.

The *mandibular foramen* is located on the medial surface of the ramus midway between the sigmoid notch and the angle of the jaw and also midway between the internal oblique line and the posterior border of the ramus. The mandibular canal begins at this point, passing downward and forward horizontally.

The anterior margin of the foramen is formed by the *lingula* or *mandibular spine*, which gives attachment to the *sphenomandibular ligament.* Coming obliquely downward from the base of the foramen beneath the spine is a decided groove, the *mylohyoid groove.* Behind this groove toward the angle of the mandible, a roughened surface for the attachment of the internal pterygoid muscle may be seen.

The Alveolar Process

The border of this process outlines the alveoli of the teeth and is very thin at its anterior portion around the roots of the incisor teeth but thicker posteriorly where it encompasses the roots of the molars. The alveolar process which composes the superior border of the body of the mandible differs from the same process in the maxillae in one very important particular: It is not so cancellous, and instead of the facial plate being thin and frail it is equally as heavy as the lingual plate. Although the bone over the anterior teeth, including the canine, is very thin and over the cervical portion of the root may be entirely missing, yet the bone which does cover the root is the compact type of bone.

The inferior border of the mandible is strong and rounded and gives to the bone the greatest portion of its strength (see Fig. 358).

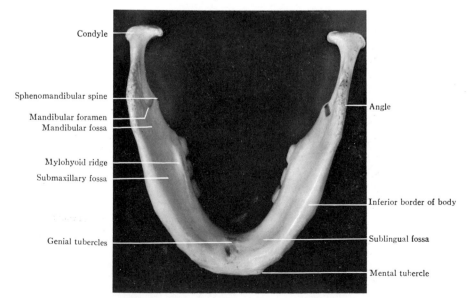

Figure 358. View of mandible from below.

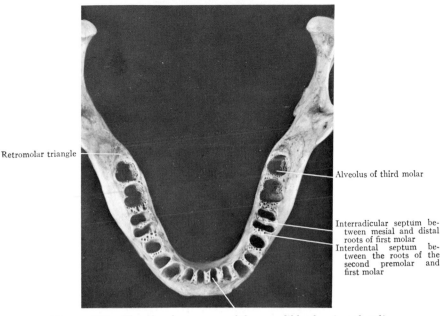

Retromolar triangle

Alveolus of third molar

Interradicular septum between mesial and distal roots of first molar

Interdental septum between the roots of the second premolar and first molar

Figure 359.   The alveolar process of the mandible showing alveoli.

When looking down on the mandible from a point above the alveoli of the first molars (Fig. 359), one may notice that, although the alveolar border may be thinner anteriorly than posteriorly, the body of the bone is uniform throughout. The lines of direction of the posterior alveoli are inclined lingually to conform to the lingual inclination of the teeth when they are in position. The anterior teeth, of course, have their alveoli tipped labially; therefore when one looks down upon the mandible from above the alveolar process, more of the bone may be seen lingual to the anterior

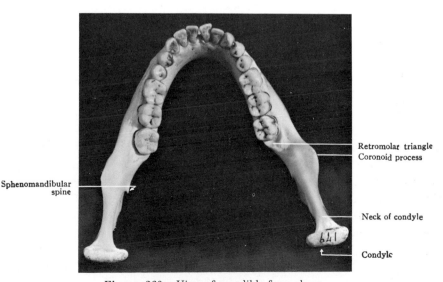

Retromolar triangle
Coronoid process

Sphenomandibular spine

Neck of condyle

Condyle

Figure 360.   View of mandible from above.

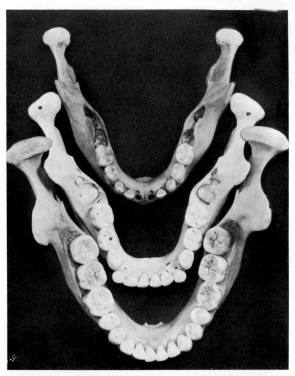

Figure 361. Comparison of size and shape of mandibles at various ages. *Top,* mandible of five-year-old. Notice the rounded bowlike form. Notice also the amount of space between the second deciduous molar and the ramus. *Middle,* mandible of nine-year-old. Notice the angular outline with constriction at the point of second permanent molar development. *Lower,* well-developed mandible of an individual approximately fifty years of age. The bone is regular in outline. The lingual constriction has lessened and has retreated to the third molar area.

teeth than lingual to the posterior teeth. In contrast posteriorly, more of the bone may be seen buccal to the teeth than lingual. *Therefore, the outline of the arch of the teeth does not correspond to the outline of the arch of the bone.* The dental arch is narrower posteriorly than the mandibular arch.

The lingual walls of the alveoli of the second and third molars are relatively thin near the bottoms of the sockets, although the bone near the periphery is somewhat thicker and very compact. If a specimen of the mandible from which the third molar has been removed is held up to the light, the bone at the bottom of the socket is so thin that light will penetrate it. This is caused by the mandible being undercut at this point for the submaxillary fossa below the mylohyoid ridge (Fig. 358).

The bone buccal to the last two molars is very heavy and thick, being reinforced by the external oblique ridge. Posterior to the third molar a triangular shallow fossa is outlined; it is called the *retromolar triangle.* The cortical plate over this fossa is not so heavy as the bone surrounding it, and it is more cancellous under the thin cortical plate covering it.

The Alveoli

The first alveolus right or left of the median line is that of the *first* or *central incisor*. The periphery of the alveolus often dips down lingually and labially and exposes the root for part of its length. This arrangement makes an interdental spine out of the interdental septum separating the alveoli of the mandibular central incisors. The central incisor alveolus is flattened on its mesial surface and is usually somewhat concave distally to accommodate the developmental groove on the root (Fig. 359).

The alveolus of the mandibular *second* or *lateral incisor* is similar to that of the central incisor. It usually has the following variations: The socket is larger and deeper to accommodate a larger and longer root; the periphery does not dip down so far on the lingual but may dip more on the labial, exposing more of the root of the lateral incisor. The interdental septum extends up just as high between the teeth as that between the central incisors.

The *canine alveolus* is quite large and oval and of course deep to accommodate the root of the mandibular canine. The lingual plate is stronger and much heavier than over the alveoli just described, although the thin labial plate may thin out at its edges and expose just as much of the canine root on the labial side. The labial outline of the alveolus is wider than the lingual outline, and the mesial and distal walls of the sockets will be irregular to accommodate developmental grooves, both mesially and distally, on the canine root.

The alveoli of the *first* and *second premolars* are similar in outline. The outline is smooth and rounded, although the dimensions are greater buccolingually than mesiodistally. The alveolus of the second premolar is usually somewhat larger than that of the first premolar. The buccal plate of the alveoli is relatively thin, but the lingual plate is heavy; the interdental septum has become heavier at this point when one compares it with the interdental septa found between the anterior teeth. The interdental septum between the canine and first premolar is relatively thin although uniform in outline. The septum between the first premolar and second premolar is nearly twice as thick.

Progressing posteriorly, one finds that the interdental septum between the second premolar socket and the alveolus of the mesial root of the *first molar* is twice as thick as that found between the first and second premolars. The socket of the first molar is divided by an interroot septum which is strong and regular. The alveolus of the mesial root is kidney-shaped, much wider buccolingually than mesiodistally and constricted in the center to accommodate developmental grooves found mesial and distal to the mesial root of the first molar. The alveolus of the distal root of the first molar is evenly oval with no constriction, conforming to the rounded shape of this root. The interdental septum between the alveoli of the mandibular first molar and the socket of the second molar is thick mesiodistally although cancellous in character.

The mandibular *second molar alveolus* may be divided into *two* alveoli, as was the case in the first molar. However, often it is found to be one compartment near the periphery of the alveolus, but divides into two compartments in the deeper portions.

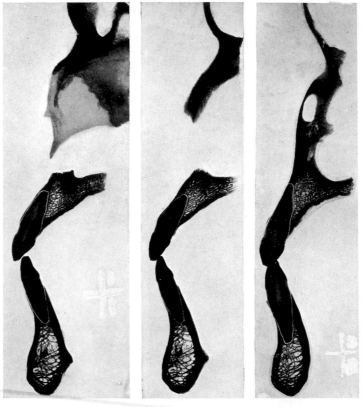

Figure 362   **Figure 363**   **Figure 364**

Figures 362 to 369. Note the axial relations of the superior and inferior teeth, the relative thickness of labial and lingual alveolar plates, the characteristics of the cancellous tissue, the relative densities and the relation of the teeth to important structures. Compare the changes in the external contour and internal architecture of the adjacent sections. The sections in this series, with the exception of Fig. 365, were taken from the same cadaver and are from the left side. A plaster cast was made before sectioning. The sections were reassembled in the cast and held in exact relation while being X-rayed.

Figure 362. The central incisor regions, showing relation of superior central incisor to inferior lateral incisor.
Figure 363. The lateral incisor regions. Note position of apex of superior lateral incisor.
Figure 364. The canine regions. Note anterior extremity of maxillary antrum.

A septal spine occurs where the developmental grooves on the root are deep enough, or an interradicular septum will appear where the roots are entirely divided. The interdental septum between the second molar sockets and the third molar sockets is not so thick mesiodistally as the two interdental septa immediately anterior.

The mandibular *third molar alveolus* is usually irregular in outline. Usually it is much narrower toward the distal than toward the mesial. It may have interradicular septa or septal spines to accommodate itself to the irregularity of the root.

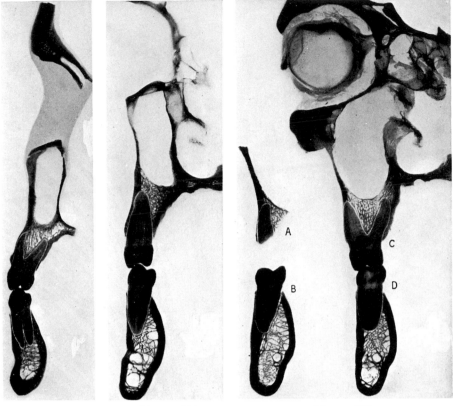

Figure 365   Figure 366   Figure 367

Figure 365. The first premolar regions.
Figure 366. The second premolar regions.
Figure 367. The first molar regions, showing relations of (*C*) mesiobuccal and lingual root with (*D*) mesial half of lower molar, (*A*) distobuccal root, (*B*) distal half.

Classical illustrations by Dr. Hugh W. MacMillan are shown in Figs. 362 to 369. The sections demonstrate the directional lines of the axes of the teeth and their alveoli. In addition, the radiographs of the sections graphically illustrate the relative densities of the teeth and supporting structures and show the outline and relative thickness of the bone over the various teeth at the site of each section.

ARTERIAL SUPPLY TO THE TEETH

The arteries and nerve branches to the teeth are mere terminals of the central systems. This book must confine itself to dental anatomy and the parts immediately associated, and references will therefore be made only to those terminals which supply the teeth and the supporting structures.

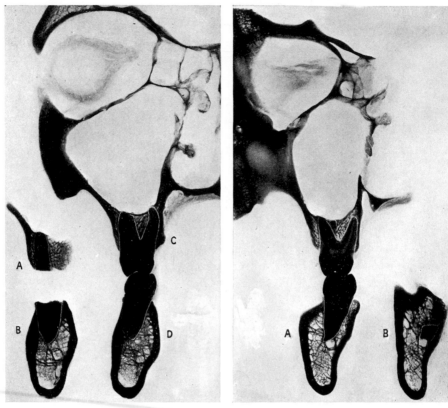

Figure 368   **Figure 369**

Figure 368. The second molar regions, showing relations of (*C*) mesiobuccal and lingual roots with (*D*) mesial half, (*A*) distobuccal root, (*B*) distal root.

Figure 369. The third molar regions, (*A*) mesial root, (*B*) apex of distal root. Note deep groove for descending palatine artery.

Internal Maxillary Artery (Fig. 370)

The arterial supply to the jaw bones and the teeth comes from the *internal maxillary artery*, which is a branch of the *external carotid artery*. The *branches* of the internal maxillary artery which feed the teeth directly are: (1) the *inferior alveolar artery* and (2) the *superior alveolar arteries*.

Inferior Alveolar Artery

The *inferior alveolar artery* branches from the internal maxillary artery medial to the ramus of the mandible. Protected by the sphenomandibular ligament, it gives off the *mylohyoid branch*, which rests in the mylohyoid groove of the mandible and continues along on the medial side under the mylohyoid ridge. After giving off the mylohyoid branch, it immediately enters the mandibular foramen and continues downward and forward through the mandibular canal, giving off branches to the

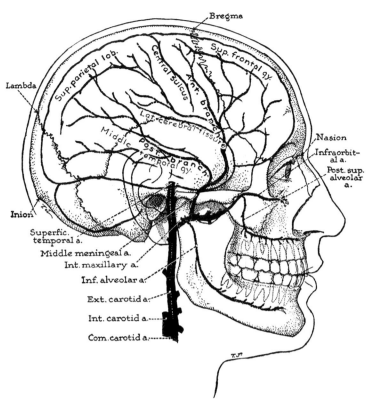

Figure 370. Projection of internal maxillary artery and its branches in relation to brain, skull and mandible, including the teeth. (Jones and Shepard, A Manual of Surgical Anatomy.)

premolar and molar teeth. In the vicinity of the mental foramen it divides into a *mental* and an *incisive branch*. The mental branch passes through the mental foramen to supply the tissues of the chin and to anastomose with the *inferior labial* and *submental arteries*. The incisive branch continues forward in the bone to supply the anterior teeth and bone and to form anastomoses with its fellows of the opposite side.

The anastomoses of the mental and incisive branches furnish a good collateral blood supply for the mandible and teeth.

In their canals, the inferior alveolar and incisive arteries give off *dental* branches to the individual tooth roots for the supply of the pulp and of the periodontal membrane at the root apex. Other branches enter the interdental septa supplying bone and adjacent periodontal membrane and terminating in the gingivae. Numerous small anastomoses connect these vessels with those supplying the neighboring alveolar mucosa.

Superior Alveolar Arteries

The *posterior superior alveolar artery* branches from the internal maxillary at the posterior of the maxillary tuberosity along with the alveolar nerves and supplies the maxillary teeth, alveolar bone and membrane of the sinus. A branch of variable size runs forward on the periosteum at the junction of the aveolar process and maxillary body supplying the gingiva, alveolar mucosa and cheek. When it is large, it may supplant in part the buccal artery.

A *middle superior alveolar branch* is usually given off by the infra-orbital branch of the internal maxillary artery somewhere along the infra-orbital groove or canal. It runs downward between the sinus mucosa and bone or in canals in the bone and joins the *posterior* and *anterior alveolar vessels*. Its main distribution is to the maxillary teeth.

Anterior superior alveolar branches arise from the infra-orbital artery just before this vessel leaves its foramen. They course down the anterior aspect of the maxilla in bony canals to supply the maxillary anterior teeth and their supporting tissues and to join the *middle* and *posterior superior alveolar branches* in completing an anastomotic plexus.

Branches to the teeth, periodontal membrane and bone are derived from the superior alveolar in the same manner as described for the inferior alveolar artery.

Descending Palatine and Sphenopalatine Arteries

The palatal blood supply comes from two sources but chiefly from the *descending palatine* artery, which descends from its origin from the internal maxillary through the pterygomandibular canal. Its *major* (greater) *palatine* branch enters the palate through the greater palatine foramen and runs forward with its accompanying vein and nerve in a groove at the junction of the palatine and alveolar processes. It is distributed to the bone, glands and mucosa of the hard palate and to the bone and mucosa of the alveolar process, in which it forms anastomoses with fine branches of the superior alveolars. Minor branches of the descending palatine pass to the soft palate through minor palatine canals in the palatine bone.

Terminal branches of the *nasopalatine* branch of the *sphenopalatine artery*: The *nasopalatine* courses obliquely forward and downward on the septum and enters the palate through the incisive canal. It has a limited distribution to the incisive papilla and adjacent palate and forms an anastomosis with the major palatine.

NERVE SUPPLY

The sensory nerve supply to the jaws and teeth is derived from the *maxillary* and *mandibular* branches of the *fifth cranial*, or *trigeminal*, nerve, whose ganglion, the *gasserian*, is located at the tip of the petrous portion of the temporal bone.

Maxillary Nerve

The *maxillary* nerve courses forward through the wall of the cavernous sinus and leaves the skull through the foramen rotundum. It crosses the pterygopalatine fossa,

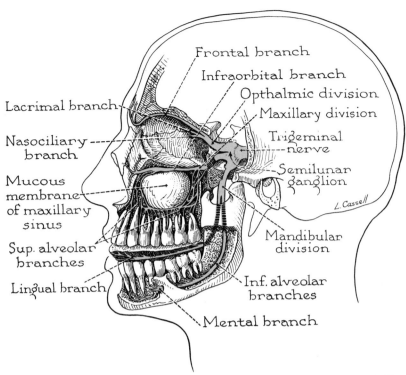

Frontal branch

Infraorbital branch

Opthalmic division

Maxillary division

Lacrimal branch

Trigeminal nerve

Nasociliary branch

Semilunar ganglion

L. Cassell

Mucous membrane of maxillary sinus

Mandibular division

Sup. alveolar branches

Lingual branch

Inf. alveolar branches

Mental branch

Figure 371. Diagram showing distribution of the trigeminal nerve. (King and Showers, Human Anatomy and Physiology, 5th Edition.)

where it gives branches to the *sphenopalatine* ganglion, a parasympathetic ganglion. This ganglion gives off several branches, now containing visceral motor as well as sensory fibers, to the mucous membrane of the mouth, nose and pharynx.

Its branches of practical significance in the mouth are the *descending palatine* branches. Of these the *anterior palatine* enters the hard palate through the major palatine foramen, to be distributed to the hard palate and palatal gingivae as far forward as the canine tooth. *Middle* and *posterior* palatine branches from the ganglion enter the soft palate through minor palatine foramina. A *nasopalatine* branch of the *sphenopalatine* branch of the ganglion runs downward and forward on the nasal septum. Entering the palate through the incisive canal, it is distributed to the incisive papilla and to the palate anterior to the anterior palatine nerve.

The maxillary nerve also has a *posterior superior alveolar* branch from its pterygopalatine portion. This nerve divides, enters foramina on the posterior surface of the maxilla and, forming a plexus, is distributed to the molar teeth and the supporting tissues.

The maxillary nerve enters the orbit and, as the *infra-orbital nerve*, runs forward in its floor first in the infra-orbital groove and then in the infra-orbital canal. It terminates at the infra-orbital foramen in branches distributed to the upper face. At a variable distance after it enters the orbit, a *middle superior alveolar* branch arises from the infra-orbital nerve and runs through the lateral wall of the maxillary sinus. It is distributed to the premolar teeth and surrounding tissues and joins the alveolar plexus. The middle alveolar nerve may be associated closely with the posterior alveolar nerve as its origin but frequently branches near the infra-orbital foramen.

An anterior alveolar branch leaves the infra-orbital nerve just inside the infra-orbital foramen and is distributed through bony canals to the incisor and canine teeth. All three superior alveolar nerves join in a plexus above the process. From the plexus *dental branches* are given off to each tooth root and *interdental branches* to the bone, periodontal membrane and gingivae; the distribution being similar to that described for the arteries.

Mandibular Nerve

The *mandibular nerve* leaves the skull through the foramen ovale and almost immediately breaks up into its several branches. The chief branch to the lower jaw is the *inferior alveolar* nerve, which at first runs directly downward across the medial surface of the external pterygoid, at the lower border of which it is directed laterally and downward across the outer surface of the internal pterygoid muscle to reach the mandibular foramen. Just before entering the foramen it releases the mylohyoid branch, which is primarily a motor branch to the mylohyoid muscle and anterior belly of the digastric muscle.

The inferior alveolar nerve continues forward through the mandibular canal beneath the roots of the molar teeth to the level of the mental foramen. During this part of its course it gives off branches to the molar and premolar teeth and their supporting bone and soft tissues. The nerve to the teeth do not arise as individual branches but as two or three larger branches which form a plexus from which *inferior dental* branches enter individual tooth roots and *interdental* branches supply alveolar bone, periodontal membrane and gingivae.

At the mental foramen the nerve divides, and a smaller incisive branch continues forward to supply the anterior teeth and bone and a larger mental branch emerges through the foramen to supply the skin of the lower lip and chin.

Other branches of the mandibular nerve contributes in some degree to the innervation of the mandible and its investing membranes. The *buccinator (long buccal) nerve*, while chiefly distributed to the mucosa of the cheek, has a branch which is usually distributed to a small area of the buccal gingiva in the first molar area, but in some cases its distribution may extend from the canine to the third molar. The *lingual nerve* as it enters the floor of the mouth lies against the body of the mandible and has mucosal branches to a variable area of lingual mucosa and gingiva. The *mylohyoid nerve* may sometimes continue its course forward on the lower surface of the mylohyoid muscle and enter the mandible through small foramina on either side of the midline. It has been implicated in the innervation of central incisor teeth and their periodontal membranes.

Chapter *XV*

TEMPOROMANDIBULAR ARTICULATION – MUSCLES OF MASTICATION AND FACIAL EXPRESSION – ORAL PHARYNX – ANALYSIS OF MANDIBULAR MOVEMENTS

THE TEMPOROMANDIBULAR ARTICULATION

THE TEMPOROMANDIBULAR articulation is closely associated with the functioning of the teeth. It receives its name from the two bones which enter into its formation, namely, the temporal bone and the mandible. The temporomandibular joint allows a wide range of motion to the mandible. Entering into its construction are bone, ligaments, cartilage and synovial membrane; these tissues are all essential to any movable articulation.

The temporomandibular joint is an example of diarthrosis, and its movements are a combination of gliding movements and a loose hinge movement. The osseous portions of the joint are the anterior portion of the *glenoid fossa* and *articular eminence* of the temporal bone and the *condyloid process* of the mandible. Both the condyle and the glenoid fossa arc covered with a layer of fibrous tissue over the usual articular cartilage. There is a cushion of interarticular fibrocartilage called the *meniscus* between the condyle and the glenoid fossa (Figs. 377, 378 and 379).

343

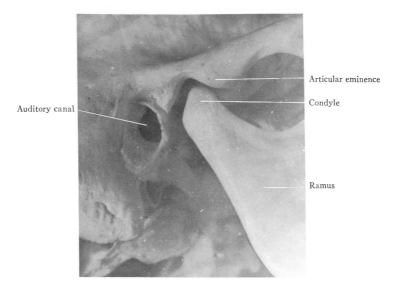

Auditory canal

Articular eminence

Condyle

Ramus

Figure 372.   The relation of the condyle of the mandible to the glenoid fossa and the articular eminence of the temporal bone when the teeth are in *centric occlusal relation.*

The Glenoid Fossa

The glenoid fossa is an oval or oblong depression in the temporal bone just anterior to the auditory canal (Fig. 373). It is bounded anteriorly by the *eminentia articularis* (articular eminence), externally by the middle root of the zygoma and the auditory process, and posteriorly by the tympanic plate of the petrous portion of this bone. The shape of the glenoid fossa conforms to some extent, though not exactly, to the posterior and superior surfaces of the condyloid process of the mandible (Fig. 372).

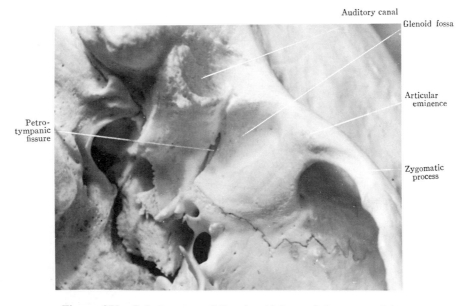

Auditory canal

Glenoid fossa

Articular eminence

Petro-tympanic fissure

Zygomatic process

Figure 373.   Inferior view of the glenoid fossa of the temporal bone.

The Condyloid Process

The condyloid process of the mandible is convex on all bearing surfaces, although somewhat flattened posteriorly, and its knoblike form is wider lateromedially than anteroposteriorly (see Fig. 360, Chapter XIV). It is perhaps two and one-half times as wide in one direction as in the other. Although the development of this condyle differs in individuals, the functional design remains the same. The long axes of the condyles are in a lateral plane, and at first sight they seem to be out of alignment, since the long axes, if the lines were prolonged, would meet at a point posterior to the condyles of the mandible (Fig. 432). However, on closer observation it is noted that the plane of the posterior surface of each condyle or a line through the long axis of the condyle is almost perpendicular to the axis of the main portion of the body of the mandible (Figs. 358, 360 and 361).

Ligaments

The temporomandibular articulation is maintained by ligaments and by the powerful muscles of mastication. The ligamentous attachments are: the *capsular* ligament, the *sphenomandibular* ligament, the *stylomandibular* ligament and accesory fibers of the stylomandibular called the *stylohyoid* ligament.

The *capsular ligament* is a synovial capsule which completely surrounds the condyle. It has fibers divided into four portions: anterior and posterior portions, and internal and external portions. The anterior portion is attached below to the anterior margin of the condyle and above to the front of the glenoid ridge. The posterior portion is attached above just in front of the glenoid fissure and is inserted into the posterior margin of the ramus of the mandible just below the neck of the condyle (Fig. 374).

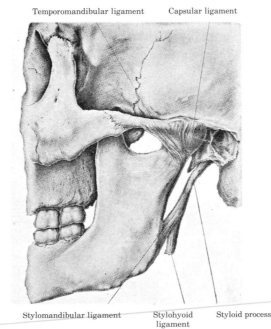

Temporomandibular ligament   Capsular ligament

Stylomandibular ligament   Stylohyoid ligament   Styloid process

Figure 374. Temporomandibular articulation—external view of the ligamentous attachment of the condyle of the mandible to the zygomatic process. Note the strong attachment of the temporomandibular ligament laterally and posteriorly to the neck of the condyle. (Deaver.)

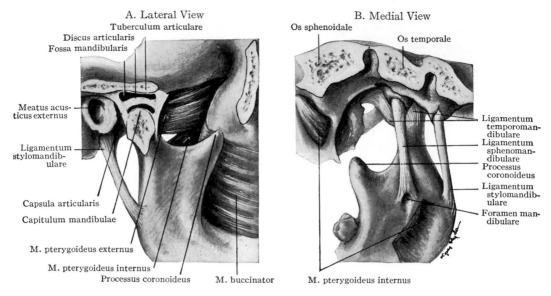

A. Lateral View   B. Medial View

Figure 375. Lateral and medial views of the region about the temporomandibular joint. (Callender, Surgical Anatomy, 2nd Edition.)

The internal portion of the capsular ligament is composed of well-defined fibers and has a broad attachment above to the inner edge of the glenoid fossa and is inserted below into the inner side of the neck of the condyle.

The *temporomandibular ligament,* which is the external portion of the capsular ligament and continuous with it, is the strongest portion of the capsular ligament. It has a broad attachment above the zygomatic process of the temporal bone, the anterior fibers attaching forward well beyond the articular eminence (Fig. 374). These fibers, slanting downward and backward, converge with more vertical fibers and are inserted into the outer side and posterior margin of the neck of the condyle. The temporomandibular ligament acts as the main suspensory ligament of the mandible during moderate opening movements, commonly referred to as the "hinge movements," when the forward movement of the condyle is very slight. With wider opening of the jaw, the condyles move forward rapidly, relaxing the external lateral ligament as the *sphenomandibular ligament* becomes taut.

The *sphenomandibular ligament* is situated some distance from the temporomandibular joint, and, as its name implies, it has its attachment above to the sphenoid bone and below to the mandible. Actually its main origin is from the spinous process of the sphenoid bone with lateral fibers from the temporal bone in the immediate vicinity. The ligament passes downward and forward and is inserted into the lingula of the mandible, with some fibers attached below the mandibular foramen and some posterior to it. The attachment of the sphenomandibular ligament is round and cordlike at its origin; it takes on more of a ribbonlike form at its insertion from the lingula backward on the inner surface of the ramus (Fig. 375B).

The *stylomandibular ligament* extends from the styloid process of the temporal bone downward and forward to be inserted into the posterior border of the ramus of the mandible just above the angle. Just before the stylomandibular ligament makes its insertion, it gives off accessory fibers which continue downward to the posterior border of the hyoid bone. This accessory ligament is called the *stylohyoid* ligament.

The temporomandibular ligament and the sphenomandibular ligament (the latter to a much smaller degree) apparently act as suspensory ligaments, whereas the stylomandibular ligament with its accessory stylohyoid ligament acts as a checkrein on the mandible and helps to prevent excessive anterior drift at the angle during the more extreme opening movements.

The *interarticular fibrocartilage* or *meniscus* is a tough fibrous disk placed between the condyle and its temporal bearing areas, the glenoid fossa and the articular eminence of the zygomatic process, adapting itself exactly to the two bony surfaces, making up for any discrepancy in these two surfaces and promoting smooth articulation and movement. It is attached at its periphery to the capsule, and a section of these tissues shows a superior joint compartment above the meniscus and an inferior joint compartment below (Figs. 377, 378 and 379). These are synovial cavities lined with synovial membrane and lubricated by synovial fluid. The upper compartment is the larger. However, neither compartment exhibits an actual space during life when there is normal articulation of the parts.

The foregoing is the usual description of the joint.

Robinson states it thus: "The inferior synovial cavity is the smaller of the two joint cavities, and it is here that the ginglymoid, or hinge, action takes place. In the larger upper synovial cavity, the arthrodial, or gliding action occurs. There are no true 'spaces' or 'cavities,' only potential cavities existing. All surfaces are in contact. These are lubricated by a small amount of synovial fluid.

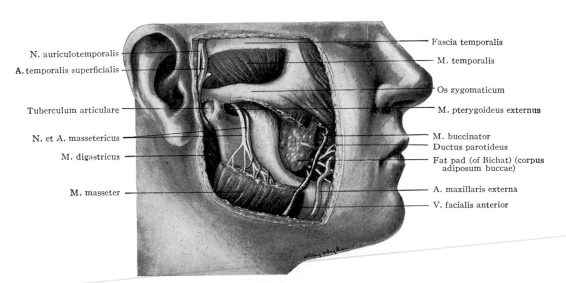

Figure 376. Deep structures of the masseter region. (Callender, Surgical Anatomy, 2nd Edition.)

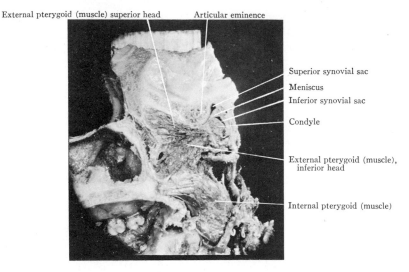

External pterygoid (muscle) superior head

Articular eminence

Superior synovial sac

Meniscus

Inferior synovial sac

Condyle

External pterygoid (muscle), inferior head

Internal pterygoid (muscle)

Figure 377. A sagittal section of a prepared anatomic specimen, sectioned through the center of the right mandibular condyle. (Courtesy of Dr. Ross Bleiker, St. Louis University.)

"The disk (meniscus) is not composed of fibrocartilage, which is known not to be repairable. It is composed of a specialized connective tissue. Fibrocartilage is characterized by oval cells with homogenous capsules arranged in groups extending lengthwise in rows. Typical fibrocartilage was not found in any of the disks examined. There are no homogenous capsules.

"A transition type between fibrocartilage and fibrous connective tissue is increasingly evident in disks of persons over twenty years of age."

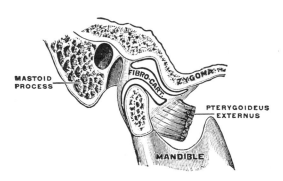

MASTOID PROCESS

FIBRO-CART.

ZYGOMA

PTERYGOIDEUS EXTERNUS

MANDIBLE

Figure 378. Temporomandibular articulation in sagittal sections. (Testut.)

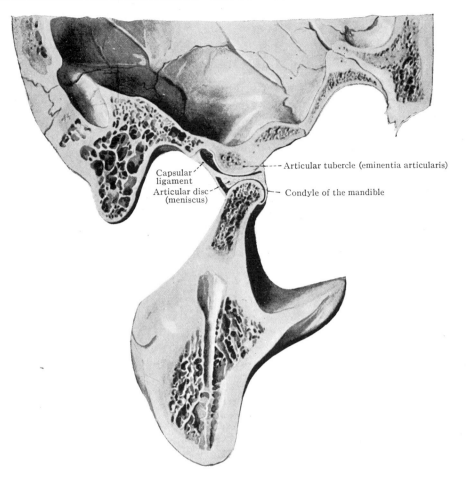

Figure 379. A cross section through the left temporomandibular joint; maximum mouth opening. (Sicher, *Oral Anatomy*, C. V. Mosby Company.)

THE MUSCLES OF MASTICATION AND FACIAL EXPRESSION

The muscles of mastication are those muscles which, through their contraction, bring about the opening and closure of the jaws. It is these muscles that apply the forces which act through the teeth of the mandibular dental arch against the teeth of the maxillary dental arch during the various movements of mastication.

The muscles of mastication comprise the following:

1. Masseter
2. Temporal
3. External pterygoid
4. Internal pterygoid

The external pterygoids aid in depressing the mandible by drawing the condyles forward so that the ramus is freed from pressures of tissues behind it and so that the hinge action in the lower joint compartment is permitted.

The suprahyoid and infrahyoid muscles, including the platysma muscle, function

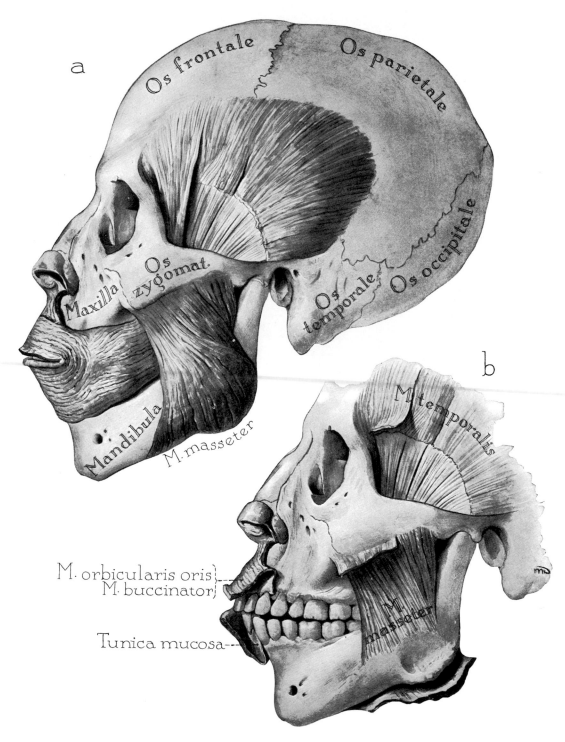

Figure 380. Muscles of mastication; lateral views. (Anson, An Atlas of Human Anatomy, 2nd Edition.)

by asserting some control over the act of mastication through their activity in applying counter forces against those greater forces which are brought to bear by the more powerful muscles of mastication. These muscles come into play during extreme depression of the mandible when the mouth is opened its widest during lateral movements of the mandible beyond the functional movements of mastication, when the mandible is attempting to close against unusual resistance, and during the act of swallowing.

Nevertheless, in the final analysis, the functional form of the teeth and their alignment in the jaws are designed to co-operate during mastication with the functional forces brought upon them by the four muscles of mastication only, in a relatively limited range of jaw movement.

For reference purposes, therefore, and to complete this text, the muscles of mastication are the only ones which will be considered, since it is not the purpose of this book to be a complete anatomic treatise on the head and neck.

The *buccinator muscle,* mentioned occasionally as a muscle of mastication, belongs to the muscles of facial expression. This muscle is located in the cheek and functions with the tongue in the placement of food between the teeth during mastication. Nevertheless, it is neither a levator nor a depressor of the mandible.

(Text continued on page 355.)

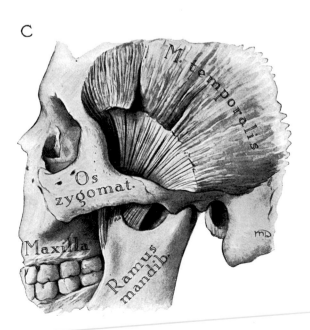

Figure 380. *Continued.*

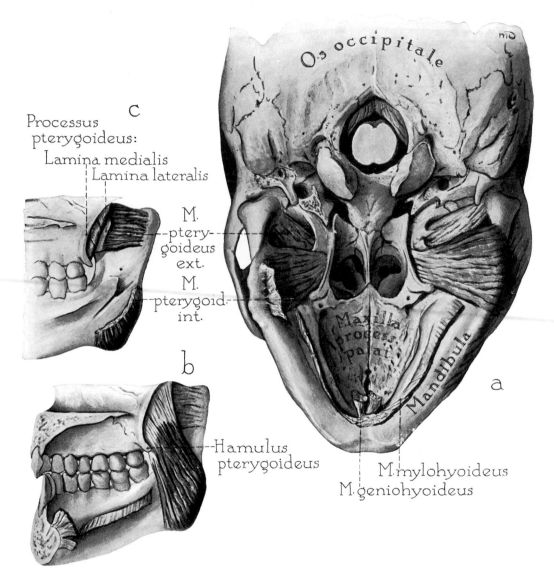

Figure 381. Muscles of mastication; pterygoid group. (Anson, An Atlas of Human Anatomy, 2nd Edition.)

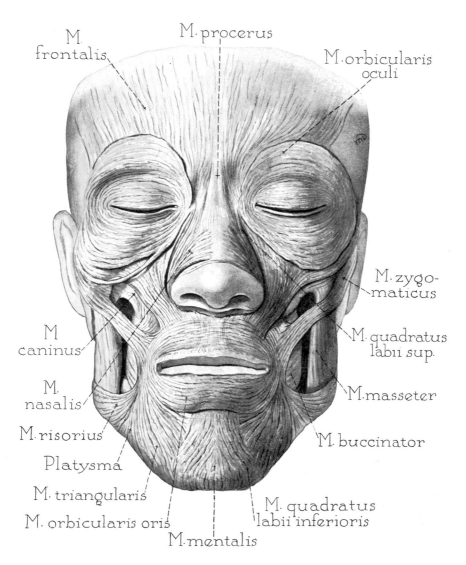

Figure 382. Muscles of facial expression; anterior view. (Anson, An Atlas of Human Anatomy, 2nd Edition.)

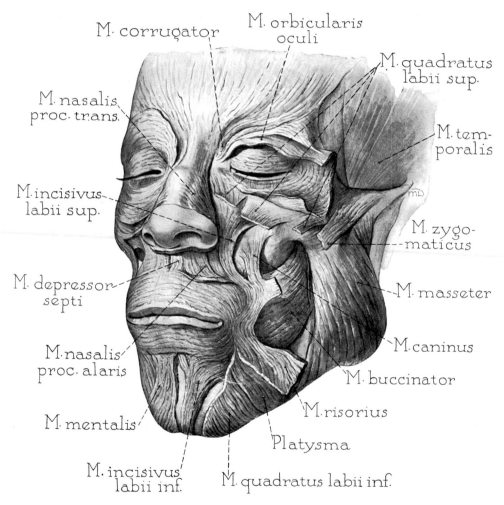

Figure 383. Muscles of facial expression; anterolateral view. (Anson, An Atlas of Human Anatomy, 2nd Edition.)

ORAL PHARYNX

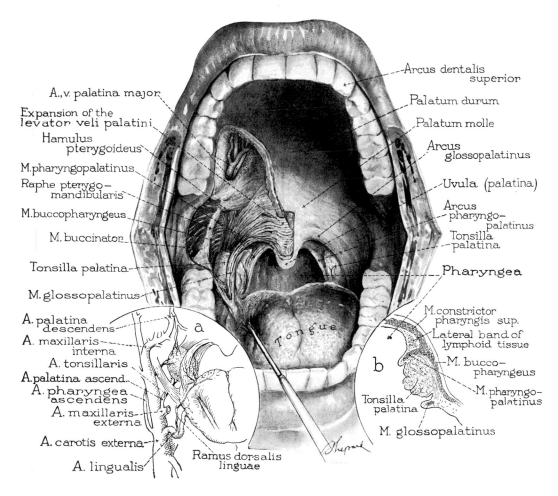

Figure 384. Oral pharynx, with special reference to the palatine tonsil and the musculature of the palate. (Anson, An Atlas of Human Anatomy, 2nd Edition.)

AN ANALYSIS OF MANDIBULAR MOVEMENTS

Anatomically or architecturally considered, the human dental mechanism consists of a fixed base, the maxillae, which bear the maxillary teeth, and a movable arm, the mandible, which bears the mandibular teeth.

The *fixed base* of the masticating mechanism, the maxillae, are supported through articulations with other bones of the skull. The maxillae are united at the median line.

The *movable arm,* or mandible, is a single bone. The teeth in the mandible are so placed that they oppose those of the fixed base when they are brought into contact during the various mandibular movements of mastication.

The teeth serve as the armament of the masticating apparatus, affording hard surfaces between which food material is reduced for assimilation by the organism. The relation of the mandibular portion of the dental apparatus to the maxillary or fixed portion is maintained by ligamentous attachments and the powerful muscles of mastication.

As mentioned heretofore, the mandible is freely moveable, the temporomandibular joint being the most flexible joint in the body. Because of its mobility, the various movements are difficult to describe. The attempt will be made to classify and explain the most obvious movements which are most important in the study of the function and occlusion of the teeth.

The mandibular movements may be classified under two headings: (1) those which are *bilaterally symmetrical* and (2) those which are *bilaterally asymmetrical*.
Those movements which are bilaterally *symmetrical* are:

Depression	Protrusion
Elevation	Retraction

The movements which are bilaterally *asymmetrical* are:

$$\text{Lateral movements} \begin{cases} \text{right} \\ \text{left} \end{cases}$$

It is the purpose in this section of the book to make an analysis of the dynamics of occlusion and occlusal relations with mandibular movements which have a bearing on the physiologic form of the teeth, their alignment and their occlusion. The mandible is capable of movements which are not related to tooth function: wide opening, excessive protrusion, etc. Repeating some lines of the functional anatomy of the teeth in Chapter IV: The anatomy is such that teeth are enabled to perform two major functions during life: they incise and reduce food material during mastication, and they help sustain themselves in the dental arches by assisting in the development and the protection of the tissues which support them. Protection of the investing tissues and stabilization of the alignment of the teeth are provided by the normal form of the individual teeth in proper alignment with the others in the same jaw, by *normal development* of the jaws, and by the *proper relation of one jaw to the other during functional movements.*

When the mandibular teeth come into contact with the maxillary teeth, they are said to be in *occlusion.* Occlusion might be defined as "the relation of the mandibular teeth to the maxillary teeth when in functional contact during the activity of the mandible."

The dental arches have several *functional relations* which are brought about by mandibular movements. They are as follows:

Centric occlusal relation (centric occlusion)
Protrusive occlusal relation
Retrusive occlusal relation
Right lateral occlusal relation
Left lateral occlusal relation

Centric occlusal relation of the dental arches (centric occlusion, central occlusion), is the concluding terminal relation of the teeth. It is the final culmination of all of the other occlusal relations. The entire dental mechanism is designed to co-operate with the design of, and to achieve finally, centric occlusion as the ultimate goal in function.

In normal centric occlusion there is an intercusping contact relation between all of the posterior teeth of both dental arches on both right and left sides. At the same time all of the anterior teeth of one arch are in contact with those of the other arch. In centric occlusion, lines of force brought to bear upon the fixed base or maxillary arch by the movable or mandibular arch are equalized and absorbed by the mutual aid of all of the teeth.

Protrusive occlusal relation is achieved by means of protrusion of the mandible. Such movement places the mandibular teeth in an anterior relation to centric occlusion. *Retrusive occlusal relation* is brought about by retrusion of the mandible. The mandibular teeth are placed by retrusion in a posterior relation to centric occlusion. Retrusion is limited by the compressibility of the tissues posterior to the condyle heads; therefore the movement is so limited it can be said to be non-functional.

Right lateral and left lateral occlusal relations are achieved by right lateral and left lateral movements of the mandible. The mandibular dental arch, through these movements, is placed in a right or a left lateral relation to centric occlusion.

Centric, protrusive and retrusive relations of the dental arches may be achieved by mandibular movements which are *symmetrical*—in short, those movements in which both condyles of the mandible make equidistant excursions in sagittal planes of the body. The symphysis of the mandible also moves in a sagittal plane. Right lateral and left lateral relations are achieved by a circular movement to right or left by one condyle of the mandible while the other condyle pivots. These movements are *asymmetrical.*

As was mentioned before, the temporomandibular articulation allows a great range of movement. The mandible is made capable of the central opening movement (so called "hinge" movement, which is an inaccurate term); the joint allows extension of the mandible forward, which movement is called "protrusion"; the mandible may be retracted to some extent in the retrusive movement and it may be rotated from side to side in the right and left lateral movements.

All of the mandibular movements have individual limitations, depending upon the ligamentous attachments and upon the functional range of the muscles of mastication, the origin and insertion of the muscles, their length, directional pull, tonus (counter tension), etc.

Quoting from Thompson and Brodie:* "It was thoroughly established by Sherrington that the same motor impulse that caused one set of muscles to contract caused an inhibition of tonus in their antagonists. Thus, the rest position of any movable part may be taken as an equilibrium between all of the forces operating upon it. If these forces happen to be entirely muscular, there is an equal pull on both sides of the part through a state of tonus. Thus, even a rest position must be viewed as a dynamic condition. Steindler points out that for every movement of the body there is a definite amount of inertia to be overcome, a definite amount of balance to be disturbed. Let us now imagine the head being held normally and motionless in the position of erect posture. Such a position is maintained by the antagonistic pull of the muscles of the back of the neck on the one hand, and the force of gravity plus the three enumerated sets working together on the other hand (muscles of mastication, suprahyoids and infrahyoids). Suppose we disturb this balance by swallowing. In deglutition, it is necessary to elevate the hyoid bone, which means the contracting of the suprahyoid muscles. If this group is contracted, it would have just as strong a tendency to depress the mandible as to elevate the hyoid. It seems obvious, therefore, that additional tension must be generated in the masticatory group to prevent the downward displacement of the mandible. The fact that this is true can be easily demonstrated by placing the fingers lightly on the temples and swallowing. At the instant of elevation of the hyoid, a pulse of contraction will be felt in the temporalis.

"A similar phenomenon may be demonstrated in mastication. In spite of the rather extensive and violent movements of the mandible, the hyoid bone is relatively stable. Indeed, it is only in wide opening movements that the hyoid bone shifts to any extent, and even this shift is unexpected. The excellent fluoroscopic moving picture, 'Physiology of Mastication,' by Klatsky, shows these points.

"Thus it is seen that the muscles lying anteriorly from the vertebral column, *i.e.,* the masticatory, suprahyoid and infrahyoid groups, have, as their roles, not only their own specific functions, but also a team play behind these which helps to maintain the posture of the head. This coordination permits of mastication, deglutition and speech without any accompanying nodding of the head.

"We have been thinking of the mandible too much as a bone concerned with a single function, rather than as a connecting link in the anterior muscle chain. The muscle tension acting on the mandible is balanced; that is, there is just as much downward pull as there is upward pull on this bone."

FUNCTIONAL MANDIBULAR MOVEMENTS

(A Description of the Association of the Activity of the Temporomandibular Articulation with the Functional Activity of the Muscles of Mastication and the Ligamentous Attachments)

When the mandible is at rest, the mandibular teeth are not in contact with the maxillary teeth. Thompson estimates an opening of 2 mm. on the average. This relation is born out by Higley, Kurth and other investigators. The relation is called the *physiologic rest position* of the mandible.

When the teeth are together in centric relation that relation is called the *physical rest position* of the mandible.

---

*Thompson, J. R., and Brodie, A. G.: Factors in the Position of the Mandible. J. Am. Dent. A. *29*:925, 1942.

All mandibular movements start with the physiologic rest position with the teeth disengaged. When the mandible is depressed, each condyle moves forward on the disk, the disk or meniscus moving with it. Since the condyles move during all manipulations, the points of rotation on the mandible are never within the condyle heads, which arrangement might be expected from the study of some other diarthrodial joints. The mandible is a single bone with bilateral joints which have to be independent of one another at times in order to allow the flexibility that is necessary for proper functional movements.

The mandible used to be regarded in function as a lever of the third class (Fig. 385). The *fulcrum* of the mandible shifts its location, however, during functional activity because of the flexibility of the bilateral joints and the independent action of all the muscles involved. The position of the fulcrum is dependent entirely on the location of the *work,* anteriorly, posteriorly or laterally.

If the mandible were regarded as a simple lever of the third class, the condyles in the glenoid fossa would have to be regarded as the fulcrum, with the muscles providing the power for force at a point between the fulcrum and the work. The work is placed at some point on the teeth over the body of the mandible.

In a lever of the third class the fulcrum absorbs a large portion of the force, depending upon (1) the location of the force between the fulcrum and the work, (2) the amount of force generated and (3) the weight or resistance of the work.

Examination of the parts of the temporomandibular joint demonstrates the fact that the area of the glenoid fossa of the temporal bone, which is situated just above the condyle of the mandible, is quite thin. This area is not designed to support the condyle as a fulcrum of a lever of the third class. In fact, any attempt to describe the activity of the mandible as a lever of any one class is oversimplification of jaw movements.

It must be remembered that the mandible is suspended by soft tissues (ligaments and muscles). The ligamentous attachments are not fixed points mechanically; in other words, the individual muscles may contract or relax independently of one another, changing the points of rotation of the mandible within certain limitation.

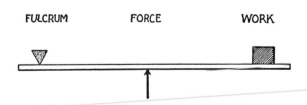

Figure 385.   An illustration of the principle of a lever of the third class.

The mandible has a "bow" form, one bone with two condyloid joints, which permits the "points of rotation," "power arms," "fulcra" or "location of the work" to be shifted from one position to another in a most flexible manner. The two temporomandibular joints may have similar movements simultaneously, as in the central opening movements, or they may work independently of each other, as in lateral movements; and each masticatory muscle of either right or left side may contract or relax independently. In addition, the point or points of rotation of the mandible change their locations according to the extent of opening and position of the jaw during depression, protrusion or right and left lateral relations. Because of the flexibility, it may be more correct to speak of rotation "areas" of the mandible rather than rotation "points," since it is impossible to locate definite points of rotation as final as in a strictly mechanical problem.

In the instances just described, the mandible approaches the second class lever in function. The components of the lever are as follows: the *fulcrum*—muscles of the left side, near the left molars; the *work*—molars and premolars of the right side; the *force*—muscles of the right side buccal to the right posterior teeth. The work is not precisely located between the fulcrum and the force, as is true in a second class lever, but the example of activity as outlined more nearly approaches a second class lever in function than it does the third class lever.

The point or points of rotation of the mandible also change their locations—a fact dependent upon the relation of the mandibular dental arch to the maxillary dental arch during depression, protrusion or right and left lateral relations, and upon the extent of depression of the symphysis of the mandible (point of chin).

Depression of the Mandible

During simple depression of the mandible (central opening movement) from its rest position, both condyles move forward, the menisci moving with them. It is generally agreed by many authorities (Prentiss, Lord, Chissin, Brodie, Higley, Stimson, Sicher and others) that both condyle heads are pulled forward in this initial opening movement by the external pterygoid muscles.

While the condyle is being pulled forward in opening the jaw by the inferior head of the external pterygoid, the meniscus is being pulled forward by the superior head of the external pterygoid muscle. When the condyle approaches the articular eminence it rides forward on the thinner portion of the meniscus—an arrangement which makes allowances for the downward protuberance of the eminence.

When in "rest position," each condyle rests upon a thick posterior portion of the meniscus which fills the space between the condyle and the deeper portion of the glenoid fossa. Anteriorly, the meniscus is much thinner at the portion which approximates the dorsal area of the articular eminence and the frontal area of the condyle (Figs. 377 and 379).

The relative thickness of the meniscus anteroposteriorly, plus the compensating activity of the two heads of the external pterygoid muscle, allows the condyles of the mandible to move forward with a gliding movement on a "single plane" regardless of the irregularity of the surface of the glenoid fossa and of that of the articular eminence. The "plane" has an inclination downward when the head is held erect. It is interesting to note that the inclined plane of the condylar glide when the mandible is depressed is seemingly parallel to the occlusal plane of the molars and the lower border of the body of the mandible when the jaws are closed.

During the central opening movement of the mandible, the axis of movement is not in the condyle heads, since these move forward immediately, even though the initial movement forward is slight. Apparently the area of rotation approaches the attachment of the temporomandibular ligament laterally and distally to the neck of the condyle. This is a logical conclusion because of the suspensory character of this strong ligament and the general direction of its fibers (Figs. 374 and 375).

The central opening movement of the mandible (depression) in conjunction with the central closing movement (elevation) provides the action commonly termed "simple hinge movement." As far as the relation of the dental arches is concerned in this opening and closing movement, the action is comparable to the action of a simple hinge. The occlusal surfaces of the maxillary teeth may be considered as the upper extension of the hinge, and the occlusal surfaces of the mandibular teeth as the lower extension in the central opening movement. However, owing to the involved design of the articulation and the support of the jaw, the rotation point or axis of the hinge is not in the condyle but below it (Fig. 374), somewhere within the area of attachment of the temporomandibular ligament in the neck of the condyle.

The truth is, however, that when the jaw is opened no more than necessary for ordinary use in mastication (10 to 12 mm. maximum), the action of placing the teeth

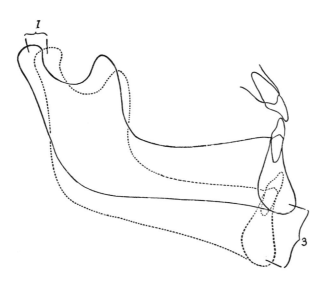

Figure 386. Outline tracings of mandible and central incisors in centric occlusal relation. The broken outline represents the relative position of the mandible and central incisor after the central opening movement. Note the relative position of the condyle and the central incisor. The condyle moves forward and downward approximately one-third the distance the symphysis of the mandible (point of chin) moves downward and backward. The position of the depressed mandible shows the approximate relation when the mandible has reached the lowest point during ordinary masticatory movement. The mandible is capable of depression much greater when the occasion makes it necessary. (Refer to Fig. 379.)

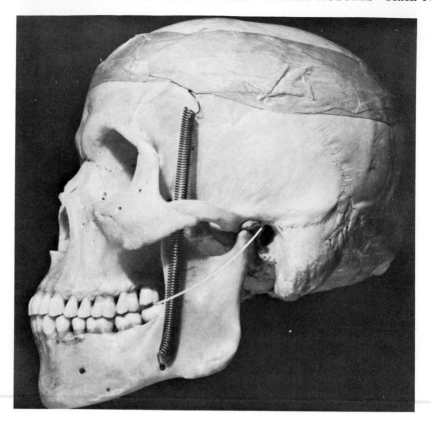

Figure 387. A curved line representing an extension of the curvature of the occlusal plane will pass laterally and slightly below the neck of the condyle. See Fig. 349. This is the area of the attachment of the temporomandibular ligament. The "point" of rotation, or "hinge axis," will be located somewhere in this area in the initial central opening movement of the mandible.

of one arch in and out of contact with the teeth of the opposing arch in a sagittal plane may be called a hinge movement, regardless of our inability to pinpoint the "hinge axis."

In the study of the individual masticatory movements to follow, make continuous reference to the illustrations of the muscles of mastication in Figures 380 and 381.

Elevation of the Mandible

The mandible is elevated by the temporal muscles, the masseter muscles and the internal pterygoid muscles.

The *temporal muscle* has anterior and posterior fibers. The anterior fibers exert an upward pull; the posterior fibers pull upward and backward.

The *masseter muscle* has two sets of fibers: superficial and deep fibers. The superficial fibers exert a pull upward and forward on the mandible. The deep fibers exert a pull vertically upward.

The *internal pterygoid muscle* has two heads, each of which pulls in the same general direction. Together they exert a pull on the mandible which is upward, forward and inward.

When the temporal, masseter and internal pterygoid muscles of the two sides contract simultaneously, the mandible is elevated and returns the teeth to occlusion.

When the teeth are brought into centric occlusion, both condyles of the mandible are moved a short distance posteriorly to their rest position.

Protrusion of the Mandible

The mandible cannot be protruded unless the cusps of the teeth are disengaged. Therefore, the mandible must be depressed slightly, the condyles moving forward before the protrusive movement is begun.

The muscles which promulgate the protrusive movement which brings about the protrusive occlusal relation of the teeth are the *external pterygoid* muscles, which are assisted by the *anterior fibers* of the *temporal muscles*. The pterygoids pull forward on the condyles and the temporals pull upward with a counter action on the coronoid processes; this prevents further depression of the mandible during the protrusive movement. The tonus and counterbalancing action of other fibers of the temporals as well as some other muscles may come into play during the protrusive movement.

During this movement the condlyes are pulled forward with their menisci, but their forward movement is quite limited (Fig. 449, Chapter XVI).

Retraction of the Mandible

In retraction, the mandible returns along the same path it traveled in the protrusive movement. The retractive movement is, therefore, just the reverse of the protrusive movement.

The jaw is pulled back by the action of the *temporal* muscle, the posterior fibers principally. The condyles with their menisci are returned to rest position.

If it is the purpose of this movement to bring the teeth back into centric occlusion, the *masseter* and *internal pterygoid* muscles join the activity of the temporals in the final culmination of the act.

The mandible may be retracted a very small degree posteriorly to centric occlusal relation of the teeth. This movement is nonfunctional and consequently very limited. Movement of the condyles distally is resisted by the posterior wall of the glenoid cavity; the movement is limited to the compressibility of the soft tissues intervening between the bony parts.

Lateral Movements of the Mandible

The lateral movements (right and left) of the mandible are *asymmetrical* movements; the right and left condyles do not follow similar paths. These movements are made possible by the ability of one temporomandibular joint to move independently of the other.

Each *internal pterygoid* muscle exerts a medial pull on the mandible, since it does not operate on a line with the forward or protrusive movement of the jaw. Its action pulls the condyle inward as well as forward.

The right lateral movement of the mandible is affected, therefore, by a slight depressive movement of the mandible, both external pterygoids operating, which action depresses the mandible and moves both condyles forward. At this point the left *internal* pterygoid contracts independently, the right internal pterygoid and other muscles relaxing. The activity of the left internal pterygoid pulls the left condyle forward and inward in a circular path which rotates about a point in the right condyle, the right condyle turning on the pivotal point. This action results in the rotation of the mandible about the pivotal point in the right condyle, moving the mandible to the right.

In the return movement, the condyles retrace their path. The mandible is returned to rest position, or the teeth into centric occlusion, through the activity of the left temporal muscle (mainly posterior fibers), other muscles of mastication of both sides joining forces as the teeth approach central occlusion with a final masticatory thrust.

The left lateral movement of the mandible is affected in the same manner. In this instance the right condyle is pulled forward and inward while the left condyle pivots. The right internal pterygoid muscle contracts and causes the movement of the mandible to the left. The right temporal is the muscle mainly operative which affects the return of the mandible to centric relation with the assistance of the other muscles in balance with it.

Chapter **XVI**

THE ARRANGEMENT OF
THE TEETH AND OCCLUSION

THE TEETH are arranged in two opposing series; one is fixed (maxillary series), and the other is movable (mandibular series). Each series is made up of sixteen teeth arranged so that they form a dental arch. Generally speaking, each dental arch conforms to a parabolic curve (Figs. 388, 389, 390, 391 and Fig. 1, Chapter I).

The mandibular arch, which is movable, operates against the maxillary arch, which is fixed. This obvious fact is sometimes overlooked. The reason for the oversight is this: Dental articulators used in dental prosthesis have the maxillary member movable, with the mandibular member fixed, just the opposite arrangement from that found in the human jaws. Mechanically, the dental articulator design simplifies the instrument for practical use in the laboratory. Nevertheless it influences the operator's thinking, without a doubt, unless he is careful to keep reminding himself of the true state of affairs. It is important in the study of occlusion that the student remember that the primary forces of occlusion are brought to bear against the *static* maxillary arch by the *dynamic* mandibular arch.

Normal tooth form (plus proper alignment) assures efficiency in the comminution of food. The form of each tooth in each dental arch must be recognized as an integral part in the total design of the arches. The form of each of the sixteen teeth, in addition to the proper position and angulation of each tooth, influences the function of each arch. If the dental arch is properly designed, through normal development and positioning of all its parts, the dental arch itself becomes an efficient unit for service. *Stability and efficiency will be assured as long as the normal arrangement is maintained.*

(Text continued on page 369.)

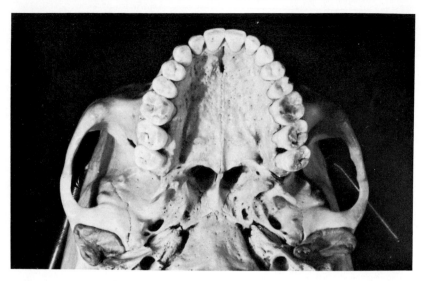

Figure 388. An occlusal view of maxillary teeth (same specimen as Figs. 389, 390 and 391). This specimen shows considerable wear of the occlusal surfaces. It demonstrates the surfaces of the maxillary teeth which are in contact during occlusal relations by the areas showing abraded facets.

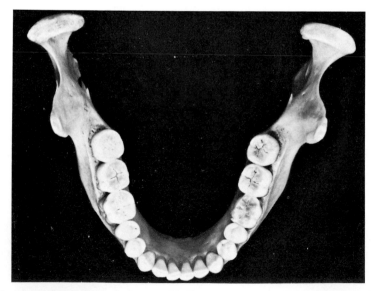

Figure 389. An occlusal view of the mandibular teeth. The facets of occlusal wear appear on the labioincisal portions of anterior teeth and the occlusal and bucco-occlusal surfaces of posterior teeth.

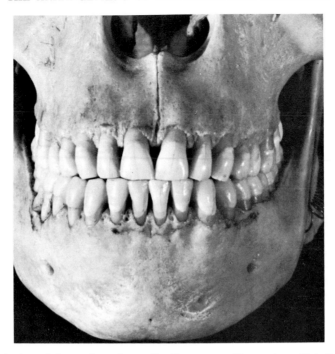

Figure 390.   A view of the teeth at the median line, or maxillary suture. Note the acute angulations of the anterior teeth to the suture. This specimen shows considerable occlusal wear, balanced occlusion and a minimum of "overbite" of the maxillary anterior teeth.

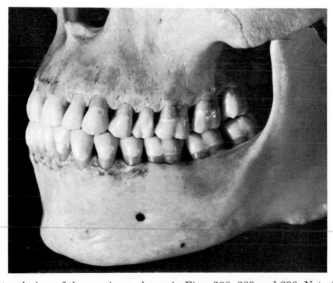

Figure 391.   Lateral view of the specimen shown in Figs. 388, 389 and 390. Note the curve of Spee.

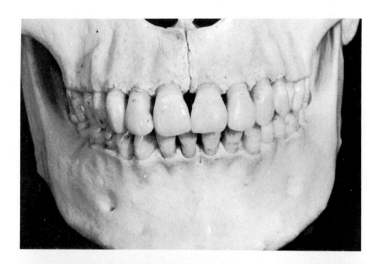

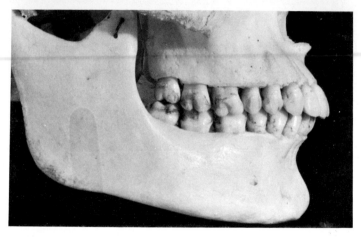

Figure 392. An illustration of normal occlusion—anterior and lateral views. This specimen demonstrates a different type of tooth and a different type of occlusion than the specimen shown in Fig. 390. These teeth show little occlusal wear and considerable "overjet"* and "overbite"† to anterior and posterior teeth. Note the extreme angulation of anterior teeth from the lateral view; this angulation is characteristic when overbite and overjet are greater than usual.

Overjet is that characteristic of the teeth in which the incisal ridges or buccal cusp ridges of the maxillary teeth extend labially or buccally to the incisal ridges or buccal cusp ridges of the mandibular teeth, when the teeth are in centric occlusal relation.

†*Overbite* is that characteristic of the teeth in which the incisal ridges of the maxillary anterior teeth extend below the incisal ridges of the mandibular anterior teeth when the teeth are placed in centric occlusal relation.

We speak of the relative degree of overbite or overjet.

Naturally, stability of the dental arches requires a healthy state of the supporting tissues in addition to normal development of the parts. If the development of the teeth and jaws has been abnormal, the result is a poorly formed apparatus capable only of *malocclusion*. Since it is not the purpose of the author to consider the pathologic; normal development, normal tissues and normal occlusion are to be taken for granted in subsequent description.

Jaw relations during function affect the directions of force which are brought to bear upon the teeth, and normal jaw relations apply the force equally in directions which the teeth in normal alignment are designed to withstand. If each tooth retains its position and remains stable, the stability and permanence of each dental arch as a functioning unit remains assured.

Definition: When the teeth in the mandibular arch come into contact with the teeth of the maxillary arch in any functional relation during the various mandibular movements, "occlusion" is accomplished.

Items for Consideration

The study of occlusion must include the following items for consideration (Fig. 393):

1. Dental arch formation (alignment of the teeth).
2. Compensating curvatures of the dental arches (curved occlusal planes).
3. Compensating curvatures of the individual teeth (curved axes).
4. Angulation of individual teeth in relation to various planes.
5. Functional form of the teeth at their incisal and occlusal thirds.
6. Facial relations of each tooth in one arch to its antagonist or antagonists in the opposing arch in centric occlusion.
7. Occlusal contact and intercusp relations of all the teeth of one arch with those in the opposing arch in centric occlusion.
8. Occlusal contact and intercusp relations of all the teeth during the various functional mandibular movements.

(Text continued on page 372.)

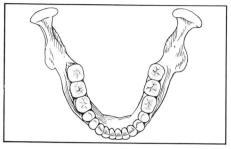

1. Dental arch formation (alignment of the teeth).

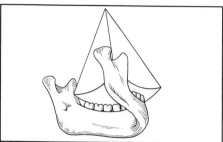

2. Compensating curvatures of the dental arches (curved occlusal planes).

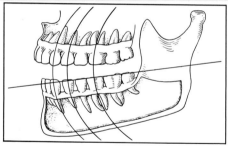

3. Compensating curvatures of the individual teeth (curved axes).

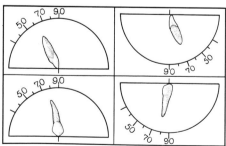

4. Angulation of individual teeth in relation to various planes.

Figure 393

5. Functional form of the teeth at their incisal and occlusal thirds.

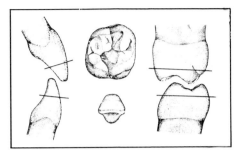

6. Facial relations of each tooth in one arch to its antagonist or antagonists in the opposing arch in centric occlusion.

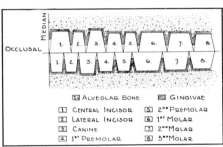

7. Occlusal contact and intercusp relations of all the teeth of one arch with those in the opposing arch in centric occlusion.

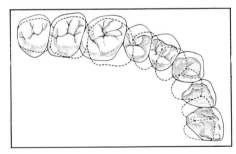

8. Occlusal contact and intercusp relations of all the teeth during the various functional mandibular movements. "Balance" in lateral occlusal relations.

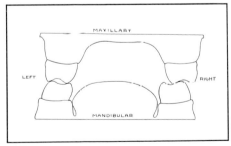

Figure 393 *(Continued).*

1. DENTAL ARCH FORMATION (ALIGNMENT OF THE TEETH)

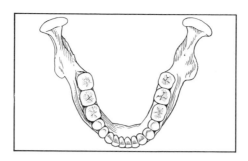

From the occlusal aspect, the outlines following the labial and buccal surfaces of the dental arches conform generally to parabolic curves (Figs. 388 and 389). The outline of the maxillary arch is somewhat larger than that of the mandibular arch. When the teeth are in centric occlusion, the maxillary arch "overhangs" labially and buccally; this arrangement is called the *overjet* of the maxillary teeth. The difference in size allows extensions in the direction of mandibular movements (Fig. 394).

This arch relation has another useful feature: during opening and closing movements of the jaws, the cheeks, lips and tongue are less likely to be clipped. Since the bucco-occlusal margins of the maxillary teeth extend beyond the bucco-occlusal margins of the mandibular teeth, and since the linguo-occlusal margins of the mandibular teeth extend lingually beyond the linguo-occlusal margins of the maxillary teeth, the soft tissues are displaced during the act of closure until the teeth have had an opportunity to come together in occlusal contact. The overjet relation facially and lingually of one dental arch to the other resembles the relation of the

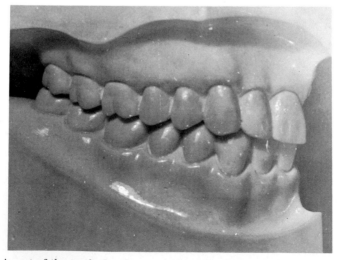

Figure 394. A cast of the teeth showing normal overjet of the maxillary arch. The lighting for the photograph was arranged for emphasis. (This is a duplicate of the cast shown in Fig. 85, Chapter IV.)

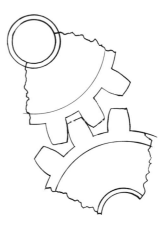

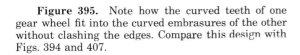

Figure 395. Note how the curved teeth of one gear wheel fit into the curved embrasures of the other without clashing the edges. Compare this design with Figs. 394 and 407.

teeth of gear wheels opposing each other. The design avoids the clashing of points and edges during contact (Fig. 395).

The teeth of each arch are arranged in an unbroken series of occlusal surfaces, each tooth being in close contact with neighboring teeth. The last molar in either arch is in contact only with the tooth mesial to it. Each of the other teeth has adjoining members in contact both mesially and distally.

The contact relation between teeth in the same arch serves two purposes: (1) it helps to protect the gingival papillae between the teeth, and (2) the collective activity of all of the teeth in contact with each other stabilizes the dental arch by helping to prevent tooth migration. (See Chapter V.)

The teeth are divided into four classifications anatomically, and they function in accordance with those classifications. The four classifications are: (1) incisors, (2) canines, (3) premolars and (4) molars.

The *incisors* are designed with broad incisal ridges, which function as shears or blades when they come in contact with opposing incisors.

The *canines* have single cusps, more or less pointed, with sloping cusp ridges. These teeth serve by piercing and holding food material, in addition to using an incising action similar to that of the incisors. The canines, by means of their structure and their excellent root anchorage, support the incisors during the stresses of incision or prehension of food which might be resistant in character.

The *premolars* have from one to three functioning cusps, and they are intermediate between canines and molars. The first premolars particularly, both maxillary and mandibular, have cusps which are long and sharp. They assist the canines in their function. The second premolars have cusps which correspond in form with those of the molars; therefore they may be considered as complementary in function to the molars. The premolars, by their intercusping relation, present more blades for the comminution of food than the incisors or canines.

The *molars* are multicusped teeth, with broad occlusal surfaces. They are the most efficient of all the teeth in chopping and reducing food material to proper consistency for assimilation. Each molar has several points or areas of occlusal contact during mastication. The molars collectively show more points of occlusal contact in centric occlusion than all of the other teeth combined (Fig. 415). Premature loss of molars presents the individual with a severe handicap in occlusal relations.

The *alignment* of the incisors, canines and first premolars, of either dental arch, is such that the labial and buccal surfaces conform generally to half of an imperfect circle. The second premolars and the mesiobuccal portion of the first molars follow straight continuations of the arc terminals in a distobuccal direction. The distobuccal portion of the first molars and the buccal surfaces of the second and third molars follow a line which is more nearly parallel to the median plane (Fig. 396).

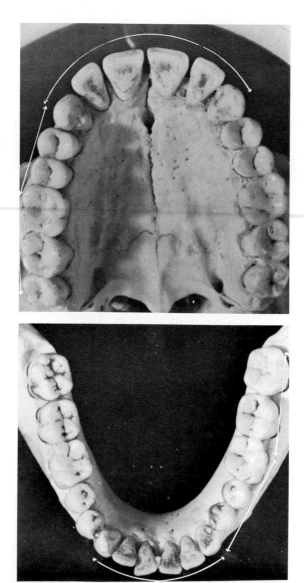

Figure 396. A photograph of the dental arches of a natural specimen. The white lines show the approximate alignment in segments of the labial and buccal surfaces of the dental arches.

The tooth alignment in the arches is divided into *three segments:* an anterior segment, a middle segment and a posterior segment. Actually, since the teeth are in close contact relation, there is an overlapping of the teeth of one segment with those of the next. The anterior segment includes the anterior teeth; the middle segment includes the first premolars, second premolars and mesial half of the first molar; the posterior segment includes the first, second and third molars.

The outline of the buccal surfaces of maxillary molars curves inward more sharply toward the median plane than do the mandibular molar buccal outlines. This alignment is caused partly by the fact that second and third molars are set somewhat lingual to first molars, and partly by the fact that buccal surfaces of maxillary molars show greater convergence distally, which convergence lessens their buccolingual measurements distally.

The arrangement and design of the *maxillary* molars allow sufficient room for the contraction of the powerful masseter muscles without interference.

The *mandibular* arch on first sight does not seem to conform to the same parabolic curvature as the maxillary arch. On close inspection, however, it may be seen that the difference in curvature is a matter of degree, the fundamental design of the arch outline remaining the same. The mandibular molars do not converge as much as the maxillary molars do, and the mandibular molars are set more nearly in a straight line, although the alignment is in a distobuccal direction. (See Chapter V, "Proximal Contact Areas.")

There are five phases of development during the process of alignment of the permanent teeth into dental arches.

First Phase

The first molars (cornerstones) take their place immediately posterior to second deciduous molars. This adds considerably to the chewing efficiency at a period of rapid development.

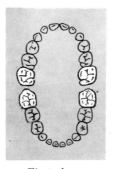

First phase

Second Phase

The placing of teeth is begun at the median line. Central incisors and then lateral incisors take arbitrary positions anteriorly near the median line. The permanent location of any of these teeth cannot be established until the final phases of development are complete.

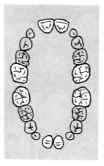

Second phase

Third Phase

The premolars come in anterior to the first molars, taking the place of deciduous molars. The individual has been able to acquire added chewing efficiency and jaw support during another period of rapid development.

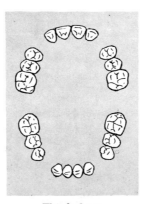

Third phase

Fourth Phase

The smooth, wedge-shaped canines (keystones), force themselves between the lateral incisors and first premolars, closing the spaces so that a dental arch is completed from the first molar forward. Simultaneously the second molar emerges distal to the first molar, backing it up so that the teeth anterior to it will not drift posteriorly during the wedging activity of the canines.

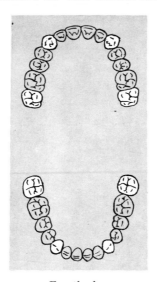

Fourth phase

Fifth Phase

As the individual approaches maturity, the jaws should develop sufficiently to accommodate third molars distal to second molars.

The late development of third molars will not permit them to take their places for several years after the eruption of second molars and canines.

Many anatomists are of the opinion that third molars may be superfluous and that the dental arches are physiologically complete without them.

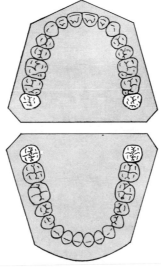

Fifth phase

2. COMPENSATING CURVATURES OF THE DENTAL ARCHES (CURVED OCCLUSAL PLANES)

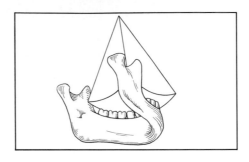

The occlusal surfaces of the dental arches do not conform to a flat plane. The mandibular arch conforms generally to a curved plane which appears concave, and the maxillary arch, to a curved plane which appears convex. When the two arches are brought together in centric occlusion, these curved planes become identical.

Because the mandible is a single bow-formed bone with two joints moving independently of one another, and because the shifting of points of rotation is quite complicated during jaw movement, the adaptation of flat planes in opposing dental arches is out of the question.

In order to achieve balance by simultaneous contact in more than one area of dental arches during mastication, only curved planes will adapt themselves.

The movement of the mandible to the right or left during mastication is called the Bennett movement. Although Bennett of England was not the first to describe the movement, his work on the activity of the condyles established the term.

Bonwill was the first to describe the mandible and mandibular arch as adapting itself in part to an equilateral triangle (Fig. 397). The angles of the triangle are placed at the centers of each condyle and at the mesial contact areas of mandibular central incisors. Bonwill was of the impression that most mandibles would conform to a 4-inch equilateral triangle. Today, anatomists realize that such measurements cannot be established arbitrarily because of variables which are always likely to be present.

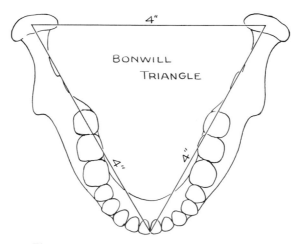

Figure 397.   The Bonwill equilateral triangle.

Nevertheless, Bonwill's theory is essentially true, and although 4 inches exactly may not be accepted as the measurement, more mandibles and mandibular arches conform to an approximation of a 4-inch equilateral triangle than to any other approximation.

Later, Von Spee noted that the cusp and incisal ridges of the teeth tended to follow a curved line when the arches were observed from a point opposite the first molars. This alignment is spoken of still as the "curve of Spee" (Fig. 90, Chapter IV). This curvature is within the sagittal planes only.

Monson, at a later date, connected the curve of Spee, or curvature in sagittal planes, with related compensating curvatures in vertical planes. Following up Bonwill's theorem, Monson originally described the normally developed mandibular arch as adapting its occlusal surfaces to the curved surface of a segment of a sphere of a 4-inch radius. Although later developments have refuted the arbitrary 4-inch measurement, the fact remains that the occlusal surfaces of mandibular teeth do conform in a general way to a curved plane which may be represented by the curved outer surface of a segment of a sphere. The radius of the segment varies considerably in different individuals. It may be less than 3 inches or more than 4 inches. Nevertheless, it is true that there is a compensating curvature of the occlusal surfaces of the teeth—a curvature which involves more than one plane (Fig. 91, Chapter IV, and Figs. 398 and 399).

The occlusal surfaces of the teeth do not conform to any one curved plane exactly. *Nothing anatomic may be reduced to the mathematical exactitude of geometrical terms.* Originally the curve of Spee was associated with the curvature followed by the cusps of maxillary teeth.

The mandibular teeth are the ones which establish the compensating occlusal curvature. The maxillary teeth adapt their occlusal surfaces to the mandibular teeth and their arrangement through forces brought to bear on them by jaw movement.

It is possible to adapt a template, or gauge, representing a segment of a sphere to the main "working" occlusal surfaces of the mandibular teeth to a close approxima-

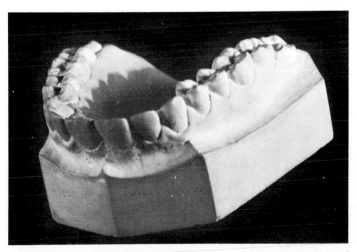

Figure 398. An accurate cast of maxillary teeth demonstrating compensating occlusal curvature.

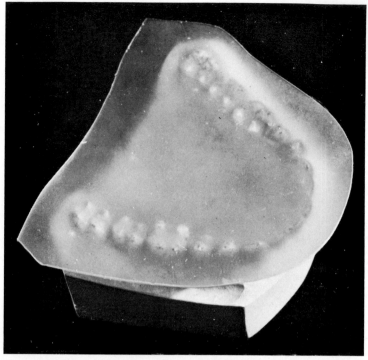

Figure 399. A curved sheet of wax adapted to buccal cusps and incisal surfaces of an accurate cast of mandibular teeth (same subject as Fig. 375). This shows the tendency of the occlusal surfaces of the mandibular arch to adapt themselves to a curved plane. See also Fig. 393, part 2.

tion (Fig. 399). These surfaces are the *buccal cusps* of the *posterior teeth,* the *cusps* of the *canines* and the *incisal ridges* of *incisors.* The lingual cusps of the mandibular posterior teeth do not touch the curved plane as a rule, although in some instances they may do so.

The template representing the curved plane adaptable to the mandibular arch cannot be adapted to the occlusal surfaces of the opposing arch, because the tips of cusps and the incisal ridges of maxillary teeth are not in the compensating occlusal plane representing centric relation, and those surfaces would prevent the template from attaining its proper level. This level would be somewhere on the lingual surfaces of maxillary anterior teeth and between the cusps of posterior teeth, within the sulci at marginal ridge levels posteriorly, where the contacting surfaces of mandibular teeth rest or glide during various occlusal relations.

Some of the occlusal surfaces of the mandibular teeth occlude with certain surfaces of the maxillary teeth when they make contact in centric occlusion. These "working surfaces" are called *morsal surfaces.* The buccal cusps of the mandibular posterior teeth fit into central sulci of maxillary posterior teeth, which sulci lie directly between the buccal and lingual cusps. The incisal ridges of mandibular canines and incisors contact the maxillary canines and incisors above their incisal and cusp ridges on lingual surfaces.

Nevertheless, the points of occlusal contact on the maxillary teeth and the points of occlusal contact on the mandibular teeth must conform to an approximation of curved planes which are identical during the occlusal relations of both arches during mastication. Several curved planes at different angulations are represented.

3. COMPENSATING CURVATURES OF THE INDIVIDUAL TEETH (CURVED AXES)

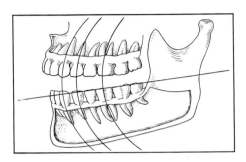

Vertical sections of the jaws with the teeth in centric occlusion demonstrate the fact that the axes of the posterior teeth, maxillary and mandibular, approach alignment with each other, but that these axes are not perpendicular to a horizontal plane (Fig. 82, Figs. 362 to 369 and Fig. 401). The sections showing the molars approach vertical planes, but as the sections are made anteriorly, the plane of the sections changes with the curvature of the dental arches until a sagittal plane is approached mesial to the central incisors.

It can be demonstrated that any line which bisects the crown and root base of a tooth from any aspect exhibits some curvature. Therefore, the design or functional activities of the dental mechanism may never be reduced to equations in plane geometry.

It is found in studying the human dental mechanism, either whole or in part, that *curvature* is the rule in its basic design. Maxwell has termed this basic phenomenon "spherical congruency." Man-made structures usually follow straight lines and definite angles considered in relation to straight lines, but Nature apparently abhors such planning—which abhorrence is clearly demonstrated in anatomic structures. The human dental mechanism is no exception in this respect.

It must be kept in mind that in the study of detail in anatomy, variations must be expected. Variations may be found in single instances as well as in the study of groups. Nevertheless, certain *tendencies* may be discovered, and those tendencies must be considered in order to acquire perspective before any conclusions may be established. Although definite rules cannot be laid down in any one direction, definite tendencies may play an important part in subsequent conclusions, which might have important practicable application.

The human dental mechanism is a complicated one and its secrets have been a challenge to those of scientific bent. In the author's opinion, one essential truth stands out in the study of occlusion, and this truth must be accepted in order to avoid confusion. In the study of the mechanism, the thought of using plane geometry as a medium for research into the intricacies must be erased from the mind. Suppositions based on planes must be accepted as a compromise only, in order to simplify the communications of ideas. Plane geometry has been used too often in the past in the actual attempt to prove the design of the mechanism. In the main, it has served only to confuse the issue.

The student must keep the following truths in mind:

1. Every segment of a tooth presents *curved* surfaces, except when the tooth is fractured or worn.

2. Lines bisecting the teeth from any aspect exhibit *curvature.*

3. The teeth are aligned to form *arches.*

4. The maxilla and mandible present *curved* outlines only.

5. The mandible operates in paths which are *curved.*

6. The occlusal and incisal surfaces of the teeth as arch units adapt themselves to *curved* planes (compensating occlusal curvature).

A common mistake is to assume that the forces of occlusion act upon the teeth in straight lines and also that the axes of the teeth are at right angles to their occlusal surfaces (Fig. 400). If the assumption were true, the arches would not be stabilized

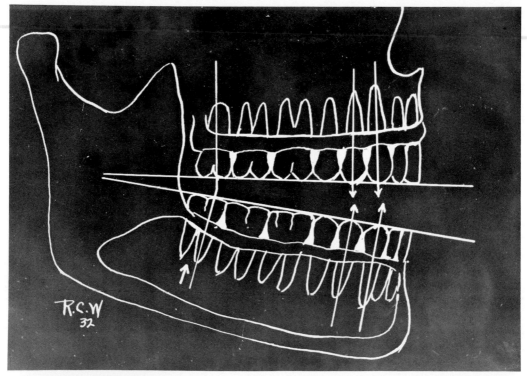

Figure 400. Schematic drawing of an imaginary occlusal relation. The occlusal surfaces have no compensating curvature, and the teeth have their axes at right angles to their occlusal surfaces. It will be noticed that as soon as the jaw is opened the axes of teeth in the upper jaw no longer coincide in direction with those of the lower jaw. A resistant bolus of food placed between the teeth at this opening will exert pressures unfavorable to stabilization of the various units.

very long, because the forces brought to bear upon the teeth would be tangent to their axes at any time the teeth of the two jaws were separated. Until the jaws and teeth were closed in centric relation, any resistant material between the teeth would put pressure upon individual teeth at angles tending to unseat them.

Another insurmountable difficulty which would be encountered is the impossibility of adapting teeth with straight axes to a compensating occlusal curvature. Any attempt in that direction overlooks proper spacing between the tooth roots— which arrangement makes normal tissue spacing and proper anchorage in the bone impossible. Some of the roots might compete with others for the same space, and the human jaws would have to be designed differently to accommodate them.

Actually, the compensating occlusal curvature of the dental arches which establishes occlusal balance could not be created unless the teeth themselves were curved individually, thereby accommodating themselves to the scheme of occlusion, a scheme based on essential curvatures. Arbitrary placement of teeth of indiscriminate form could not achieve the same result. An interesting comment might be made at this point: Practicing dentists, and dental students also, are too likely to be influenced in their considerations of occlusion by prosthetic technical procedure in which they "set up" manufactured artifical teeth into dental arch forms. It must be realized that in such procedures the operator is dealing with tooth crowns only, with no roots or foundation tissues to be considered. In addition, the artificial crowns may not conform to known anatomic values. Observations made on dissected human jaws showing the teeth *in situ* with their roots exposed prove without doubt the presence of axial curvatures in the individual teeth and the apparent co-ordination of these curvatures with the occlusal curvatures of the arches.

A dissected specimen is shown in Figure 401. The line of vision is at right angles to the buccal surface of the mandibular first molar. The anterior teeth are seen from a distal aspect and the posterior teeth from a buccal aspect.

It is readily apparent that the long axes of the teeth are all curved; consequently a line bisecting any one of them describes an arc. Arcs passing through the teeth of one dental arch seem to be parallel to those passing through the teeth of the opposite arch. It just happens that in the specimen under consideration the extent of jaw opening places the axes of the teeth in one jaw in the same curved plane with their namesakes in the opposite jaw. We know that such a situation does not obtain when the teeth are in centric occlusion, because the teeth then have an offset relationship with each other. Nevertheless, *the axial arcs would have a tendency toward parallelism or concentricity with each other regardless of the extent of jaw opening.*

Evidently the axial curvature is necessary in order to stabilize each tooth in its relative position in the arches. Apparently curved lines passing through the first molars (if viewed from the buccal aspect), and any of the teeth anterior to them, describe arcs of concentric circles of equal radii (the central and lateral incisors viewed from distal aspects). The axes of these circles are on a line parallel with the occlusal surface of the mandibular first molar.

The second and third molar axes are arc segments of smaller circles. *It is interesting to note in this connection that the position and design of the second and third molars are such that they act as braces to the rest of the arch, forbidding any tendency*

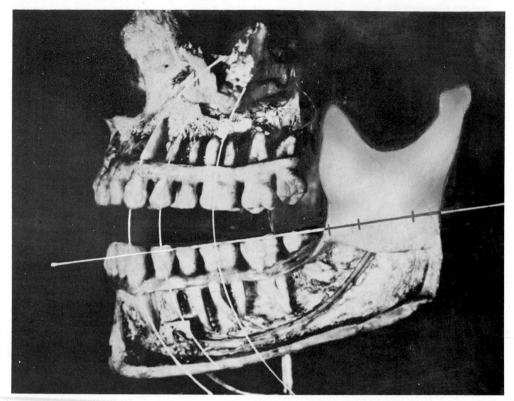

Figure 401. A dissected specimen with the roots of the teeth exposed. The axes of the teeth show curvature. The axes of the arcs of the tooth axes for this specimen are on a line with the occlusal plane of the mandibular first molars. The marks on the ramus of the mandible represent the axes of the arcs shown.

of the posterior teeth to drift in a distal direction. The mandibular second and third molars have an extra inclination mesially. During mandibular activity, they strike the maxillary second and third molars with a mesial inclination of force. This may explain the tendency of molars to drift mesially as age advances, especially when space is created anteriorly to them.

It is a known fact that any one point in the mandibular arch follows a curved path during normal masticatory movements of the mandible, masticatory forces traveling in curved paths. Therefore, the axial curvatures of the individual teeth conform to the physical laws when one considers them as part of the dental mechanism.

Photographs of individual teeth placed within a protractor prove their axial relation to compensating occlusal curvature (Figs. 402, 403 and 404). In these illustrations the anterior teeth were posed in the approximate positions they assume in the jaws. The posterior teeth were posed with their marginal ridges (mesial and distal) parallel with the horizontal plane, or 0 degrees. The horizontal plane is taken as an approximation of the occlusal plane for each tooth.

The illustrations, as shown, must be accepted as experiments only, made to

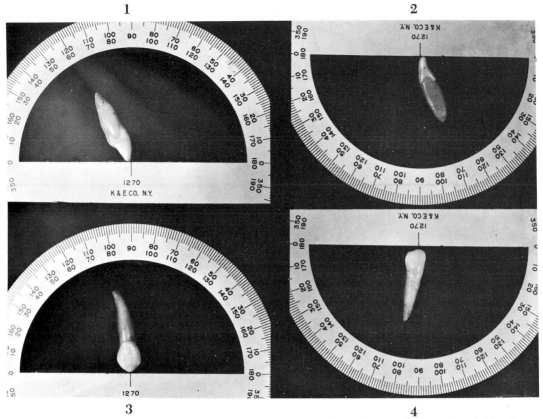

Figure 402. Individual teeth placed within a protractor to show their axial inclinations. 1, Maxillary central incisor. 2, Mandibular central incisor. 3, Maxillary canine. 4, Mandibular canine.

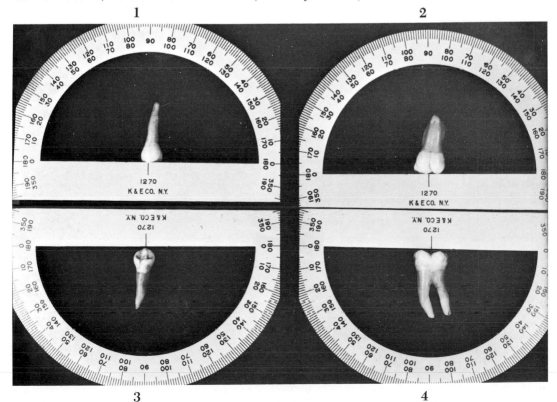

Figure 403. Individual teeth placed within a protractor to show their axial inclinations. 1, Maxillary first premolar. 2, Mandibular first premolar. 3, Maxillary first molar. 4, Mandibular first molar.

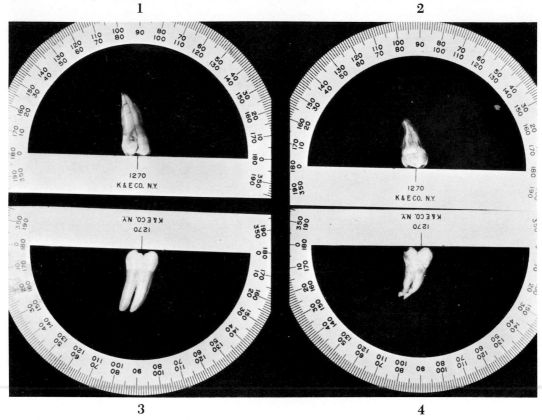

Figure 404.   Individual teeth placed within a protractor to show their axial inclinations. 1, Maxillary second molar. 2, Mandibular second molar. 3, Maxillary third molar. 4, Mandibular third molar.

prove the adaptability of axes of the teeth to various angulations as part of the compensating dental mechanism. The experiments do not prove angulations of any certain degree. This subject requires further research.

4. ANGULATION OF THE INDIVIDUAL TEETH IN RELATION TO VARIOUS PLANES

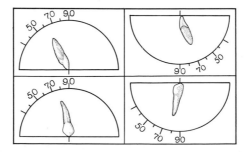

The relations of the axes of maxillary and mandibular teeth to each other vary and depend upon which tooth group or anatomic classification is to be considered.

Sections through the jaws with the teeth in centric occlusion, made to show the mesial aspect of each tooth in either arch, are shown in MacMillan's illustrations in Figs. 362 to 369, Chapter XIV. It may be noted that the incisors are placed with their axes at about 60 degrees to the horizontal plane at the occlusal contact, the axis of the maxillary tooth being placed at an acute angle to the axis of the mandibular tooth. The canines are placed so that the axes form angles less acute, followed by the first premolars, which resemble the canines in their placement.

The second premolars and the first molars differ from the teeth anterior to them in their axial relations to each other and in their angulations to a horizontal plane. The axes of these maxillary and mandibular teeth are nearly parallel. A line drawn through the center of the mandibular tooth forms an acute angle of approximately 80 degrees buccally with a horizontal line drawn at the occlusal contact.

A line drawn through the center of the crown and roots of the maxillary teeth (crown and bifurcation in the first maxillary molar) forms an obtuse angle buccally of about 100 degrees with the horizontal line. These angulations place the axes of maxillary and mandibular teeth on a line with each other approximately.

The second and third mandibular molars have their axes at angles somewhat more acute in relation to the horizontal than the first molar axis. Prolongations of the lines bisecting the mandibular second and third molars tend to bisect the lingual roots of the maxillary second and third molars. The axis line of the mandibular first molar, when prolonged, would tend to pass between the buccal and lingual roots of the maxillary first molar.

No definite rules may be assumed when describing the axial relations of maxillary and mandibular teeth in centric occlusion. Nevertheless, even though skulls and specimens show some variations in degree of angulations, normally developed specimens show angulations of crowns and roots which conform to the generalizations just described.

Each tooth must be placed at the angle that best withstands the forces brought against it during function. The angle at which it is placed depends also upon the function the tooth has to perform. If the tooth is placed at a disadvantage, its functional efficiency is limited and the permanency of its position is not assured. The dental arch naturally can be only as efficient and as permanent as the various component parts of which it is comprised.

The anterior teeth, seem to be placed at a disadvantage when one views them from mesial or distal aspects. The lines of force during mastication tend to be tangent to the long axes of the teeth (Fig. 405). Actually they are *shearing* teeth. The mandibular teeth are brought against the fixed maxillary teeth in a forward position, and the shearing action as the mandible is retruded applies the forces against the maxillary teeth in line with their long axes. The axes of the mandibular anterior teeth are in line with resultants of forces brought against them by the angulation of the maxillary anterior teeth. *The full force of the jaws is not brought to bear on any of the anterior teeth until the posterior teeth have had an opportunity to assume the load.* The anterior teeth assume a disadvantage if for any reason they lack posterior tooth support.

The greatest amount of force which the jaws are capable of applying against the

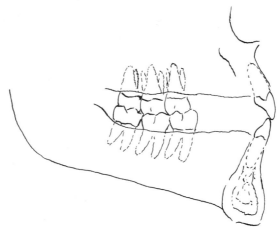

Figure 405. This illustration, which emphasizes the contrast in placement and angulation between molars and incisors, also emphasizes the "power ratio" of the two segments of the dental arch. It is obvious that the molars are designed to be the principal jaw support and that anterior teeth, both in design and in placement, are not capable substitutes when the molars are lost.

teeth does not culminate until centric occlusion is approached. As the teeth come into centric occlusion, the posterior teeth, and the molars especially, assume the full force of the load, supported by the arch form and all of the compensating curvatures of the dental arches. The molars are able to withstand the maximum forces during masticatory function by virtue of their form, structure, anchorage and placement (Figs. 405 and 416).

Loss of support, through damage or loss of molars, seriously handicaps the entire dental mechanism. The teeth anterior to the molars are not designed or placed in a manner conducive to total dental arch support.

The anterior teeth, when observed from directly in front of the median line, demonstrate their axial inclinations in relation to vertical or horizontal lines. The degree of their inclinations varies, of course, but it may be readily seen that there is some inclination of the axes and that the long axes of the teeth are never at right angles to the horizontal plane.

The teeth are placed so that their axes on either right or left side are at acute angles to the median line or median plane (sagittal plane) (Fig. 390). This arrangement makes the anterior teeth of each side of the mouth point, with their crowns, in the direction of the median line. The arrangement therefore favors the stabilization of the contact relationship of these teeth.

The teeth are inclined at angles of from 5 to 10 degrees to the median plane — which is in effect angulations of 85 to 80 degrees to the horizontal plane.

Items 5, 6, 7 and 8 in the study of tooth form, arrangement and occlusion have to do with crown forms and their arrangement: practical aspects of occlusion as observed in the mouth.

5. THE FUNCTIONAL FORM OF THE TEETH AT THEIR INCISAL AND OCCLUSAL THIRDS

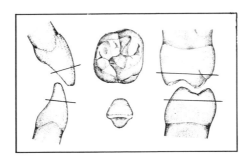

However some of the basic concepts of design, which have just been described under items 1, 2, 3 and 4, must be realized and respected, in order for one to understand certain fundamentals of form which contribute to stability. These stabilizing principles are reflected in the crown forms also.

The incisal and occlusal thirds of the tooth crowns present convex or concave surfaces at all contacting occlusal areas (Fig. 406). When the teeth of one jaw come into occlusal contact with their antagonists in the opposite jaw during the various

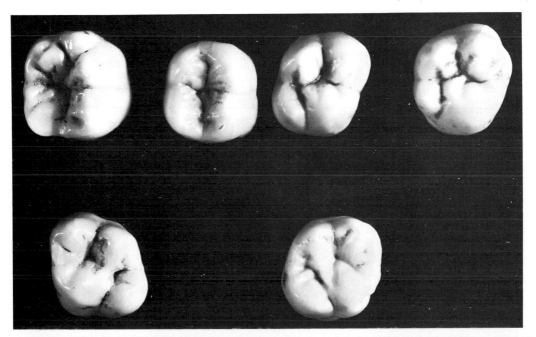

Figure 406. Occlusal views of molars, showing curvature of their surfaces. It should be noted that no flat planes are in evidence even though these specimens had been subject to daily use for many years.

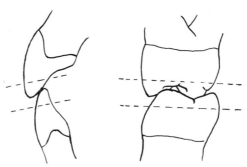

Figure 407. The incisal or occlusal thirds of the tooth crowns present convex or concave surfaces at all contacting occlusal areas.

mandibular movements, curved surfaces come into contact with curved surfaces. These curved surfaces may be convex or concave. A convex surface, representing a segment of the occlusal third of one tooth, may come into contact with a convex or a concave segment of another tooth; always, however, curved segments contact curved segments, large or small (Fig. 407).

There are no flat planes on the incisal or occlusal surfaces of any of the teeth unless there are some created by wear or accident. When such planes are created, the efficiency of the occlusal form is lessened in direct proportion to the extent of the deterioration.

Every segment of a cusp, marginal ridge or incisal ridge is a segment of a spheroid regardless of the size of the segment (Fig. 408).

Lingual surfaces of maxillary incisors present some concave surfaces where convex portions of the incisal ridges of mandibular incisors come into occlusal contact.

The posterior teeth show depressions in the depths of sulci and developmental grooves; nevertheless, the enamel sides of the sulci are formed by convexities which point into the developmental grooves. Until the cusps are worn flat, the deeper por-

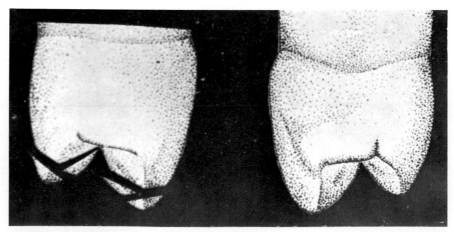

Figure 408. A diagrammatic representation of spheroidal segments sectioned from the occlusal portion of a maxillary premolar.

tions of the sulci and grooves act as escapements for food, since the convex surfaces of opposing teeth are prevented from fitting into them perfectly by the curved sides of the sulci (Figs. 365 to 369, 409 and 411).

The crown of a human tooth, with its occlusal form, is at its most efficient period immediately following its eruption and its occlusion with its antagonists. *The curved hard surfaces, coming into contact with like surfaces, permit the teeth to be used as cutters, because, when convexities come into contact with other convexities or with concavities, they touch in points or in small circumscribed areas only. When the con-*

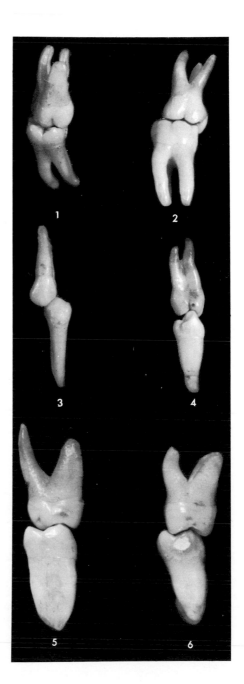

Figure 409. Maxillary and mandibular first molars and maxillary and mandibular first premolars, placed in centric occlusal relation. 1, Lingual aspect of first molars in occlusion, showing occlusal relations and escapement spaces in centric relation. 2, Buccal aspect of first molars in occlusion, showing occlusal relations and escapement spaces in centric relation. 3, Buccal aspect of first premolars in centric occlusal relation. 4, Mesial aspect of first premolars in centric occlusal relation. Note the approximation of cusps to marginal ridges. 5, Mesial aspect of first molars in centric occlusion. 6, Distal aspect of first molars in centric occlusion. Note the escapement design.

tacting areas are hard and unyielding, they cut or shred any penetrable material when, in addition to their contact, they are moved over each other with considerable force.

The cusps, marginal ridges and sulci on multicusped posterior teeth may be compared favorably with the eminences and spillways of the schematic drawings in Figs. 410, 411 and 412.

The cusps of the schematic tooth are made to resemble spheres which approximate each other. The opposing tooth is similarly drawn and placed in occlusal contact. One may see that the cusps touch in circumscribed areas or points, with spillways appearing where the spheres of one tooth fail to penetrate the deeper portions of the sulci of the other.

Although the cusps and rounded eminences of the occlusal surfaces of natural teeth are not comparable to spheres, the various segments of the rounded eminences are comparable to spheroids of greater or lesser dimensions; their comparison with the schematic cusps is therefore a logical one. The curvatures formed at the occlusal portions of the teeth conform to the physiologic entity of the entire dental mechanism, which, as has been mentioned before, is based on curvature.

Another aspect of importance is this: *Curved contacting surfaces of opposing teeth allow greater facility of adjustment to changing conditions involving the dental mechanism with less sacrifice of efficiency than any design which might include flat planes.* Any mechanism, to be practicable in use, allows ease of adjustment of parts during its assembly, and the completed mechanism allows proper facilities for adjustment to changing conditions which are brought about by wear or accident. The design of the human tooth forms and the design of the temporomandibular articulation make such allowances in a most complete manner. The articulation allows the maximum adjustment; it adjusts itself with limitations to movement in various planes, flat or curved. The curved occlusal surfaces allow the individual teeth to be adjusted to various angulations of their long axes with the minimum of variance in their placement and, simultaneously, with the minimum of loss of occlusal efficiency.

The occlusal design of the crowns of the permanent teeth is established several years before the teeth have an opportunity to complete occlusal relations with their antagonists. In the meantime, the bones of the jaws and the temporomandibular articulation are developing and are subject to changes which must take place during the years when the teeth are erupting and establishing their relations to each other.

Pointing to the chronology of the development of the parts and the fact that the occlusal design of all of the teeth is permanently fixed in unchangeable form years before the investing tissues of the teeth are completed, the student logically concludes that the jaws and their articulation will tend to coincide with the requirements of the occlusal design of the teeth.

Paradoxically, the occlusal curvatures of the tooth crowns are the *foundation* of occlusion, and the *investing tissues* of the teeth, which include the alveolar process of the jaw bones and the temporomandibular articulation, are the *superstructure* of occlusion.

Jaw relation, as has been pointed out, is dependent upon the form and alignment of the teeth. Loss of one or more teeth ultimately changes the jaw relation and the

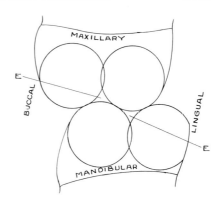

Figure 410. Schematic drawing of the mesial aspect of first molars in occlusion, illustrating the cusp forms as perfect circles. With this arrangement, escapement spaces would be larger, but the centric occlusal relation would be too unstable and the cusps would be too flat. Also, "mortar and pestle" activity, where indicated for efficiency, would be absent. *E,* escapement spaces.

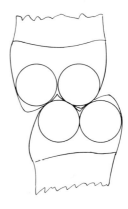

Figure 411. Schematic drawing of the mesial aspect of maxillary and mandibular first molar crowns in centric relation. Circles have been placed within the outlines of cusp forms to emphasize the curvatures.

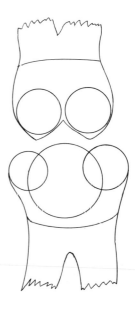

Figure 412. Schematic drawing of the buccal aspect of maxillary and mandibular first molar crowns, separated as in jaw opening. Circles have been placed within the outlines of cusp forms to emphasize curvatures. Note the adaptability of the circles to the actual occlusal outline of the mandibular first molar.

compensatory action of the temporomandibular articulation. The occlusal relations of the dental arches change in direct proportion to the number of dental arch units which are lost or damaged. Each unit plays its part as a stabilizer of occlusion; naturally the stability of the occlusion is affected in direct ratio to the number of stabilizers lost. The temporomandibular articulation is capable of the adjustment within limitations) which is required in order to accommodate the damaged arches, and by virtue of this adaptability, the maximum efficiency of which the damaged masticatory mechanism is capable is maintained.

The movements of the condyles over the meniscus in the glenoid fossa are regulated by the alignment and the occlusion of the teeth.

The ligamentous attachments to the condyles allow a greater range of movement than the occlusion of the teeth usually requires.

When all of the teeth are lost, the mandible loses the terminals of movement which are established by the teeth. The limitations of mandibular movement after loss of the teeth are governed by the extent of the *flexibility* and *elasticity* of the ligamentous attachments and muscle tonus.

The curved surfaces of the occlusal surfaces of tooth crowns allow adjustment with a minimum of placement and displacement of the individual teeth during the development of the jaws and the alignment of the dental arches.

If occlusal thirds possessed plane surfaces, these plane surfaces would require the teeth to be placed in one position only. If that position were not attained, *i.e.*, if the plane surfaces of one tooth did not adapt themselves perfectly to the plane surfaces of its antagonists in the opposite jaw, the position of the tooth would not be stabilized until the counterplanes became parallel to each other. No flexibility of adjustment would be permitted. Plane surfaces would adapt themselves to each other so closely that there would be little or no spacing between cusps and marginal ridges. This arrangement would produce a mashing rather than a cutting effect, decreasing the efficiency for our purposes, not to mention the tremendous increase in occlusal pressure which would have to be accommodated by a more secure periodontal anchorage and attachment.

Escapement spaces are absolute requisites to efficient occlusion because of the nature of the duties the teeth must perform during mastication.

The human being is omnivorous. His teeth are designed to reduce the varied food material to a consistency which fits the requirements of his digestive system. His dental mechanism does not reduce food material to a pulpy mass. The teeth cut, shred or crush food into particles which are small enough to enable the digestive system to continue the reduction without strain and within a normal time limit for proper nourishment of the individual.

The cusps and incisal ridges of the teeth act as cutting blades when they are brought into contact with opposing cusps and incisal ridges or into contact with the concave surfaces of opposing teeth. These concavities may be natural or they may be created by wear. When curved surfaces of different planes come together at any point, they touch in circumscribed points or areas, and spaces appear all around the points of contact where the curved surfaces do not fit together (Figs. 413 and 414). These spaces, when relating the process to the occlusal surfaces of the teeth, act as escapement spaces or spillways.

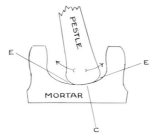

Figure 413. Sectional drawing of a typical mortar and pestle. The convex end of the pestle is in contact with the concave floor of the mortar chamber. The surfaces are in contact in a small circumscribed area, with escapement space appearing around the area of contact. Some of the occlusal contacts of the human teeth resemble this working arrangment. *C*, contact; *E*, escapement.

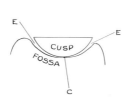

Figure 414. Schematic drawing of "mortar and pestle" design of some of the occlusal contacts of the teeth. Examples: buccal cusps of mandibular molars in contact with central sulci of maxillary molars; incisal ridges of mandibular incisors in contact with lingual fossae of maxillary incisors. *C*, contact; *E*, escapement.

Escapement space is provided in the teeth by the form of the cusps and ridges, the sulci and developmental grooves, and the interdental spaces or embrasures. (See "Embrasures," Chapter V.)

Although the teeth when in centric occlusion seem to intercuspate rather closely, on examination it is found that escapements have been provided. Some escapement spaces are so slight that light is scarcely admitted through them; they vary in degree of opening from such small ones to generous ones of a millimeter or more at the widest points of embrasure (Fig. 409).

The *location* and *form* of the escapement spaces are immediately changed when the occlusal relation is changed. When the occlusion is normal, the teeth fit together or intercuspate with less escapement space available in centric occlusion than in any other occlusal relation. As soon as the mandibular teeth are moved out of centric relation with the maxillary teeth, the escapements are enlarged, since the intercusping relation is not so complete.

When the teeth are occluding in the lateral relation or in protrusive relation, the escapement space is increased but the number of spotted areas or points of occlusal contact between the teeth of the two arches is decreased. This variation in the number of contacting areas of the teeth during the various occlusal relations may be demonstrated by markings made by the teeth of one jaw on the teeth of the opposing jaw, registered by carbon paper held between the teeth during the movements (Fig. 415). As the teeth are brought back from lateral or protrusive toward centric occlusion, the spotted areas of contact increase in number as the teeth approach centric. Simultaneously the escapement space is reduced in direct ratio to the increase in occlusal contact.

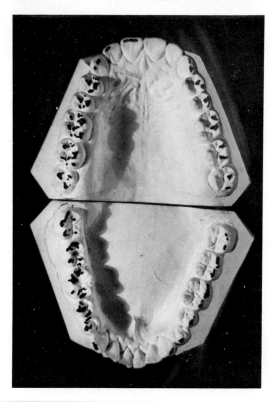

Figure 415. Casts of maxillary and mandibular teeth showing the occlusal contacts. The side showing buccal markings only demonstrates the contacting areas in left lateral relation for this individual. The opposite side with many more registered markings shows the contacting areas in centric occlusal relation. Note all of the unmarked areas on occlusal surfaces. These areas represent escapement spaces existing at the same time spotted areas were in contact.

The functional value of the system just described is obvious: *The number of cutting blades is reduced when the position of the teeth places them at a greater disadvantage to the resistance of force, as experienced in a lateral relation; and at the same time the escapement spaces, which serve to decrease pressure, are multiplied or enlarged. The opposite arrangement is countenanced only as the teeth return to centric occlusion, where their form and their alignment with each other offer combined resistance to the maximum forces of mastication.*

6. THE FACIAL RELATIONS OF EACH TOOTH IN ONE ARCH TO ITS ANTAGONIST OR ANTAGONISTS IN THE OPPOSING ARCH IN CENTRIC OCCLUSION

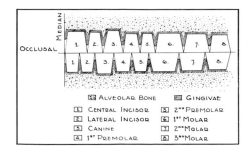

In the centric occlusal relation, facial views of the normal denture show each tooth of one arch in occlusal contact with portions of two others in the opposing arch with the exception of the mandibular central incisors and the maxillary third molars. Each of the exceptions named has one antagonist only in the opposing jaw (Fig. 416).

This scheme serves to equalize the forces of impact in occlusion and to distribute the work of the teeth more evenly. Each tooth helps to support the next. This arrangement helps in another way to preserve the integrity of the denture: The loss of

A

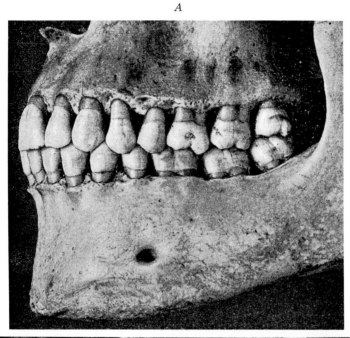

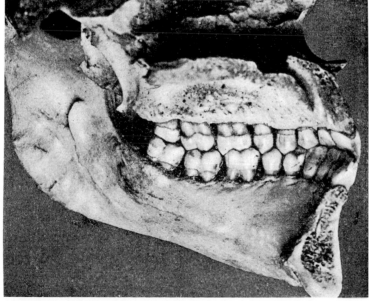

B

Figure 416. *A,* Occlusion of the teeth — facial view. *B,* Occlusion of the teeth — medial view. The teeth in centric occlusal relation. (After specimen in possession of Dr. F. A. Peeso. From Turner, *American Textbook of Prosthetic Dentistry,* Lea & Febiger.)

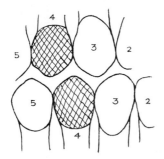

Figure 417. Buccal view of first premolars, showing relation of one tooth to two in apposition as they come together in occlusal contact. 2, Lateral incisors. 3, Canines. 4, First premolars. 5, Second premolars.

one tooth does not throw another tooth in the opposing arch out of function. Since each tooth has two antagonists, the loss of one still leaves one antagonist remaining which will keep the tooth in occlusal contact with the opposing arch and keep it in its own arch relation at the same time by preventing elongation and displacement through the lack of antagonism. Actually, the loss of one or more teeth ultimately precipitates a gradual disintegration of the occlusal relation of the dental arches unless a prosthetic replacement is made. The permanency of the arch forms depends upon the mutual support of the teeth in contact with each other. The original tooth arrangement minimizes the loss, however, and serves to resist *immediate* disintegration of the alignment.

When a tooth is lost, the adjoining teeth in the same arch finally *migrate* and tend to fill the space. The migration of adjoining teeth destroys the contact relations of the teeth in the same arch in that vicinity. In the meantime, migration of these teeth changes their occlusal relations with their antagonists in the opposing arch. This usually causes elongation of the tooth in the opposing arch immediately opposite the space left by the absent tooth. Elongation of one or more of these teeth breaks up the contact relation in the second arch also and results in a collapse of the occlusal relation of an entire side. The ultimate result of the loss is a gradual breakdown of the mechanism, which, if uninterrupted, ends in complete destruction through mechanical and pathologic changes (Fig. 418).

The only way to avoid possible premature loss of all of the teeth is to avoid any permanent change in the original normal arrangement of them.

If one of the maxillary central incisors is lost, the mandibular central incisor on the same side is left without an opposing tooth. The same situation exists regarding the maxillary third molar if the mandibular third molar is lost.

The offset arrangement of the teeth, showing one against two (alternating from one arch to the other), is attained by an ingenious manipulation of the dimensions of the individual teeth (Figs. 419, and 420). The dental arches are composed of pairs of teeth starting at the median line, right and left. These pairs consist of two units of equal dimensions; they differ from other pairs and, except in the instance of central incisors, maxillary and mandibular, the components of the pairs are not set in contact with each other in the arches, since each tooth is a unit of the right or left side. The right and left central incisors are together at the median line; right and left lateral incisors are placed distal to them; right and left canines are distal to the lateral incisors, etc.

Each arch is bilaterally symmetrical, with central incisors coming into contact with each other at the median line. These points of contact with their embrasures are

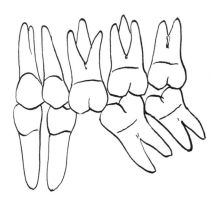

First 418. This illustration demonstrates a typical clinical picture showing elongation, migration and improper contact and occlusal relation resulting from neglect after the loss of a mandibular first molar.

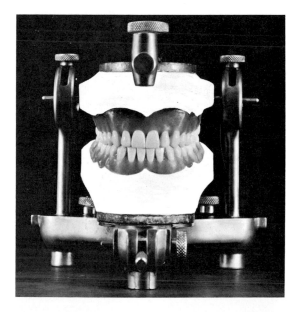

Figure 419. Carvings in ivorine of individual teeth set up into complete dental arches on an anatomic articulator.

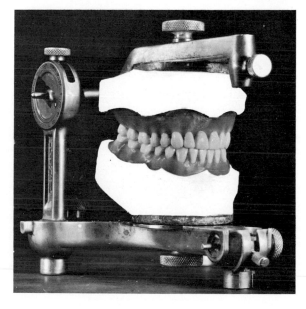

Figure 420. Another view of the carvings shown in Fig. 419.

the only ones directly above or below each other; or, to put it another way, the only ones in line with each other when the teeth are in centric occlusion. All the other points of contact with associated embrasures, when located in one arch, are offset mesially or distally from the closing contact and embrasure form in the opposing arch.

The contacts and embrasures of one arch are not equidistant from those in the opposing arch at any one location, since the teeth are varied in size.

The maxillary arch is larger in outside measurement than the mandibular arch, yet the difference in arch length is slight, the distal margins of maxillary and mandibular third molars appearing almost flush with each other when the teeth are in centric occlusion.

The mandibular arch is narrower when calibrated at the buccal surfaces of posterior teeth than is the maxillary arch. This relation is brought about by the differences in mesiodistal width between mandibular and maxillary anterior teeth (particularly the incisors) and by the lingual projection of mandibular posterior teeth crowns, an arrangement which is necessary for proper intercusping with the maxillary posterior teeth.

7. THE OCCLUSAL CONTACT AND INTERCUSP RELATIONS OF ALL THE TEETH OF ONE ARCH WITH THOSE IN THE OPPOSING ARCH IN CENTRIC OCCLUSION

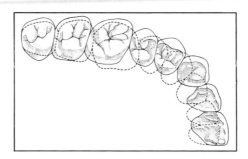

In order to obtain a clear understanding of the occlusal contact and the intercusping relation of the teeth in centric occlusion, the teeth must be observed while in the centric relation from three aspects:

A. Facial aspect (Figs. 421 to 424).

B. Lingual aspect (Figs. 416, *B*, and 427).

C. Occlusal aspect (Figs. 427, 428 and 431).

The occlusal aspect can be studied only by superimposing the outlines of the teeth of one arch over those of the other in centric relation.

Figures 421 to 424, inclusive, illustrate the teeth in centric occlusion from their facial aspects. It is suggested that, during the reading of the following text, the student should refer to illustrations continuously, in order to clarify in his own mind the description of occlusion.

The *key* to occlusion lies in the proper occlusal relation of the first molars (maxillary and mandibular) to each other. It is taken for granted that the development

Figure 421

Figure 422

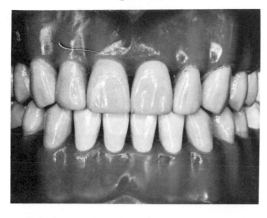

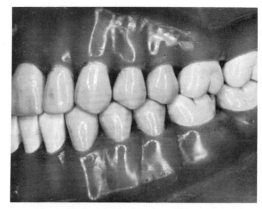

Figure 423

Figure 424

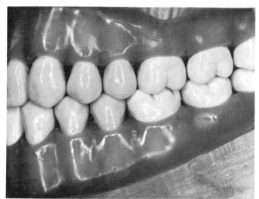

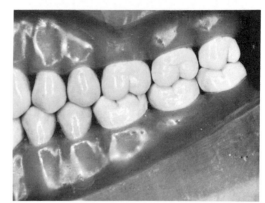

Figure 421. Labial aspect of the teeth in centric occlusion. This aspect is taken from a position directly in alignment with the median line. (These photographs are of sections of the carved model shown in Fig. 18.)

Figure 422. Labiobuccal aspect of the teeth in centric occlusion. This aspect is taken from a position directly in line with the labial surface of the maxillary canine.

Figure 423. Buccal aspect of the teeth in centric occlusion. This aspect is taken from a position directly buccal to the contact of maxillary premolars.

Figure 424. Buccal aspect of the teeth in centric occlusion. This aspect is taken from a position directly buccal to the mesiobuccal cusp of the maxillary first molar.

of the teeth and jaws is normal, so that the teeth have proper dimensions and so that the development allows their placement in proper relation to each other.

The occlusion of the *first molars* must be considered first: The first molars are the first permanent teeth to emerge into the oral cavity. The take their places immediately posterior to second deciduous molars, apparently using them as a guide in determining their original position in the developing jaws. The mandibular molar erupts first, and the maxillary molar moves down against it to establish the *initial occlusal relation of the permanent dentition.*

If the first molars attain normal occlusal contact and intercusping relation, and if the jaws develop normally, the teeth anterior to the first molars and posterior to them are enabled to take their normal positions; *the final result should be normal placement and occlusion of all of the teeth.*

A. Centric Occlusal Relation—Facial Aspect

Detailed Description

The occlusion of the molars will be described first because they show the most intricate occlusal relation of all of the teeth and they accomplish the most in the stabilization of the occlusion.

The Molars, Facial or Buccal Aspect (Figs. 409,2 and 424)

All maxillary molars bear a distal relation to the mandibular molars. The maxillary molars are somewhat smaller in mesiodistal dimensions that are the mandibular molars, but their buccolingual dimensions are greater. (See Table of Measurements, Chapter I.)

From the buccal aspect it is apparent that the facial portions of the posterior teeth in contact in centric occlusion are the occlusal slopes of the buccal cusps of maxillary teeth and the occlusal third portions of the buccal cusps of mandibular teeth. It must be remembered that maxillary teeth always have an overjet facially in relation to the mandibular teeth.

The *maxillary first molar,* from the buccal aspect, has the *triangular ridge* of the *mesiobuccal cusp* resting in the *mesiobuccal sulcus* of the *mandibular first molar* just above the *mesiobuccal developmental groove.* The *triangular ridge* of the *distobuucal cusp* of the *maxillary first molar* rests in the *sulcus* of the *distobuccal developmental groove* of the *mandibular first molar.*

The distal relation of maxillary molar to mandibular molar is repeated in the arrangement of *second* and *third molars.* However, distobuccal triangular ridges of distobuccal cusps of *maxillary second* and *third* molars rest on distal slopes of distobuccal cusps of corresponding *mandibular molars,* since the latter do not have distobuccal developmental grooves.

The Premolars, Buccal Aspect (Fig. 423)

The tip of the buccal cusp of the *maxillary first premolar* is free of contact, but the slopes of its *triangular ridge* rest within the *buccal* and *occlusal embrasures* formed by the contact of *mandibular first* and *second premolars.* From the buccal aspect the buccal cusp of the maxillary first premolar seems to be resting between the cusps of the two mandibular premolars.

The arrangement of the *second maxillary premolar* is similar except that the buccal cusp fits within the *embrasure* formed by the *distal slope* of the *buccal cusp* of the *mandibular second premolar* and the *mesiobuccal cusp* of the *mandibular first molar.*

The buccal portion of the *mandibular first premolar* cusp may be seen within the *embrasure* formed by the *distal cusp slope* of the *maxillary canine* and the *maxillary first premolar*.

The *mandibular second premolar* buccal cusp fits with the *embrasure* formed by the *two maxillary premolars*.

The Canines (Fig. 422)

The cusp of the *maxillary canine* is placed in the embrasure formed by the *distal cusp slope* of the *mandibular canine* and the *mesial cusp slope* of the *mandibular first premolar*.

The *mandibular canine* takes its place with the embrasure formed by the *maxillary lateral incisor* and the *maxillary canine*.

The Incisors (Fig. 421)

The *maxillary lateral incisor* is placed over the *distal half* of the *mandibular lateral incisor* and the *mesial portion* of the *mandibular canine*.

The *maxillary central incisor* has its *mesial surface* at the *median line* and is superimposed over the *entire width* of the *mandibular central incisor* and the *mesial half*, approximately, of the mandibular lateral incisor.

The alignment of the *mandibular incisors* in centric relation from the facial aspect has been indicated in the description of the alignment of the maxillary incisors.

Summary

The facial aspect of the alignment of the teeth of both arches in centric relation has just been described, beginning with the molars and working forward toward the median line.

The teeth of one arch have an offset arrangement in relation to the teeth of the opposing arch (Fig. 101).

Generally speaking the plan indicates one tooth against two antagonists except for the mandibular central incisor and the maxillary third molar (or the maxillary second molar, when third molars are non-existent).

In review, the reader should check this arrangement again, beginning at the median line this time and working distally (Figs. 419 and 420). Note the following features:

1. The overjet of maxillary teeth
2. The offset arrangement
3. The distal relation of all maxillary teeth to counterparts in the mandible
4. The mesial relation of all mandibular teeth to counterparts in the maxilla, excepting the mandibular central incisor

B. Centric Occlusal Relation — Lingual Aspect

Figure 416, *B*, is photograph of a sectioned specimen which portrays graphically the alignment of the teeth in centric relation. It might be a help also to refer to Figures 405, 407, 409, 427 and 428.

The alignment of the teeth in one arch in relation to the other is of course the same as that described under "Facial Aspect." However some details of the arrangment that are to be seen from the lingual aspect only should be noted.

Observe the angulation and contact of the incisal surfaces of the mandibular anterior teeth against lingual surfaces of the maxillary anterior teeth. Observe the overjet and overbite of maxillary anterior teeth, and the lingual projection of mandibular posterior teeth in relation to maxillary posterior teeth. Study the apposition of lingual cusps of maxillary posterior teeth to the occlusal surfaces of mandibular posterior teeth.

C. Centric Occlusal Relation — Occlusal Aspect

Under this heading, emphasis will be placed on the large number of occlusal contacts to be noted when the teeth come together in centric occlusal relation in comparison with other occlusal relations. As mentioned under item 5, more of the functional form of the teeth at occlusal thirds in both arches comes into contact in centric relation than in any other.

When the teeth are in centric occlusal relation the mandible is said to be in its *physical rest position* (Chapter XV, page 359).

The surfaces of the tooth crowns which represent the areas where occlusal contact may be expected in centric occlusal relation are as follows, and may be studied in figures 392, 425, 426, 427 and 428.

1. Maxillary anterior teeth
    a. Linguoincisal ridges
    b. Incisal half of lingual surfaces
2. Maxillary posterior teeth
    a. Occlusal slopes of buccal cusps
    b. Occlusal slopes of lingual cusps
    c. Lingual slopes of lingual cusps
3. Mandibular anterior teeth
    a. Labioincisal ridges
    b. Incisal third of labial surfaces
4. Mandibular posterior teeth
    a. Buccal slopes of buccal cusps
    b. Occlusal slopes of buccal cusps
    c. Occlusal slopes of lingual cusps

Before studying the details in the text to follow on occlusion, the reader should have a good model or skull for additional reference. The study of occlusion involves

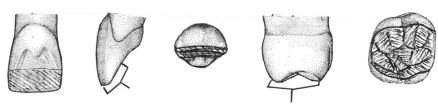

Figure 425. Maxillary teeth.

Figure 426. Mandibular teeth.

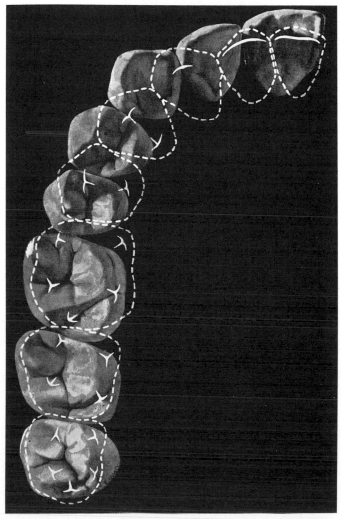

Figure 427. Contact relation of human teeth—maxillary teeth with dotted lines of mandibular teeth superposed in occlusion. Heavy lines and T's within dotted outlines denote incisal ridges and summits of cusps. (Courtesy of Sheldon Freil, Dublin.)

405

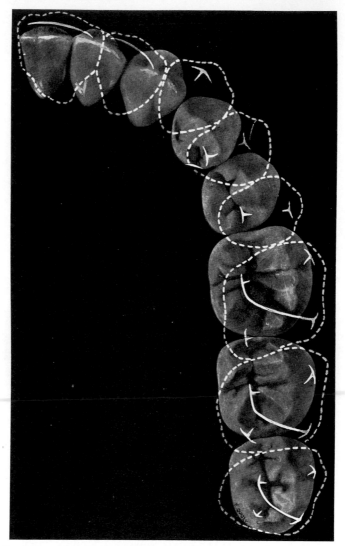

Figure 428. Contact relation of human teeth—mandibular teeth with dotted lines of maxillary teeth superposed in occlusion. (Courtesy of Sheldon Freil, Dublin.)

three dimensions. The best arrangement of text and illustrations is hardly sufficient without a three-dimensional reference at hand.

Returning now to the study of centric relation, the occlusal aspect can be studied only by superimposing the outlines of the occlusal aspect of the teeth of one arch over those of the other in centric relation (Figs. 427 and 428).

The description of occlusal relations assumes an idealized arrangement to conform to the apparent aim in development; such perfection in natural dental arches is seldom attained. Nevertheless, close approximations may be found (Figs. 427, 428, etc.).

The first approach to this study should be made by locating the relation of incisal ridges and cusp tips of mandibular teeth to the maxillary teeth when in occlusal contact in centric relation. This will be followed by a study of the same relations of maxillary to mandibular teeth. The plan is to fix in the mind the location of the highest points of contour topographically on the occlusal surfaces of the teeth and to compare the positions of these points on the teeth of one arch with the relative positions on the teeth of the opposing arch while they are in centric relation.

In the meantime, while *checking the text against a three-dimensional model*, the reader is supposed to connect the rest of the occlusal form of each tooth with the high points described, so that simultaneously he may note the relations of occlusal slopes, slopes of sulci, and relations of cusps and occlusal slopes to marginal ridges, fossae, triangular ridges, etc. By this means he may note the most likely points of contact and escapement during occlusal relations. *To read text describing every slope, sulcus and possible contact and escapement in monotonous detail would be confusing and futile.*

The next six pages of text are without graphic illustrations. The reader must have a three-dimensional model at hand to follow descriptions. This arrangement was deliberately planned because it was found through years of experience that drawings and photos would not suffice.

Example

In the following text, under "Maxillary First Molar," the mesiobuccal *cusp tip* is described as being out of contact, which it is. Nevertheless, it must be recognized that the mesiobuccal cusp of a first molar includes much more than a *tip*. At the same time the reader is apprised of the location and relation of this cusp tip, he must continue his observations to include all the ramifications of the mesiobuccal cusp and must note the contacts or lack of contact of all of its cusp ridges and slopes with the occlusal contours of the mandibular first molar.

Centric Relation of Incisal Ridges and Cusp Tips of Mandibular Teeth to Maxillary Teeth

A good exercise, which would help considerably to fix details in the mind, would be to make a *tissue tracing* of dotted lines in Freil's illustration in Figure 427, which lines portray the outline of mandibular teeth superposed over maxillary teeth, and then add the lines and T's to the tracing indicating incisal ridges and cusp tips. *Details of the tracing might be made simultaneously with the assimilation of the same details in the following text.*

MANDIBULAR CENTRAL INCISOR

Beginning at the median line, the *labioincisal portion* of the *incisal ridge* of the *mandibular central incisor* strikes the *maxillary central incisor lingually* near the *junction* of *incisal* and *middle thirds*. The incisal ridge of the mandibular central will extend over more than half the mesiodistal width of the maxillary central when both teeth have their mesial surfaces in alignment at the median line. The incisal ridge of the mandibular tooth is in contact for most of its mesiodistal width.

MANDIBULAR LATERAL INCISOR

The labioincisal portion of the *incisal ridge* of the *mandibular lateral incisor* contacts the *maxillary central incisor* and the *lateral incisor* as well. The ridge contact crosses the marginal ridges of the maxillary teeth just lingual to their proximal contact areas at a level which approximates the incisal and middle thirds. The contact relation of the mandibular tooth is rather evenly divided in extent between the maxillary central and lateral incisors.

MANDIBULAR CANINE

The tip of the mandibular canine cusp contacts the maxillary lateral incisor and the maxillary canine at the junction of their marginal ridges just lingual to contact areas. When cusp ridges are in occlusal contact, the mesial cusp ridge contacts the maxillary lateral incisor and the distal cusp ridge (a little longer) contacts the maxillary canine.

MANDIBULAR FIRST PREMOLAR

The point of the *buccal cusp* of the *mandibular first premolar* contacts the *mesial marginal ridge* of the *maxillary first premolar* approximately in line with its central groove. When cusp ridges of the buccal cusp are in contact, the *mesial cusp ridge* will be in contact with the linguoincisal portion of the maxillary canine, and the distal cusp ridge will be centered over the mesial portion of the occlusal surface of the maxillary first premolar, near the site of the central groove.

The *lingual cusp* of the *mandibular first premolar* is short and free of contact.

MANDIBULAR SECOND PREMOLAR

The point of the buccal cusp of the *mandibular second premolar* contacts the *mesial marginal ridge* of the *maxillary second premolar* in alignment with its central groove.

When *cusp ridges* of the *buccal cusp* are in contact, the *mesial cusp* ridge is in contact with the *disto-occlusal slope* of the *buccal cusp* of the maxillary first *premolar* and the *distal cusp ridge* is in contact with the *mesio-occlusal cusp slope* of the *maxillary second premolar*.

In centric relation the *lingual cusp tip* or *tips* of the *mandibular second premolar* is out of *occlusion*. Lingual cusps are located lingual to the embrasure formed by the contours of the lingual cusps of the maxillary first and second premolars.

MANDIBULAR FIRST MOLAR

The occlusal relations of first molars establish the plan of occlusion of the dental arches. They are the largest teeth in the jaws and are the first to be located in functional relation to each other in the second dentition.

The tip of the *mesiobuccal cusp* of the *mandibular first molar* contacts the *maxil-*

lary teeth at the junction of the *marginal ridges* of the *maxillary second premolar* and the *maxillary first molar* near the contact areas.

The tip of the *distobuccal cusp* of the mandibular first molar rests in the *sulcus* of the *buccal groove* of the *central fossa* on the occlusal surface of the *maxillary first molar* buccal to the central pit.

The tip of the *distal cusp* of the mandibular first molar lies *distal* to the *oblique ridge* in the *distal triangular fossa* of the occlusal surface of the maxillary first molar.

When cusp ridges are in contact, the surfaces in contact are as follows:

Mandibular first molar:

1. Mesiobuccal cusp
   a. Mesial cusp ridge
      In contact with the disto-occlusal slope of the buccal cusp of the maxillary second premolar
   b. Distal cusp ridge
      In contact with the mesio-occlusal slope of the mesiobuccal cusp of the maxillary first molar
2. Distobuccal cusp
   a. Mesial cusp ridge
      In contact with the disto-occlusal slope of the mesiobuccal cusp of the maxillary first molar mesial to the buccal groove of the central fossa
   b. Distal cusp ridge
      In contact with the mesio-occlusal slope of the distobuccal cusp of the maxillary first molar, distal to the buccal groove of the central fossa
3. Distal cusp
   a. Mesial cusp ridge
      In contact with the disto-occlusal slope of the distobuccal cusp of the maxillary first molar near the distal triangular fossa
   b. Distal cusp ridge
      Not in contact

The summits of lingual cusps of the mandibular first molar are out of contact in centric relation.

The mesiolingual cusp will be located in the large lingual embrasure formed by the distolingual contour of the maxillary second premolar and the mesiolingual contour of the maxillary first molar.

The distolingual cusp will be near (but lingual to) the sulcus of the lingual developmental groove of the maxillary first molar.

MANDIBULAR SECOND MOLAR

The tip of the mesiobuccal cusp of the mandibular second molar contacts the maxillary second molar at the mesial marginal ridge area near the mesial triangular fossa.

The tip of the distobuccal cusp of the mandibular second molar is centered within the central fossa of the occlusal surface of the maxillary second molar.

When cusp ridges are in contact, the surfaces in contact are as follows:

Mandibular second molar:

1. Mesiobuccal cusp
   a. Mesial cusp ridge

      In contact with the disto-occlusal slope of the distobuccal cusp of the maxillary first molar
   b. Distal cusp ridge

      In contact with the mesio-occlusal slope of the mesiobuccal cusp of the maxillary second molar
2. Distobuccal cusp
   a. Mesial cusp ridge

      In contact with the disto-occlusal slope of the mesiobuccal cusp of the maxillary second molar
   b. Distal cusp ridge

      In contact with the mesio-occlusal slope of the distobuccal cusp of the maxillary second molar

The tips of lingual cusps of the mandibular second molar are out of contact in centric relation.

The mesiolingual cusp is located lingual to the embrasure formed by the distolingual contour of the maxillary first molar and the mesiolingual contour of the maxillary second molar.

The distolingual cusp is located lingual to the sulcus containing the lingual developmental groove of the maxillary second molar.

MANDIBULAR THIRD MOLAR

When third molar development and alignment are normal, the relation of the mandibular third molar to the maxillary molars is almost identical to the arrangement as described for the mandibular second molar. The only change in the description would be to mention maxillary second and third molars as contacting members instead of maxillary first and second molars.

Centric Relation of Incisal Ridges and Cusp Tips of Maxillary Teeth to Mandibular Teeth

Because the reader has just learned the relation of cusps and ridges of mandibular teeth to maxillary teeth and therefore has learned the procedure in observation of those relations, outline form will be used to describe the centric relations of cusp tips and ridges of maxillary teeth to mandibular teeth (Fig. 428).

It should be emphasized again that the study should be assisted by the use of a good skull or model demonstrating occlusion of the teeth in three dimensions.

MAXILLARY CENTRAL INCISOR

1. Incisal ridge
   a. Labial to mandibular central and lateral incisors
   b. No contact

MAXILLARY LATERAL INCISOR

1. Incisal ridge
   a. Labial to mandibular lateral incisor and canine
   b. No contact

MAXILLARY CANINE

1. Cusp tip
   a. Labial to mandibular canine and first premolar
   b. Centered over labial embrasure formed by the mandibular canine and first premolar

MAXILLARY FIRST PREMOLAR

1. Buccal cusp tip
   a. Above buccal embrasure formed by the mandibular first and second premolars
   b. No contact
2. Lingual cusp tip
   a. Contacts the distal fossa, just mesial to the distal marginal ridge of the occlusal surface of the mandibular first premolar

MAXILLARY SECOND PREMOLAR

1. Buccal cusp tip
   a. Above the buccal embrasure formed by the mandibular second premolar and the first molar
   b. No contact
2. Lingual cusp tip
   a. Contacts the distal fossa (resting within it) of the occlusal surface of the mandibular second premolar

MAXILLARY FIRST MOLAR

1. Mesiobuccal cusp tip
   a. Buccal to sulcus of mesiobuccal groove of the mandibular first molar
   b. No contact
2. Distobuccal cusp tip
   a. Buccal to sulcus of distobuccal groove of the mandibular first molar
   b. No contact
3. Mesiolingual cusp tip
   a. Located a trifle buccal to center of the central fossa of the occlusal surface of the mandibular first molar
4. Distolingual cusp tip
   a. Contacts the mesial marginal ridge of the occlusal surface of the mandibular second molar approaching the mesial triangular fossa

MAXILLARY SECOND MOLAR

1. Mesiobuccal cusp tip
   a. Buccal to sulcus of mesiobuccal groove of the mandibular second molar
   b. No contact
2. Distobuccal cusp tip
   a. Buccal to distal slope of the distobuccal cusp ridge of the mandibular second molar
   b. No contact
3. Mesiolingual cusp tip
   a. Centered in central fossa of occlusal surface of the mandibular second molar, directly over the central pit
4. Distolingual cusp tip
   a. In contact with the distal marginal ridge of the mandibular second molar and near the lingual border of the distal traingular fossa

MAXILLARY THIRD MOLAR

When third molar development and alignment are normal, the relation of the maxillary third molar cusp tips to the mandibular third molar is practically the same as that described for maxillary and mandibular second molars.

8. THE OCCLUSAL CONTACT AND INTERCUSP RELATIONS OF ALL THE TEETH DURING THE VARIOUS FUNCTIONAL MANDIBULAR MOVEMENTS

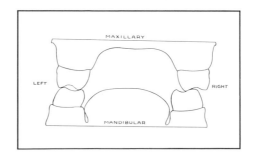

Centric occlusal relation, just described, is the terminus of all functional jaw movements. Rarely, however, is the jaw opened from centric relation and closed in centric with a perfectly straight hinge movement. The normal activity of the mandible is a rotating movement to the right or left before a return to centric relation, or a forward movement and return. These masticatory movements of the mandible are named as follows:

1. Right lateral movement
2. Left lateral movement
3. Protrusive movement

Each of these movements is but part of a cycle which has centric relation as starting point and terminus.

Therefore the functional occlusal contact relation of the teeth of one arch with those of the other have been named according to the relative position of the mandible which governs the relations. They are:

1. Centric occlusal relation
2. Right lateral occlusal relation
3. Left lateral occlusal relation
4. Protrusive occlusal relation

Although the mandible is capable of a wide range of movements, and the possible extent of the motion in any one direction can be considerable when the teeth are separated; when the teeth are brought together in any of the occlusal relations, the extent of the movements of the teeth over each other while in contact is extremely limited. Therefore *the physiologic form of the teeth, their alignment and their anchorage are concerned with final short arcs of movement only, near the terminus of centric relation.*

During the *right lateral movement,* the mandible is depressed and the dental arches are separated, the jaw moves to the right and brings the teeth together at points to the right of centric relation, called *right lateral occlusal relation.* The return movement bears left, sliding the teeth over each other until centric relation is re-established.

The *left lateral movement* is similar, except that the initial action is to the left, causing the teeth to come into contact in a *left lateral occlusal relation,* and the return movement to centric bears right.

During the *protrusive movement,* the mandible is depressed, then moves directly

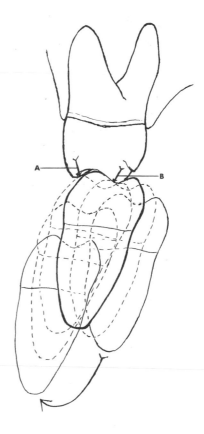

Figure 429. The cycle of occlusal movements, represented by a schematic drawing of first molar relations—mesial aspect. The heavy outline of the mandibular molar represents it in centric occlusal relation to the maxillary molar. The shadow outlines represent the mandibular molar in various relations during the cycle of mandibular movement during mastication. The two short arrows, A and B, at right angles to the occlusal surface of the maxillary molar, measure the extent of movement over the occlusal surface from the first contact of the mandibular molar to the last contact before continuing another cycle.

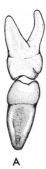 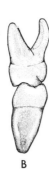 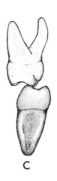

A   B   C

Figure 430. Occlusal relations of first molars during the cycle of occlusal movements. (See also Fig. 429.) *A,* Initial occlusal contact in *right lateral occlusal relation. B, centric occlusal relation. C,* Final contact after leaving centric relation before the mandible drops away to begin another cycle. This is also the balancing contact for the left lateral occlusal relation.

forward, bringing the anterior teeth together at points most favorable for the incision of food. After contact has been established, the jaw is retruded, returning to centric occlusion. Protrusive movement is followed by a retrusive movement to centric.

It is possible to retrude the mandible to a point slightly posterior to centric relation, dependent entirely upon the compressibility of the soft tissues posterior to the condyle heads. Since this places the teeth in a nonfunctional occlusal relation, *retrusive relation* is not considered as an occlusal relation.

To repeat: The range of movement of the mandible may appear quite extensive while one is watching the complete displacement during lateral excursions, but, from the time the opposing teeth come into contact, the extent of movement of the mandibular teeth over the maxillary teeth is very limited (Fig. 429 A and B).

The teeth do not mill together from side to side in the manner of small millstones.

The *curved* occlusal surfaces come into contact during a rotary movement of the mandible with a cutting thrust as the teeth approach centric relation; then there is a momentary *mortar and pestle* action in a narrow range before the mandibular teeth drop away to begin another excursion.

The compensating curvature of the dental arches is intended to achieve *occlusal balance* throughout the range of mandibular movements. Occlusal balance is apparently a definite part of the plan in occlusion of the teeth, but ideal occlusal balance as anatomists conceive it is rare. Nevertheless, many people may be found who have teeth in good alignment and occlusion, passing all of the requirements necessary for use and permanence including balanced occlusal contacts.

Occlusal balance is achieved when one section of the arch is supported by one or more other sections, each section having some contact simultaneously. The more nearly these sections are opposite one another in the arch, the more nearly perfect the balance. As an example, if the molars on one side of the jaws are at some point of occlusal contact during lateral mandibular movement, the occlusion is balanced by simultaneous contact at some points in the molar areas on the opposite side of the jaws. If, at the same moment, some contact is made anteriorly in the region of anterior teeth, or even in the region of the premolars, the occlusal balance is made more complete. During the approach to centric occlusion, the more rapidly all teeth come into contact with antagonists, the more perfect the occlusal balance is said to be for that individual (Figs. 441 and 442).

When the mandible is making a protrusive movement during incisive action of the anterior teeth, good balance requires simultaneous contact of posterior teeth on each side at the same moment the anterior teeth make actual contact; some balancing contacts on each side are maintained until centric occlusion is re-established.

Lateral Occlusal Relations of the Teeth

When the mandibular teeth make their initial contact with the maxillary teeth in right or left lateral occlusal relation, they bear a right or left lateral relation to centric position. The canines, premolars and molars of one side of the mandible make their occlusal contact facial (labial or buccal) to their facial cusp ridges at some portion of their occlusal thirds. Those points on the mandibular teeth make contact with maxillary teeth at points just lingual to their facial cusp ridges (Fig. 442). The central and lateral incisors of the working side may also be in contact at the same time; if they are, the labioincisal portions of the mandibular teeth of that side are in contact with the linguoincisal portions of the maxillary teeth of the same side.

During the sliding contact action, from the most facial contact points to centric relation, the teeth intercuspate and slide over each other in a *directional line approximately parallel with the oblique ridge of the upper first molar* (Fig. 431). The combined sulci of the distobuccal and lingual developmental grooves of the occlusal surface of the mandibular first molar are counter in form generally to the oblique ridge of the maxillary first molar. The sulci and ridge fit together loosely, the sulci encompassing the ridge during the lateral occlusal movement in line with the oblique ridge longitudinally (Figs. 431 and 432).

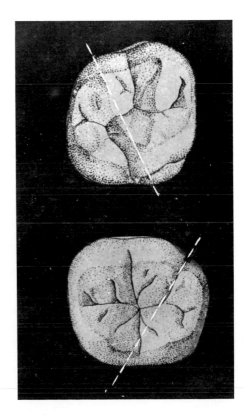

Figure 431. Drawings of the occlusal surfaces of the first molars, showing the directional path traveled by the teeth during lateral occlusal movements. The path follows the general direction of the alignment of the oblique ridge of the maxillary first molar and the occlusal sulci of the distobuccal and lingual developmental grooves of the mandibular first molar.

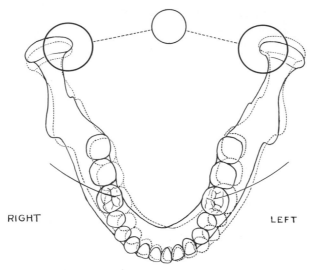

RIGHT   LEFT

Figure 432. Tracing of actual photograph of a mandible (from Fig. 389) taken from a point directly above the first molar. The heavy outline denotes centric occlusal relation; the dotted outline denotes the approximate position of the mandible during left lateral occlusal relation. The dotted outline represents a tracing which was superposed over the other drawing in centric relation, then rotated in such a manner that the *heavy arc lines to central fossae of first molars,* of both the drawings, *were kept in the same arc of rotation.* The pivotal center of the first molars is somewhere within the area of the small circle between, and posterior to, the condyles. The pivotal center of either condyle in right or left lateral relation is somewhere within the circles drawn over the medial portion of the condyles. Evidently all points on the mandible or on the teeth move in concentric circular motions which make it difficult if not impossible to locate pivotal points in single planes.

From the foregoing it is evident that the *mandibular teeth do not ride over the maxillary teeth at right angles to the buccal surfaces but at an acute angle to them.*

At this point the reader must have his three-dimensional model of occlusion at hand in order properly to study the subsequent details of tooth relations during the mandibular movements.

As the teeth move from lateral relation to centric relation, the cusps and incisal ridges bear an interrelation to each other; the cusps of the canines and posterior teeth of the mandibular arch have an intercusping relation to the cusps of the teeth of the maxillary arch.

The cusp tip of the mandibular canine moves through the linguoincisal embrasure of the maxillary lateral incisor and canine. Its mesial cusp ridge contacts the distal portion of the linguoincisal ridge of the maxillary lateral incisor. Its distal cusp ridge contacts the mesial cusp ridge of the maxillary canine.

The cusp tip of the mandibular first premolar moves through the occlusal embrasure of the maxillary canine and first premolar (Figs. 433, A, and 434). Its mesiobuccal ridge contacts the distal cusp ridge of the maxillary canine, its distobuccal cusp ridge the mesio-occlusal slope of the buccal cusp of the maxillary first premolar.

The mandibular second premolar cusp tip moves through the occlusal embrasure of the maxillary first and second premolars. Its mesiobuccal cusp ridge contacts the disto-occlusal slope of the buccal cusp of the maxillary first premolar, its distobuccal cusp ridge the mesio-occlusal slope of the buccal cusp of the upper second premolar.

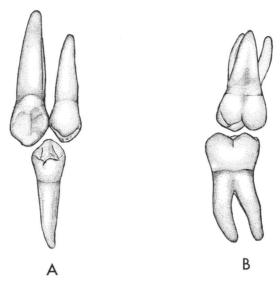

Figure 433. Cusps and cusp ridges, embrasures, etc., bear an interrelationship to each other. *A,* Mandibular first premolar relation to maxillary canine and first premolar on the verge of occlusal contact. Lingual aspect. *B,* Mandibular first molar relation to the maxillary first molar on the verge of occlusal contact. Lingual aspect.

The lingual cusps of all premolars are out of contact until centric relation is attained. Then the only lingual cusps in contact are those of the maxillary premolars, with the possible addition of the distolingual cusp of a mandibular second premolar of the three-cusp type.

The molars have a more involved lateral occlusal relation because of their complex design. Their occlusal form and their other occlusal relations have been described in detail under other headings.

It has just been determined, in studying the lateral occlusal relations of canines and premolars, that cusps, cusp ridges, sulci, and embrasures, bear an interrelationship to each other. Cusps and elevations on the teeth of one arch pass between cusps or through embrasures or sulci. The individual teeth are formed and situated to make this possible. The cusps of the teeth of one jaw, simply do not ride up and down the cusp slopes of the teeth in the opposing jaw. This situation is the one most often

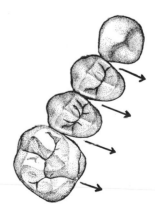

Figure 434. Assembly of the maxillary canine, first and second premolars and the first molar as they appear in the maxillary arch. The arrows indicate the direction of movement of the mandibular teeth over the maxillary teeth during the masticatory cycle. The major embrasures of canines and premolars are above marginal ridges occlusally. The arrows are on a line, approximately, parallel to the oblique ridge of the maxillary first molar.

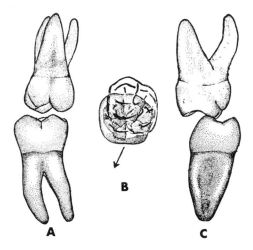

Figure 435. *A,* Maxillary and mandibular first molars as they are related just before contact during the occlusal cycle. *B,* Shadowed maxillary molar superimposed over the mandibular molar in the relation they bear to each other in centric relation contact. *C,* The final contact relation upon completion of the occlusal cycle.

misunderstood by students of occlusion. Normal occlusion will not allow teeth to clash or interfere with one another during any functional occlusal relation (Fig. 433, *A* and *B*, and Fig. 434).

A Description of the Occlusal Cycle in the Molar Areas during Right or Left Lateral Occlusal Relations

In lateral movements during mastication (*Bennett movements*), the mandible drops downward and to the right or left of centric relation. As it continues the cycle of movement and returns toward centric relation, the bucco-occlusal portions of mandibular molars come into contact with the occlusal portions of the maxillary molars lingual to the summits of buccal cusps on buccal slopes of their central sulci (Figs. 429 and 430).

From these first contacts the mandibular molars slide into centric relation with maxillary molars, coming to a momentary rest following a mortar and pestle action (Fig. 436), and then pass centric relation, continuing the cycle in a lingual direction. The movement continues with occlusal surfaces in a sliding contact until the bucco-occlusal slopes of mandibular teeth pass the final points of contact on the linguo-occlusal slopes of the maxillary teeth. As the molars lose contact the mandible drops away in a circular movement to begin another cycle.

The actual distance traveled by mandibular molars across the occlusal surfaces of maxillary molars, from first contacts to final contacts at the time of separation, is very short, probably not more than 3 or 4 mm. in most instances. The measurement on the maxillary molars from first to final contacts may be a little more than this, but it must be noted that the first contacts on lower molars are buccal to the summits of buccal cusps, whereas final contacts are lingual to the same summits. The lower molars, which are the moving antagonists, are taken out of contact before the first contact location on their buccal cusps reaches the final points of contact on the maxillary molars (Fig. 430).

Figure 436. Shadow drawings of opposing first molars superposed so that centric relation may be studied in detail. The arrows show the angle at which the mandibular molar crosses over the maxillary molar in a lingual direction. *A,* Centric relation of mandibular first molar to maxillary first molar. *B,* Centric relation of maxillary first molar to mandibular first molar.

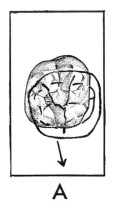
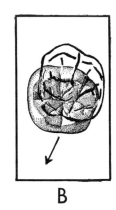

A   **B**

Mechanism of Mastication

During the process of mastication of food, the individual chews in one location of the dental arches only at any one chewing stroke. Most of the chewing is done by shifting from one side to the other in the molar and premolar regions. Occasionally the shift is toward the anterior region. However, the posterior teeth of the right or left side do the major portion of the work of mastication. The food is manipulated by the tongue, lips and cheeks so that it is thrown between the teeth continuously during mandibular movements which bring the teeth together in their various relations. The major portion of the work is accomplished in the *premolar* and *molar* regions while the mandible is making right lateral and left lateral movements, bringing the teeth into right lateral and left lateral occlusal relations, finishing the strokes in centric relation.

Most persons enjoy considerable tactile sense in the teeth, by which sense they are enabled to place the teeth in their most efficient relation to each other during mastication, although most of the time the act of mastication is carried on subconsciously. When a bolus of food is placed between the teeth, the food separates the teeth of one jaw from those of the other. As long as the teeth are out of contact relation, occlusal balance is unnecessary. As soon as the bolus of food is penetrated, the teeth come into lateral contact relation in the area occupied by the food on one side of the mouth (working side), and at the instant the contact is operative on that side, occlusal balance requires an occlusal contact relation on the opposite side (balancing side). Without such bilateral contact, producing jaw balance, the stresses and strains of masticatory force, on one side only, would tend to unseat the teeth on the working side and produce torsion in the temporomandibular joints.

Occlusal Balance

Normal dental arches in good alignment with good occlusion demonstrate occlusal balance during right and left lateral occlusal relations (Figs. 441 to 445). Normal cases may not demonstrate ideal relations.

Figure 437

Figure 438

Figure 439

Figure 440

Figure 437. Centric occlusal relation—anterior view.
Figure 438. Centric occlusal relation—lateral view.
Figure 439. Casts of the person's teeth shown in Figs. 437 and 438. Centric occlusal relation—right side.
Figure 440. Looking at the casts from the lingual on the left, one may see normal intercusping in centric relation.

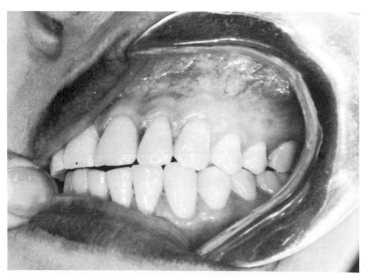

Figure 441. Left lateral occlusal relation. Note the contact from the lateral incisor posteriorly. In this instance the left central incisor and all of the *right* anterior teeth are out of contact.

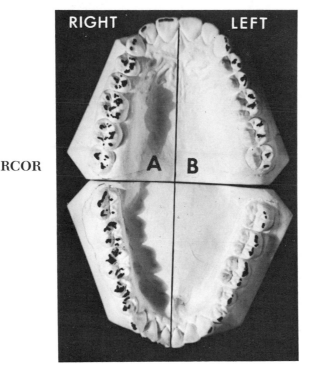

Figure 442. A, right side, and B, left side. This is a photograph of the casts of the individual shown in Figure 441 and 450. LLOR, *left lateral occlusal relation* in contrast with RCOR, *right centric occlusal relation.* In any lateral relation the occlusal contacts are reduced markedly. Black spots represent the markings of occlusal contacts.

The most perfect balancing relation is as follows: When the posterior teeth of one side (working side), achieve their lateral occlusal relation (Fig. 442, the occlusal slopes of the lingual cusps of the maxillary posterior teeth of the opposite side (balancing side) contact the occlusal slopes of the buccal cusps of the posterior mandibular teeth of that side (Fig. 443, *A* and *B*). All of the premolars and molars of both sides are in occlusal contact simultaneously.

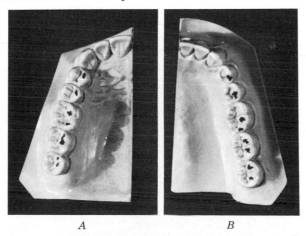

A   *B*

Figure 443. The spotted contacts on lingual cusps of right maxillary teeth and the buccal cusps of right mandibular teeth represent the approximate balancing contacts for the left lateral occlusal relation. *A,* Right maxillary teeth. *B,* Right mandibular teeth. Compare these balancing occlusal contacts on the right side with the preceding figure showing the left lateral occlusal relation.

In most cases which may be classified as normal, occlusal balance is present, but all of the premolars or all of the molars may not take part on the balancing side. The molars are the most important balancing members because of their superiority in size and anchorage and because they are situated to greater advantage as balancers. They are placed closer to points of rotation of the mandible, and their location posteriorly makes them better able to withstand the forces brought to bear by the powerful muscles of mastication.

Occlusal Cycle of the Posterior Teeth

The *occlusal cycle* of the *posterior* teeth during right or left lateral relations, with the accompanying occlusal balance, may be summarized as follows:

1. There are right lateral and left lateral occlusal relations, depending upon which side is being used.

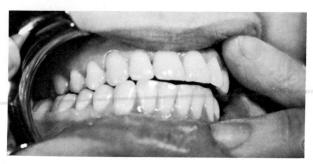

Figure 444.   Right lateral occlusal relation. Balancing contacts on the left side shown in a cast of the individual below in Fig. 445.

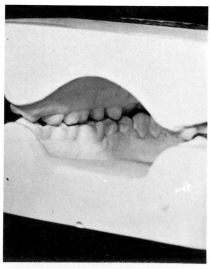

Figure 445.   Balancing contacts on the left side shown from the lingual aspect. The casts were made from accurate impressions of the teeth shown in Figure 444.

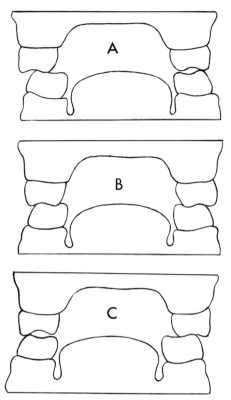

Figure 446. Schematic drawing of posterior view of molars. *A,* Right lateral occlusal relation. *B,* Centric occlusal relation. *C,* Left lateral occlusal relation.

2. When the right side is the working side, the teeth of that side are in right lateral occlusal relation first, with buccal cusps in contact; the lingual cusps of maxillary teeth of the left side are in balancing relation with the buccal cusps of the mandibular teeth of the left side (Fig. 446, *A*).

3. The teeth slide into centric occlusal relation of both sides (Fig. 446, *B*).

4. In left lateral occlusal relation, the buccal cusps of the posterior teeth of that side have their buccal cusps in contact; the lingual cusps of the maxillary posterior teeth of the right side are in contact with the buccal cusps of the mandibular teeth of the right side (Fig. 446, *C*).

Protrusive Occlusal Relations of the Teeth

The process of *biting* or *shearing* food material is negotiated by the *protrusive occlusal relation.*

Although the mandible may be lowered and retracted considerably in producing a wide opening of the mouth, just as in any other occlusal relation, the occlusion of the anterior teeth is not concerned with any position that is very far removed from centric relation.

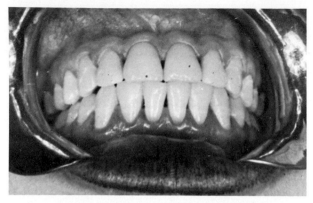

Figure 447. Protrusive occlusal relation. Anterior view of natural teeth.

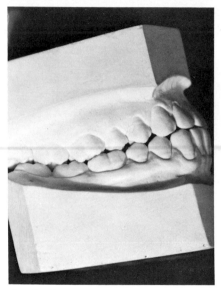

Figure 448. Protrusive occlusal relation. Lateral view of all of the teeth of one side as shown by a cast of the individual in Figure 447.

When the jaw is opened and moved straight forward to the normal protrusive relation, the mandibular arch bears a forward, or anterior, relation of only 1 or 2 mm. in most cases to its centric relation with the maxillary arch (Fig. 449).

The protrusive occlusal relation places the labioincisal areas of the incisal ridges of the mandibular incisors in contact with the linguoincisal areas of the incisal ridges of the maxillary incisors. The mesiolabial portion of the mesial cusp ridge of the mandibular canine is in contact with the maxillary lateral incisors distolinguoincisally.

As soon as food has been penetrated during the incisive movement, the anterior teeth come into contact in the protrusive occlusal relation which has just been noted. At the same moment occlusal balance requires instantaneous occlusal contact of the posterior teeth. The buccal cusps of posterior teeth furnish the balancing contacts

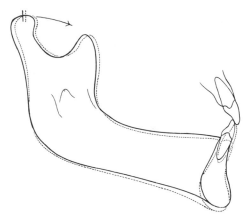

Figure 449. Outline tracing of the left portion of a human mandible sectioned at the median line. The maxillary central incisor is also outlined. The unbroken outlines illustrate the central incisors in centric occlusal relation. The broken outline illustrates the approximate relation of the central incisors in protrusive relation. Note the relative positions of the condyle, the coronoid process and the body of the mandible on the two outline drawings.

posteriorly, although rarely does one find all of the posterior teeth co-operating in protrusive balance. Naturally, in the occlusal balance relation during protrusion, the mandibular posterior teeth bear an anterior relation to their centric relation with the maxillary posterior teeth.

From the protrusive occlusal relation the teeth glide over each other in a *retrusive* movement of the mandible, a movement which ends at centric occlusal relation. During this final shearing action, the incisal ridges of the lower incisors are in continuous contact with the linguoincisal third portions of the maxillary incisors, from the position of protrusive occlusal relation to the return to centric occlusal relation.

The maxillary canines may assist in the balancing relation by having their distal cusp ridges in contact with the mesial cusp ridge of the mandibular first premolar. They do not assist in the incisive action; however, they pierce food material when their mesial cusp ridges come into contact with the distal cusp ridges of the mandibular canines at the moment centric relation is attained.

Occlusal balance posteriorly during the protrusive relation is requisite in order to insure the stability of the incisors. It must be remembered that their angulation in the jaws makes them unable to withstand the forces of occlusion without the assistance of the posterior teeth. Therefore, any lack of posterior support, such as premature loss of posterior teeth, affects the permanence of the anterior teeth, the incisors in particular (Fig. 405).

Occlusal Cycle of Anterior Teeth

The occlusal cycle of the anterior teeth (protrusive relation to centric relation) with the accompanying occlusal balance may be summarized as follows:

1. The anterior teeth come together with the mandibular arch a bit depressed and a bit forward to its centric relation with the maxillary arch.

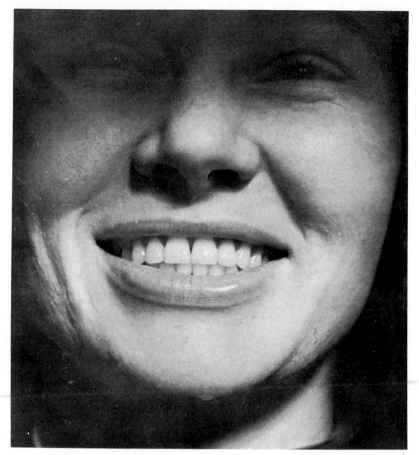

Figure 450. A smiling portrait of a person with normally functioning teeth and jaws. The development and preservation of properly functioning natural teeth should be the dental practitioner's primary interest, because he is the only one capable of assuming the responsibility.

2. When the anterior teeth come into contact, the mandibular arch is in protrusive occlusal relation; the posterior teeth furnish a balancing contact on both sides with their buccal cusps.

3. The mandible is retruded and slides the teeth over each other in a movement which is upward and backward, ending at centric relation.

4. The opening movement downward and forward to the protrusive relation, combined with the closing movement backward and upward to centric relation, makes a cycle of rotation which is a protrusive and retrusive cycle.

G. V. Black's
Measurements of the Teeth

EVIDENTLY many teeth were measured by Dr. Black in formulating the tables of measurements that appear on this and the following page. Although the averages given in the tables will not demonstrate teeth that are in good proportion to each other in a single dental arch (which must be expected), so far as the author knows there are no other published tables equivalent to these, giving the dimensions of human teeth and listing them as average, greatest, and least.

Measurements of the Maxillary Teeth

Measurements of the Maxillary Teeth of Man, Given in Millimeters and Tenths of Millimeters*		Length over all	Length of crown	Length of root	Mesio-distal diameter of crown	Mesio-distal diameter of neck	Labio- or bucco-lingual diameter	Curvature of the gingival line
Central Incisor	Average	22.5	10.0	12.0	9.0	6.3	7.0	3.0
	Greatest	27.0	12.0	16.0	10.0	7.0	8.0	4.0
	Least	18.0	8.0	8.0	8.0	5.5	7.0	2.0
Lateral Incisor	Average	22.0	8.8	13.0	6.4	4.4	6.0	2.8
	Greatest	26.0	10.5	16.0	7.0	5.0	7.0	4.0
	Least	17.0	8.0	8.0	5.0	4.0	5.0	2.0
Cuspid	Average	26.5	9.5	17.3	7.6	5.2	8.0	2.5
	Greatest	32.0	12.0	20.5	9.0	6.0	9.0	3.5
	Least	20.0	8.0	11.0	7.0	4.0	7.0	1.0
First Bicuspid	Average	20.6	8.2	12.4	7.2	4.9	9.1	1.1
	Greatest	22.5	9.0	14.0	8.0	6.0	10.0	2.0
	Least	17.0	7.0	10.0	7.0	4.0	8.0	0.0
Second Bicuspid	Average	21.5	7.5	14.0	6.8	5.3	8.8	0.8
	Greatest	27.0	9.0	19.0	8.0	6.5	10.0	1.5
	Least	16.0	7.0	10.0	6.0	4.5	7.5	0.0
First Molar	Average	20.8	7.7	13.2	10.7	7.5	11.8	2.2
	Greatest	24.0	9.0	16.0	12.0	8.0	12.0	3.0
	Least	17.0	7.0	10.0	9.0	7.0	11.0	1.0
Second Molar	Average	20.0	7.2	13.0	9.2	6.7	11.5	1.6
	Greatest	24.0	8.0	17.0	10.0	8.0	12.5	4.0
	Least	16.0	6.0	9.0	7.0	6.0	10.0	0.0
Third Molar	Average	17.1	6.3	11.4	8.6	6.1	10.6	0.7
	Greatest	22.0	8.0	15.0	11.0	8.0	14.5	2.5
	Least	14.0	5.0	8.0	7.0	5.0	8.0	0.0

* There are 25.4 millimeters to the inch.

Measurements of the Mandibular Teeth

Measurements of the Mandibular Teeth of Man, Given in Millimeters and Tenths of Millimeters		Length over all	Length of crown	Length of root	Mesio-distal diam-eter of crown	Mesio-distal diam-eter of neck	Labio- or bucco-lingual diam-eter	Curva-ture of the gingival line
Central Incisor	Average	20.7	8.8	11.8	5.4	3.5	6.0	2.5
	Greatest	24.0	10.5	16.0	6.0	5.0	6.5	3.0
	Least	16.0	7.0	9.0	5.0	2.5	5.5	1.5
Lateral Incisor	Average	21.1	9.6	12.7	5.9	3.8	6.4	2.5
	Greatest	27.0	12.0	17.0	6.5	5.0	7.5	3.5
	Least	18.0	7.0	11.0	5.0	3.0	6.0	2.0
Cuspid	Average	25.6	10.3	15.3	6.9	5.2	7.9	2.9
	Greatest	32.5	12.0	21.0	9.0	7.0	10.0	4.0
	Least	20.0	8.0	11.0	5.0	3.0	6.0	2.0
First Bicuspid	Average	21.6	7.8	14.0	6.9	4.7	7.7	0.8
	Greatest	26.0	9.0	18.0	8.0	5.0	8.0	1.5
	Least	18.0	6.5	11.0	6.0	4.5	7.0	0.5
Second Bicuspid	Average	22.3	7.9	14.4	7.1	4.8	8.0	0.6
	Greatest	26.0	10.0	17.5	8.0	6.5	9.0	2.0
	Least	18.0	6.0	11.5	6.5	4.0	7.0	0.0
First Molar	Average	21.0	7.7	13.2	11.2	8.5	10.3	1.1
	Greatest	24.0	10.0	15.0	12.0	9.5	11.5	2.0
	Least	18.0	7.0	11.0	11.0	7.5	10.0	0.0
Second Molar	Average	19.8	6.9	12.9	10.7	8.1	10.1	0.2
	Greatest	22.0	8.0	14.0	11.0	8.5	10.5	1.0
	Least	18.0	6.0	12.0	10.0	8.0	9.5.	0.0
Third Molar	Average	18.5	6.7	11.8	10.7	8.3	9.8	0.2
	Greatest	20.0	8.0	17.0	12.0	9.5	10.5	1.5
	Least	16.0	6.0	8.0	8.0	5.0	9.0	0.0

BIBLIOGRAPHY

Black, G. V.: Dental Anatomy. S. S. White Mfg. Co., Philadelphia, 1902.

Bonwill, W. G. A.: Scientific Articulation of Human Teeth as Founded on Geometrical Mathematical Laws. Dental Items of Interest 21:817, 1889.

Brauer, J. C., Higley, L. B., Massler, M., and Schour, I.: Dentistry for Children. The Blakiston Co., Philadelphia, 1947.

Brodie, A. G.: Temporomandibular Joint. Illinois Dent. J. 8:2, 1939.

Carabelli, G.: Anatomie des Mundes. Braumuller & Seidel, Vienna, 1842.

Chissin, C.: Ueber die Offhungbewegung des Unterkiefers und die Beteiligung der ausseren ptergoidmuskein bei derselben. Arch. f. Anat. u. Entwickelungsgesch, 1906.

Cunningham, D. S.: Textbook of Anatomy, 8th Ed. Oxford University Press, London, 1943.

Deaver, J. B.: Surgical Anatomy of the Human Body, 2nd Ed. P. Blakiston's Son & Co., Philadelphia, 1926.

Dewey, M.: Dental Anatomy. C. V. Mosby Co., St. Louis, 1916.

Dewey, M., and Thompson, A. H.: Comparative Dental Anatomy, 2nd Ed., C. V. Mosby Co., St. Louis, 1920.

Diamond, M.: Dental Anatomy. The Macmillan Co., New York, 1929.

Easlick, K., and Moyers, R. E.: Chapter XII in Watson, E. H., and Lowery, G. H.: Growth and Development of Children, 2nd Ed. Year Book Publishers, Inc., Chicago, 1954.

Freil, S.: Occlusion — Observations on Its Development from Infancy to Old Age. Internat. J. Orthodontia and Oral Surgery 13:322, 1927.

Gottlieb, B.: Tissue Changes in Pyorrhea. J. Am. Dent. A. 14:2178, 1927.

———: The Gingival Margin (Pathological, Normal). Odonto. Sec. Royal Soc. Med. Trans. 20:51, 1926–27.

Gregory, W. K.: The Origin and Evolution of the Human Dentition. Williams and Wilkins Co., Baltimore, 1922.

Grossman, L. I.: Root Canal Therapy. Lea & Febiger, Philadelphia, 1946.

Hemley, S.: Fundamentals of Occlusion. W. B. Saunders Co., Philadelphia, 1944.

Hess, W., and Zürcher, E.: The Anatomy of Root Canals. William Wood & Co., Baltimore, 1928.

Higley, L. B.: Some Controversies Over the Temporomandibular Joint. J. Am. Dent. A. 27:594, 1940.

Hogeboom, F. E.: Practical Pedondontia, 5th Ed. C. V. Mosby Co., St. Louis, 1946.

Klatsky, M.: A Cinefluorographic Study of the Human Masticatory Apparatus in Function. Am. J. Orthodontics 26:664, 1940.

Kronfeld, R.: Dental Histology and Comparative Dental Anatomy. Lea & Febiger, Philadelphia, 1937.

Kurth, L. E.: Mandibular Movements in Mastication. J. Am. Dent. A. 29:1769, 1942.

Logan, W. H. G., and Kronfeld, R.: Development of the Human Jaws and Surrounding Structures from Birth to the Age of Fifteen Years. J. Am. Dent. A. 20:379, 1933.

Lord, F. P.: Movements of the Jaw and How They Are Effected. Internat. J. Ortho. 23:557, 1937.

MacMillan, H. W.: Foundations of Mandibular Movement. J. Am. Dent. A. 21:429, 1934.

McBride, W. C.: Juvenile Dentistry, 4th Ed. Lea & Febiger, Philadelphia, 1945.

McCall, J. O., and Wald, S. S.: Clinical Dental Roentgenology, 2nd Ed. W. B. Saunders Co., Philadelphia, 1947, Chaps. XI, XII, and XIII.

Massler, M., and Schour, I.: Atlas of the Mouth. Bureau of Public Relations and Council on Dental Health, American Dental Association, Chicago.

429

Maximow, A. A., and Bloom, W.: Textbook of Histology, 7th Ed. W. B. Saunders Co., Philadelphia, 1957.

Monson, G. S.: Architectural Bone Changes of Face and Cranium. J. Am. Dent. A. *14*:828, 1927.

Morris, H.: Human Anatomy, 10th Ed. The Blakiston Co., Philadelphia, 1942.

Mueller, E., and Orban, B.: The Gingival Crevice. J. Am. Dent. A. *16*:1206, 1929.

Nolla, C.: Studies, Child Development Laboratories, University of Michigan, University Elementary School, Ann Abor, Michigan.

Noyes, F. B., Schour, I., and Noyes, H. J.: Dental Histology and Embryology. 5th Ed. Lea & Febiger, Philadelphia, 1938.

Orban, B.: Dental Histology and Embryology. P. Blakiston's Son Co., Philadelphia, 1930.

Prentiss, H. L.: Regional Anatomy Emphasizing Mandibular Movements with Specific Reference to Full Denture Construction. J. Am. Dent. A. *15*:1085, 1923.

Prinz, H.: The Etiology of Pyorrhea Alveolaris. Dental Cosmos *68*:1, 1926.

Riethmüller, R. H.: The Filling of Root Canals with Prinz' Paraffin Compound. Dental Cosmos *56*:490, 1914.

Robinson, M.: The Temporomandibular Joint: Theory of Reflex Controlled Nonlever Action of the Mandible. J. Am. Dent. A. *33*:1260, 1946.

Sherrington, C. S.: Proc. Royal Soc. London *92*:245, 1921.

Sicher, H., and Tandler, J.: Anatomie für Zahnärzte. Julius Springer, Vienna and Berlin, 1928.

Simpson, C. O.: Advanced Radiodontic Interpretation, 3rd Ed. C. V. Mosby Co., St. Louis, 1947.

Skillen, W. G.: Normal Characteristics of the Gingiva and Their Relation to Pathology. J. Am. Dent. A. *17*:1088, 1930.

Skillen, W. G., and Lundquist, G. R.: An Experimental Study of Peridental Membrane Re-attachment in Healthy and Pathologic Tissue. J. Am. Dent. A. and Dental Cosmos *24*:175, 1937.

Spee, F. Graf von: Die Verschiebungsbahn des Unterkiefers am Shadel. Arch. f. Anat. u. Physiol., 1890.

Stimson, L. A.: Treatise on Dislocations. Lea Brothers & Co., 1907.

Thompson, J. R.: Cephalometric Study of Movements of the Mandible. J. Am. Dent. A. *28*:750, 1941.

Thompson, J. R., and Brodie, A. G.: Factors in the Position of the Mandible. J. Am. Dent. A. *29*:925, 1942.

Tims, H. W., and Henry, C. B.: Tomes' Dental Anatomy. The Macmillan Co., New York, 1923.

Turner, C. R.: American Textbook of Prosthetic Dentistry. Lea & Febiger, Philadelphia, 1913.

Wheeler, R. C.: Some Fundamentals in Tooth Form. Dental Cosmos *70*·889, 1928.

———: Restoration of Gingival or Cervical Margins in Full Crowns. Dental Cosmos *73*:238, 1931.

———: A Comparison of Periodontal Attachment Levels. Dental Digest *41*:261, 1935.

———: Tooth Form, Drawing and Carving, 2nd Ed. W. B. Saunders Co., Philadelphia, 1954.

GLOSSARY

Abrasion. *n.* In dentistry, the normal wearing away of tooth substance under the stress of mastication (occlusal abrasion).

Alignment. Also **Alinement.** The act of arranging in a line; the state of being arranged in a line.

Alveolar process. That part of the bone which surrounds and supports the teeth in the maxilla and the mandible.

Alveolus, *pl.* **Alveoli.** *n.* The cavity or socket in the alveolar process in which the root of the tooth is held.

Anomaly, *pl.* **Anomalies.** *n.* Any marked deviation from that which is ordinary or normal.

Anterior. *a.* Situated in front of; a term commonly used to denote the incisor and canine teeth, or forward region of the mouth.

Apex, *pl.* **Apices.** *n.* The point or extremity of a conical object, as of the tooth root.

Apical foramen. An aperture at or near the apex of a tooth, through which the blood and nerve supply of the pulp enters the tooth.

Arch, dental. The ensemble of teeth in either jaw in the form of an arch.

Atrophic. *a.* Pertaining to or characterized by atrophy.

Atrophy. *n.* The wasting away of a tissue, organ or part from disease or defective nutrition.

Bennett movement. The movement of the mandible during normal right and left lateral occlusal relations of the teeth during mastication.

Bifurcation. *n.* Division into two parts or branches, as any two roots of a tooth.

Bonwill triangle. An equilateral triangle with the base of the triangle composed of a line from centers of the two condyles of the mandible, the apex of the triangle being located at the contact of mandibular central incisors.

Buccal. *a.* Pertaining to the cheek; towards the cheek or next to the cheek.

Calcification. *n.* The process by which organic tissue becomes hardened by a deposit of calcium salts within its substance. The term, calcification, is used in dentistry with a liberal interpretation to denote the deposition of any mineral salts which contribute toward the hardening and maturation of tooth tissue.

Canine eminence. The prominence in the labial aspect of the maxilla overlying the root of the canine tooth.

Cemento-enamel junction. The junction of enamel on the crown and the cementum of the root. This junction forms the cervical line.

Cementum. *n.* The layer of bony tissue covering the root of a tooth.

Centric occlusion (central occlusion). The relation of the occlusal surfaces of the teeth of one arch to those of the other when the jaws are closed and the teeth are said to be in the position of physical rest.

Cervical. *a.* Pertaining to the neck or to any cervix, i.e., that portion of a tooth near the junction of crown and root.

Cervical line.   The line formed by the junction of the enamel and cementum on a tooth.

Cervical third.   That portion of crown or root of a tooth approximating the cervical line.

Cervico-enamel ridge.   Any prominent ridge of enamel immediately above the cervical line on the crown of a tooth.

Cervix. *n.*   A neck or constricted portion. The narrowed region near the junction of the crown with the root of the tooth.

Cingulum. *n.*   The lingual lobe of incisor teeth; a bandlike enamel ridge rising crownwise from the cervix and often accentuated to a blunt point or rudimentary cusp.

Comminution. *n.*   The process of crushing into small pieces.

Compensating occlusal curvature.   The occlusal curvature of the teeth, singly or in series, which helps to achieve occlusal balance during jaw movements.

Contact area.   The area of contact of one tooth with another in the same arch.

Crown. *n.*   A name applied to that part of a tooth which is covered with enamel.

Curve of Spee.   The line beginning at the tip of the canines and following the buccal cusps of premolars and molars when viewed from a point opposite the buccal aspect of first molars.

Cusp. *n.*   A notably pointed or rounded eminence on or near the masticating surface of a tooth.

Deciduous. *a.*   That which will be shed; specifically, the first dentition of man or animal.

Dental arch.   See *Arch, dental.*

Dentin, Dentine. *n.*   The calcific tissue forming the body of a tooth, underlying the cementum and the enamel.

Dentino-enamel junction.   The line marking the junction of the dentin with the enamel.

Dentition. *n.*   Used by anatomists and palaeontologists to designate the general character and arrangement of the teeth, taken as a whole, as in carnivorous, herbivorous and omnivorous dentitions. *Primary dentition* refers to the deciduous teeth; *secondary dentition* refers to the permanent teeth.

Developmental grooves.   Fine depressed lines in the enamel of a tooth which mark the union of the lobes or primitive elements of the crown in its development.

Diastema. *n.*   A cleft or space such as that between the maxillary lateral and canine, into which the lower canine occludes in the carnivora. Sometimes used to denote any spacing between teeth.

Distal. *a.*   Distant or farthest from a central point; away from the median line of the face, following the curve of the dental arch.

Edge, incisal.   Term used to denote the edge formed at the labio-incisal line angle of an anterior tooth after an incisal surface has been created through wear.

Embrasure. *n.*   The open space between the proximal surfaces of two teeth where they diverge buccally, labially, or lingually and occlusally from the areas of contact.

Enamel. *n.*   The hard calcified tissue which covers the dentin of the crown portion of a tooth.

Enamel cuticle.   Nasmyth's membrane; the thin membrane, the remains of the enamel organ, which covers the crown of a tooth at the time of its eruption.

Epithelial attachment.   The attachment of the soft tissue of the mouth to the tooth by means of epithelium.

Exfoliation. *n.*   The process of casting or throwing off from the surface.

Facial. *a.*   Term used to designate the outer surfaces of the teeth collectively (buccal and labial).

Fissure. *n.*   A deep ditch or cleft; a developmental linear fault found usually in the occlusal or the buccal surface of a tooth; commonly the result of the imperfect fusion of the enamel of the adjoining dental lobes.

Follicle. *n.*   A small sac or crypt enclosing a developing tooth.

Fossa. *n.*   A rounded, wide, relatively shallow depression in the surface of a tooth, as seen commonly in the lingual surfaces of the maxillary incisors.

Gingiva. *n.*   That part of the gum tissue and mucous membrane which immediately surrounds a tooth.

Gingival crevice.   The subgingival space which, under normal conditions, lies between the gingival crest and the epithelial attachment.

Gingival line, gingival margin, gingival crest.   The line which marks the limit of the gingival crest about the tooth.

Gingival papillae. The portion of the gingiva found between the teeth in the interproximal spaces below the contact areas. Also called *interdental papillae.*

Gingivitis. *n.* Inflammation involving the gingival tissue only.

Hyperemia. *n.* Congestion of blood.

Incisal edge. See *Edge, incisal.*

Incisal ridge. The entire ridge form of the incisal portion of an anterior tooth.

Intercusping relation. The relation of the cusps of the premolars and molars of one jaw with those of the opposing jaw during any of the occlusal relations.

Interdental. *a.* Situated between the teeth.

Interproximal. *a.* Between the proximal surfaces of adjoining teeth.

Interproximal space. An anatomical triangular space between contacting teeth; the proximal surfaces of the teeth making the sides of the triangle, the alveolar bone, the base, and the contact of the teeth, the apex.

Labial. *a.* Of or pertaining to the lips. Toward the lips.

Line angle. The angle formed by two surfaces, as mesial and buccal; the junction is called the *mesiobuccal line angle.*

Lingual. *a.* Pertaining to or affecting the tongue. Next to, or toward the tongue.

Lobe. *n.* The part of a tooth formed by any one of the separate points of the beginning of calcification.

Malocclusion. *n.* Abnormal occlusion of the teeth.

Mamelon. *n.* One of the three rounded protuberances on the cutting edge of a newly erupted incisor tooth.

Marginal ridge. A ridge or elevation of enamel forming the margin of a surface of a tooth; specifically, at the mesial and distal margins of the occlusal surfaces of premolars and molars and the mesial and distal margins of the lingual surfaces of incisors and canines.

Mastication. *n.* The act of chewing.

Median line. *a.* The periphery of the median plane; the vertical, central line dividing the body into right and left. (Dentally, the median line of the face.)

Mesial. *a.* Toward or situated in the middle, as toward the median line of the dental arch.

Morsal. *a.* Taking part in mastication; a term applied to the masticating surface of a premolar or molar.

Nasmyth's membrane. The thin epithelial membrane which is the remains of the enamel organ and envelops the enamel of a tooth during development and eruption. *Enamel cuticle.*

Oblique ridge. A ridge running obliquely across the occlusal surface of the upper molars. It is formed by the union of the triangular ridge of the distobuccal cusp with the distal portion of the ridge forming the mesiolingual cusp.

Occlusal. *a.* The surface of a premolar or molar tooth that meets the opposing teeth in the closure of the jaws. Term used also to include incisal and occlusal surfaces when spoken of collectively.

Occlusal trauma. Injury brought about by malocclusion.

Occlusion. *n.* The natural closure and fitting together of upper and lower teeth; the relation of the mandibular and maxillary teeth, when closed or during those excursive movements of the mandible whereby masticating efficiency is obtained.

Definition. *When the teeth of the mandibular arch come into contact with the teeth of the maxillary arch in any functional relation, occlusion is established.*

Overbite. *n.* That characteristic of the teeth in which the incisal ridges of the maxillary anterior teeth extend below the incisal edges of the mandibular anterior teeth when the teeth are placed in centric occlusal relation.

Overjet. *n.* That characteristic of the teeth in which the incisal ridges or buccal cusp ridges of the maxillary teeth extend labially or buccally to the incisal ridges or buccal cusp ridges of the mandibular teeth when the teeth are in centric occlusal relation.

Periodontal. *a.* Surrounding a tooth.

Periodontal membrane. Periosteal tissue attached to both tooth root and alveolar bone, serving as tooth attachment. Also called *alveolo-dental periosteum.*

Periodontium. *n.* The supporting tissues adjacent to the teeth.

Periodontoclasia. *n.* A general term to include those degenerative changes which affect the supporting tissues of the teeth.

Periphery. *n.* The circumferential boundary.

Pit. *n.* A small, pointed depression in dental enamel, usually at the junction of two or more developmental grooves.

Pit fault. A developmental fault due to improper fusion of enamel in a pit.

Point angles. The meeting of three surfaces at a point, forming a corner. Those angles formed by the junction of three surfaces, as the mesio-buccal-occlusal point angle.

Posterior teeth. Those teeth of either jaw to the rear of the incisors and canines.

Protrusion. *n.* The condition of being thrust forward, as the protrusion of the incisor teeth.

Proximal, proximate. *a.* Nearest, next, immediately preceding or following.

Pulp canal. That canal in the root of a tooth which leads from the apex to the pulp chamber. Under normal conditions it contains a portion of the dental pulp.

Pulp cavity. The entire cavity within the tooth including the pulp canal and pulp chamber.

Pulp chamber. That cavity or chamber in the center of the crown of a tooth which normally contains the major portion of the dental pulp and into which the root canals open.

Pulp, dental. The highly vascular and innervated connective tissue contained by the pulp cavity of the tooth.

Pulp horn (horn of pulp). Extension of pulp tissue into the horn-like extension of the pulp chamber in the tooth crown.

Radiogram, radiograph, roentgenogram. *n.* The photographic representation of opaque objects produced by the action of roentgen rays upon a sensitized plate or film.

Resorption. *n.* Physiological removal of tissues or body products, as of the roots of deciduous teeth, or of some of the alveolar process after the loss of the adult teeth.

Retrusion. *n.* The act or process of retraction, as when the mandibular teeth are placed in a posterior occlusal relation to the maxillary teeth.

Ridge. *n.* A narrow elongated elevation or crest, as on the surface of a tooth or a bone.

Root. *n.* That portion of a tooth embedded in the alveolar process and covered with cementum.

Root trunk. That portion of a multi-rooted posterior tooth found between the cervical line and the points of bifurcation or trifurcation of roots.

Secondary dentin. That dentin which is often formed within the original limits of the pulp chamber of a tooth in an attempt by nature to protect the pulp from irritation or caries.

Succedaneous. *a.* The teeth which succeed to, or take the place of, the deciduous teeth after the latter have been shed: the incisors, canines and premolars.

Sulcus. *n.* A notable long-shaped depression in the surface of a tooth, the inclines of which meet at an angle.

Supplemental grooves. A shallow linear groove in the enamel of a tooth. It differs from a developmental groove in that it does not mark the junction of lobes.

Supplementary canal. A root canal which is an extra branch supplemental to the typical single canal in the tooth root.

Transverse ridge. A ridge formed by the union of two triangular ridges and crossing transversely the surface of a posterior tooth.

Trauma. *n.* An injury; damage; impairment; external violence producing bodily injury or degeneration.

Triangular ridge. Any ridge on the occlusal surface of a posterior tooth, which extends from the point of a cusp to the approximate center of the crown occlusally.

Trifurcation. *n.* The division of three tooth roots at their point of junction with the root trunk.

Tubercle. *n.* A small cusp-like elevation on some portion of a tooth crown produced by an overcalcification of enamel. A tubercle is a deviation from typical form.

INDEX

Nasal meatus, inferior, 318
middle, 318
Nasal process, 315
Nasmyth's membrane, 41
Nasopalatine nerve, 341
Nerve(s), 340-342
alveolar, 342
buccinator, 342
infra-orbital, 341
lingual, 342
mandibular, 342
maxillary, 340
mylohyoid, 342
nasopalatine, 341
palatine, 341
sphenopalatine, 341
trigeminal, 340
Nomenclature, 3-26
Notch, sigmoid, 330

Oblique groove, distal, 243
Oblique ridge, 11, 67, 69, 242
external, 329
internal, 331
transverse groove of, 243
Occlusal balance, 414, 419-422
Occlusal cycle, in molar areas during occlusal
relations, 418
of anterior teeth, 425
of posterior teeth, 422
Occlusal embrasures, 100
Occlusal planes, curved, 378-381
Occlusal relations of teeth, lateral, 415-418
molar occlusal cycle in, 418
protrusive, 423
Occlusal surfaces, 8
Occlusal trauma, 98
Occlusion, 8
arrangement of teeth and, 365-426
centric. See *Centric occlusion.*
deterioration of teeth and, 390
dynamics of, 356
foundation of, 392
migration of teeth and, 77
movements of condyles and, 394
of deciduous teeth, 75-77
superstructure of, 392
use of carbon paper to demonstrate, 395
Overbite, 368
Overjet, 368
normal, 372

Palatine nerve, 341
Palatine process, 315
of maxilla, 319
Papilla(e), gingival, 79- 98
interdental, 79
Periodontium, protection, tooth form in, 95-123
Permanent dental formula, 5
Permanent dentition, 29-44
physiology of, 78-94
Permanent teeth, 5. See also under specific teeth.
calcification, chart, 35, 36, 37
deciduous teeth and, differences, 49
development appraisal, 34

Pit(s), 12
central, 69, 72, 224, 275
developmental, distal, 198, 225
mesial, 198, 225
mesial, 72, 275
Planes, curved occlusal, 378-381
Platysma muscles, 349
Point angle(s), 13, 15
Posterior teeth, 10
calibration, 25-26
contact areas, 106
line angles, 15
mandibular, curvatures, 118
mesial and distal aspects, 93
maxillary, mesial and distal aspects, 92
occlusal cycle, 422
point angles, 15
Premolar(s), 3, 31, 373
first, 31, 46
lobes of, 88, 206
mandibular, 206-227
cusps of, 206
first, alveolus, 335
aspects of, 104, 110, 208-215
chronology of development, 207
contact areas, 104
incisal and occlusal embrasures, 104
labial, buccal and lingual embrasures, 110
measurements of, 207
occlusal relations, 402, 408
lateral, 416
pulp cavities, 308
second, 215
alveoli, 335
aspects of, 105, 110, 220-227
chronology of development, 215
contact areas, 105
cusps of, 215
forms, 215
incisal and occlusal embrasures, 105
labial, buccal and lingual embrasures, 110
measurements of, 215
occlusal relations, 402, 408
lateral, 416
root of, 215
maxillary, 184-205
crown of, 185
curvatures, 116
maxillary, first, alveolus, 322
aspects of, 103, 107, 186-199
chronology of development, 185
contact areas, 103
crown of, 197
incisal and occlusal embrasures, 103
labial, buccal and lingual embrasures, 107
measurements of, 185
occlusal relations, 402, 411
lateral, 416
pulp cavities of, 299
lobes of, 184
marginal ridge of, 185
roots of, 185
second, 199
alveolus, 322
aspects of, 103, 107
chronology of development, 199
contact areas, 103